Praise

'Chris Kresser is the mo ͺ
Paleo/ancestral he   ͺf
people, often   ͺnal
Paleo Di   ͺnical
experience ͺͺͺp you look, feel and perfoͺͺ ͺest'

> Robb Wolf, *New York Times*
> bestselling author of *The Paleo Solution*

'We humans might all run on the same basic physiological
equipment and follow the same laws of biochemistry, but our
varied experiences and journeys and choices throughout life
change our relationship to those foundations. With *Your
Personal Paleo Diet,* Kresser heeds the evolutionary ties that
bind us together while showing us how to design a healthy,
personalized lifestyle that acknowledges our differences'

> Mark Sisson, author of *The Primal Blueprint*

'Chris Kresser is a leading voice within the Paleo nutrition
community for his objective, balanced and evidence-based
approach. In *Your Personal Paleo Diet,* Chris has done the
heavy-lifting for you by pulling together all of his best advice
in one place. Whether this is the first you're hearing of it, or
you already follow a Paleo type of diet, this book will support
your deeper understanding of the approach and outline a clear-
cut plan for your transition'

> Diane Sanfilippo, *New York Times*
> bestselling author of *Practical Paleo*

'There is no "one-size-fits-all" approach to health, but how do
you know what works best for you? Thanks to Chris Kresser's
Personal Paleo Diet, now your ideal health plan is easy to create
and implement. Kresser's detailed step-by-step action plan will
teach you how to eat better, sleep better, move more and stress
less – and helps you tweak your approach until it's just right'

> Dallas & Melissa Hartwig, *New York Times*
> bestselling authors, *It Starts With Food*

CHRIS KRESSER

YOUR PERSONAL
PALEO
DIET

Feel and look great by eating the foods
that are ideal for your body

piatkus

PIATKUS

First published in the US in 2013 by Little, Brown and Company,
Hachette Book Group

First published in Great Britain in 2013 by Piatkus

A CIP catalogue record for this book
is available from the British Library.

ISBN 978-0-349-40202-4

Typeset in Sabon by M Rules
Printed and bound in Great Britain by
Clays Ltd, St Ives plc

Papers used by Piatkus are from well-managed forests
and other responsible sources.

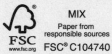

MIX
Paper from
responsible sources
FSC® C104740

Piatkus
An imprint of
Little, Brown Book Group
100 Victoria Embankment
London EC4Y 0DY

An Hachette UK Company
www.hachette.co.uk

www.piatkus.co.uk

This book is intended to supplement, not replace, the advice of a
trained health professional. If you know or suspect that you have a
health problem, you should consult a health professional. The
information given in this book is solely intended as education and
information and should not be taken as medical advice.

To all who struggle with chronic illness: may this book
be a catalyst for healing and self-discovery.

ABOUT THE AUTHOR

Chris Kresser, MS, LAc, is a practitioner of integrative and functional medicine and the creator of ChrisKresser.com, one of the most respected natural health sites in the world. He is widely known for his in-depth research uncovering myths and misconceptions in modern medicine and providing natural health solutions with proven results. He developed the Personal Paleo Diet – or the Personal Paleo Code as it is known in the US – based on more than ten years of research, his own recovery from a debilitating, decade-long illness and his clinical work with patients. Chris maintains a private practice in Berkeley, California, where he lives with his wife and daughter.

CONTENTS

Step 2: Rebuild Your Life

Step 3: Revive Your Health

ACKNOWLEDGEMENTS

Writing a book is a monumental task, and not something I could have done on my own. It emerged out of a thriving community of readers, patients, colleagues, teachers, friends, family and other supporters, both past and present. Although my name is on the cover, this book was truly a collaborative effort.

I am grateful for the contribution of pioneering scientists, physicians and bloggers whose work continually inspired and enlightened me. This book wouldn't have been possible without their willingness to challenge mainstream dogma and blaze new trails. I especially want to thank Dr Chris Masterjohn, Dr Stephan Guyenet, Dan Pardi, Dr Mat Lalonde, Robb Wolf, Dr Kurt Harris and Dr Emily Deans for their input and feedback on the manuscript and their ongoing advocacy, support and friendship.

My patients continue to be my greatest teachers. Thank you for putting your trust in me, and allowing me to bear witness to your healing journey.

To the fantastic team (Diane, Shannon, Keith, Jon, Kelsey, Laura, Aidan, Andrew, Michelle, Jordan, Steve and many more) behind my private practice and ChrisKresser.com: thank you for all of the ways you have supported this endeavour, both seen and unseen, and for your help in making the world a healthier place, one person at a time.

I'd like to thank the incredible group of people that helped transform this book from an idea into reality. Betsy Rapoport's keen insight and belief in my vision were instrumental in developing the proposal and initial structure of the book. Becky Cabaza helped me wrangle 165,000 words into a polished final draft. My editor, Tracy Behar, took a chance on a new author and was a source of constant support and encouragement. Carolyn O'Keefe, Miriam Parker and countless others at Little, Brown were tireless advocates of the book, and worked hard to ensure its success; I couldn't have asked for a better first experience with a publisher. My agent, Richard Pine, shepherded the book through each stage of the publishing process with wisdom, clarity and candour.

Finally, my deepest gratitude goes to my family and friends for their unconditional love, selfless support and enduring belief in me. I wish there was room to name you all; you know who you are, and I am thankful for your presence in my life.

I can't finish without mentioning four very special people specifically. Mom and Dad, you provided the foundation that made all of this possible, and have always been there when I needed you. Elanne and Sylvie, the joy and light of my life, thank you for putting up with the long hours, hectic schedule and time away. Sharing my life with you both is the most precious gift I could have ever imagined, and you've made me the luckiest man in the world.

JOIN THE PERSONAL PALEO DIET COMMUNITY

My website is an important extension of this book, an additional resource to enrich your quest for optimal health. Throughout the book I'll refer you to the website for additional information on a particular topic, programme-enhancing tools, helpful resources, ongoing education and, perhaps most importantly, support. Making significant dietary and lifestyle changes can be challenging, and I've found over the years that community is essential to success.

Visit ChrisKresser.com/PPC to find:

- Bonus chapters with more than 150 pages of additional information about customising your diet and lifestyle to address common health conditions. I'll refer to these bonus chapters throughout the book.
- A user forum with people from around the world following the Personal Paleo Diet approach, moderated by my approved 'Paleo Ambassadors'.
- An additional three weeks of delicious meal plans and recipes, including snacks and side dishes.
- Handy shopping lists.
- A supplement guide with specific recommendations mentioned throughout the book, updated regularly so that you

can order the ones that meet my strictest guidelines for safety and efficacy.

- A guide to finding and working with a Paleo-oriented clinician and much more ...

Note The website pages refer to *The Personal Paleo Code*, which is the US version of *The Personal Paleo Diet*. With a few exceptions, most of the information is relevant to readers from the UK, Australia and elsewhere.

You'll also find links to over 700 original studies I have cited within the book, as well as detailed chapter notes and references.

Head over to ChrisKresser.com/PPC now to connect with others creating their own Personal Paleo Diet and taking charge of their own health and well-being. I hope you'll love becoming part of this supportive community.

FOREWORD

We live in extraordinary times. Human ingenuity has given us flight, space travel, lasers, the internet and amazing medical technologies that can help the deaf hear or surgeries to give the blind sight again. Bio-hackers and tech folks talk of uploading the consciousness before death, looking for a second (and presumably very lengthy) existence as a program. So much is possible, yet the highly modern *Homo sapiens* is struggling with debilitating and chronic health conditions: obesity, depression, diabetes, autoimmune disease and cancer, among others.

A number of doctors, laypeople and scientists have come to rely on the mismatch hypothesis to explain much of modern chronic disease. Our bodies, having had only a few hundred generations to cope with agriculture, much less the light bulb and the digital age, are simply not equipped to handle industrial processed food, endless artificial light and a sedentary modern life. As a psychiatrist – a medical doctor specialising in mental illness – I deal with the emotional and neurological consequences of this mismatch all the time in my clinical practice. We might label the low mood, crying spells, anxiety and insomnia as a 'depressive disorder', but in truth it is a breakdown of resiliency. Our hardy species can take only so much stress before we begin to experience anxiety, depression and other consequences of our frenetic lives. Before we go forwards into the future, we have to come to terms with our biology and its limitations. We must rebuild our resiliency to recover our health.

The prescription seems simple enough. Eat wholesome, real foods. Get plenty of sleep along with appropriate play and activity. But as a physician and working mother, I know far too well how difficult it can be to find that balance between the pace of modern life, the needs of family and having the time and patience to keep yourself truly well and functioning at your best. In addition, despite the fact that we are all members of the same species, we have very individual needs based on current health conditions and activity.

Chris Kresser struggled with serious, disabling health problems that modern medicine seemed to have no solution for. He used science, wisdom and trial and error to heal himself, and from that experience decided to pursue acupuncture (in California, a four-year master's programme that combines Western and traditional medical arts), because he felt the holistic model it offered gave him a better way to understand and help the ill than the fragmented, speciality model of conventional medicine. His clinical experience, curiosity and scientific savvy helped him to become enormously successful. His private practice has thrived, while his website and podcasts reach hundreds of thousands of eager readers and listeners around the world.

With *Your Personal Paleo Diet*, Chris sets out the basic prescription for health and resiliency, and then backs it up with techniques to tailor it for *your* needs and to make it work on a personal level. His three-step programme steers you to diet and lifestyle changes that will have you feeling better than you have in years – perhaps better than you've ever felt. Chris gives you everything you need – not just recipes but a recipe for living – to achieve that improvement in health and functioning that anyone would get from a positive lifestyle change, but then he takes it a step further to address the complexities of your personal situation. Everything is spelled out in this book, plus his website offers bonus chapters, more details on the science behind the Paleo movement and copious online tools to ease your transition to good health.

By uncovering your own Personal Paleo Diet, you can benefit from Chris's experience, clinical acumen, wisdom and common sense to find that state of lasting health that can be so elusive in the modern world. Recover your natural human resiliency and thrive.

Emily Deans, MD
Board Certified Psychiatrist
Clinical Instructor of Psychiatry
Harvard Medical School

How *Your Personal Paleo Diet* Can Change Your Life

You may have picked up this book for several reasons. You may want to lose weight, boost your energy, or improve your overall health. You may be looking for ways to treat a particular health problem naturally, such as irritable bowel syndrome (IBS), hypothyroidism or high blood pressure. You may already feel well, but want to optimise your athletic performance, feel sharper at work or increase your longevity.

What if you could create your own personalised approach to nutrition, one that is designed exactly for your body, to create the results you want? An approach that respects the wisdom of your genetic template but also acknowledges your own unique circumstances and needs? This is exactly what I'm going to teach you how to do in this book. I call it *Your Personal Paleo Diet* – it's your 'code' for living, your unique prescription for optimal health.

WHAT IS A PERSONAL PALEO DIET?

Perhaps you've heard of the Paleo movement. Millions of people around the world are joining this health revolution based on the latest cutting-edge science, seeking to eat and live in closer harmony with our genetics and biology. This development has come just in time. We're in a health crisis, getting sicker and fatter every year, dying from chronic diseases our ancestors never faced. We thrive when we eat and live a certain way, and our profound sickness stems directly from contemporary choices that are far from that ideal way of living. We were never meant to eat the sugar, refined flour and industrial seed oils that are the mainstays of the modern diet that most of us eat today. In the US it's called the Standard American Diet (SAD) – and what an apt acronym that is! – but it's applicable to people in the UK and Australia as well as countries worldwide who have adopted a similar Western diet. We were never meant to work around the clock under the glare of artificial lights, or spend half our lives sitting and staring at computer screens, or live in relative isolation, with Facebook and Twitter standing in for genuine human contact.

Both the fossil record and studies of contemporary hunter-gatherer cultures suggest that our Palaeolithic forebears enjoyed excellent health: they were lean, fit and apparently free of chronic disease. The benefits of mimicking their lifestyle are undeniable. Those who walk the Paleo road report near-effortless weight loss, new-found vitality and often miraculous resolution of the most dire health issues; however, even the most dedicated 'Paleo purists' hit a wall. Weight loss stalls. Symptoms persist. Energy flags. People tire of restricted eating.

As a licensed clinician who practises functional medicine (which is different from conventional medicine), I specialise in helping seriously ill patients find natural solutions to overcome their health challenges. Through deep research, personal experience and clinical investigation, I developed a three-step process to help them. The first step is the 30-Day Reset Diet, which follows a typical Paleo approach very closely. The results from Step 1 are amazing. 'I'm medication free after just 30 days,' one patient told me; 'I feel like a new man!' another said; 'I've never felt or looked better in my life ... Energy levels more even, tennis elbow inflammation disappeared, asthma improved, waistline shrunk,' reported another. My file of testimonials speaks for itself: Paleo works.

As I tracked the experiences of people who adhered to the typical Paleo approach, however, including some of my patients, I began to notice certain drawbacks. Sometimes the benefits don't go far enough – or they're not sustainable.

I don't stop with my patients after Step 1 for exactly this reason. I've discovered that Paleo functions best as a general template, not a rigid prescription. Think of it as a starting point, not a destination. Even though we each share so much of the same DNA, we have unique circumstances and needs. We need a programme that addresses our specific health issues. A more flexible, dynamic approach that recognises the joys of eating, yet goes far beyond food, taking into account how we like to move, live, love. My goal is to help people discover what works for them, individual by individual, not adhere to a dogmatic regimen because it sounds more 'authentic'.

We don't live in the Palaeolithic anymore. We're not cavemen, so why should we follow a strict caveman diet? Why should we cut out foods we love and might thrive on, simply because our ancestors didn't eat them? We've evolved and we need a plan that's evolved to meet our individual needs and preferences. (Some of my patients are even vegetarians – anathema to hard-core meat-eating Paleo purists.) Why not combine the best of ancient wisdom and the best of modern nutrition?

That's why I created the three-step Personal Paleo Diet: an approach that is custom-made to your individual genetic blueprint, one that enables you to enjoy lifelong health and vitality.

A note to readers outside the US

Although the Paleo concept is spreading beyond the US, it is still relatively new in the UK, Australia and other parts of the world. For this reason I wanted to make this book as approachable to those people who have never heard of Paleo before as to those who may already be following it. This book is called *Your Personal Paleo Diet*, but it embraces much more than diet alone, as you will see as you work through the chapters. In the US, the book is called *Your Personal Paleo Code*. This is also the name you will find on the website pages, but you will also discover that the information on the website will be relevant to you, wherever you live, with only a very few pieces of information that relate only to people in the US.

ONE SIZE DOESN'T FIT ALL

If you're like most of my patients, you will have tried a lot of diets over the years. Some diets did nothing at all, some made you worse and some may have even worked – at least for a little while. Or perhaps the diets solved some problems (being overweight) but caused others (you were exhausted all the time, your hair fell out and your hands and feet turned into ice cubes).

Perhaps you've already tried a Paleo-style diet: eating the same kinds of natural foods our ancestors enjoyed. At first, you were ecstatic. You lost weight and felt so much better, but after a while you noticed some of your old problems creeping back in. Or perhaps you hit a plateau and just couldn't lose those last 10 pounds (4.5kg) no matter what you did. Or perhaps you just got tired of special diets in general and wanted to find a better approach to nutrition that would be more sustainable over the long term.

You set out to find some help. You searched some of the popular health websites, posted a few messages in discussion forums and emailed your friend who's trying the same thing.

They're all happy to help – you got a ton of advice. The problem is – it's all different! A new study just proclaimed that the Mediterranean diet is 'the best'. 'Very low-carb is the way to go' you hear on that morning radio programme; didn't another expert on that same show say exactly the same thing about vegan diets last week? 'No, you've got to eliminate nightshades and eggs,' your friend says. 'Doctor Google' says that if you've got a thyroid problem, you need to eat a lot more starchy vegetables and fruit. One website says yoghurt helps with digestion; another says you should avoid dairy entirely.

It's enough to make you go crazy.

You want to feel better, lose weight and fix your health problems, but how do you know you're making the right choice? And how do you ensure that the next diet you try doesn't end up being yet another failed experiment?

Here's the truth: there is no single formula for you to follow that would guarantee your perfect health in three weeks – or seven days, or any other arbitrary number you find on the bestseller list. As seductive as that sounds, it just doesn't work that way. The only formula I want to give you is the formula for working out how not to follow a formula! If my clinical experience from treating patients has taught me one thing, it's this: there's no one-size-fits-all approach when it comes to diet and lifestyle. After all, the fossil record indicates that not even all Palaeolithic people ate the same way, so why should we expect a single programme to be 'the perfect fit' for everybody?

Personalisation is the missing ingredient. I've found that even two people who come to my office with exactly the same health condition might need different solutions; for example, I recently saw two patients with ulcerative colitis. Eating even a small amount of dairy sent one running to the bathroom in three seconds flat. For the other, fermented dairy (for example, yoghurt or kefir) was a crucial component of the healing process. This is why so many typical 'diets' – even very good ones like the Paleo diet – often fail in the long run, and it's why I teach all my clients how to discover their own unique Personal Paleo Diet. Because no two patients are alike, no two walk out of my office with the same plan.

Case studies

- When Tina, aged 54, visited my office, she was almost 3 stone 3lb (20.4kg) overweight, with high blood pressure and early stage type-2 diabetes. She was fed up with feeling so sluggish and hated the way her clothes fitted. 'I've tried every low-fat diet out there, but nothing works,' she told me. As part of her Personal Paleo Diet, I put her on a lower-carbohydrate version of my Step 1 Reset Diet, with a few additional tweaks because of her blood sugar problems. She began to lose weight immediately while enjoying the foods her doctors had forbidden, such as red meat and butter.

  I can't get over it,' she said, 'I'm never hungry and I don't feel deprived!' After three months, Tina had lost 2½ stone (15.8kg), her skin glowed, her digestive system ran smoothly and there was no sign of diabetes. 'I've never felt better', she told me, 'and my doctor is amazed by my test results.'

- When Mark, aged 33, came to see me, he was virtually crippled by Crohn's disease, spending much of his day fleeing to the bathroom. He was on a cocktail of medications, including steroids and mesalamine. 'I'm scared,' he told me. 'My gastroenterologist wants to remove part of my colon.' Mark was desperate to avoid surgery. I determined that his Personal Paleo Diet would include an intensive gut-healing element, along with some stress-reducing measures. Mark felt dramatically better in just a week. Within a month, he felt like a new person. Six months later, Mark was in complete clinical remission – no surgery necessary!

- At 38, Sam couldn't seem to control his blood pressure. His doctor wanted him to go on medication to lower it. During my intake examination, I asked Sam about his diet. 'It's funny', he told me, 'but I went on one of those very low-carb diets to lose weight and my blood pressure shot up.' I suspected that Sam might be potassium deficient, which can contribute to high blood pressure. His Personal Paleo Diet included potassium-rich foods such as potatoes, plantains and cold-water fish, along with two cups of hibiscus tea a day, which has been shown to decrease blood pressure. Three months later, Sam's blood pressure was back to normal – without medication.

In all these cases, and hundreds of others like them, I worked closely with my clients to determine their unique formula for vibrant good health. Now I'm going to teach you how to do the same. First, though, I'd like to give you some background on why I'm such an ardent believer in this lifestyle. My personal experience is what motivates me to share my knowledge with others, because finding my own Personal Paleo Diet changed – and even saved – my life.

CRACKING THE CODE FOR HEALTH: MY STORY

My own journey into the Personal Paleo Diet lifestyle began with a devastating illness – one that dogged me for more than a decade.

In 1998, not long after I graduated from college, I quit my job, sold off my possessions and took off to see the world. Thailand was the first stop on my trip. I studied traditional Thai massage, kriya yoga and vipassana meditation, deepening the practice I'd begun as an 18-year-old.

The next stop on my trip was Indonesia. I'm a lifelong surfer, so I was drawn to this Mecca for its perfect waves and warm water. Then one day I woke up delirious with a high temperature, chills, vomiting and severe diarrhoea. (I later found out that I, along with several other surfers, had become ill because some locals had dug a trench that allowed stagnant water polluted with cow faeces to drain into the surf break.) An Australian friend gradually nursed me back to health with some antibiotics he had in his medical kit.

After recuperating, I tried to continue my world tour, but my recurring illness forced me to return to the US. The first doctor I saw, suspecting parasites, gave me powerful antibiotics that initially worked, but eventually I felt worse again: exhausted and listless with almost continuous digestive distress. Unfortunately, my illness lingered, and over the next few years I saw at least 15 doctors; nobody could tell me what was wrong and nothing they told me to do worked.

I decided to attend graduate school to study traditional Chinese medicine. Perhaps herbal medicine and dietary changes might help where conventional doctors and antibiotics had failed. I tried vegetarian and macrobiotic vegan diets and I consulted with several different professors at my school with expertise in treating digestive problems. Nothing helped. After two years, determined to find a cure, I dropped out of school and moved to the Esalen Institute, a residential community and retreat centre in Big Sur, California, that offers holistic educational and personal development programmes. I'd begun to wonder whether there might be an emotional, psychological, or even a spiritual, element to my illness.

My time at Esalen was transformative, mind- and heart-opening and healing at the deepest levels. My experiences there helped me to accept my illness and find peace in the midst of the intense struggles I was going through, but unfortunately, they didn't heal my body. I was still suffering from severe digestive distress and fatigue, and developing new symptoms such as muscle and joint pain, brain fog and insomnia.

The next few years were the most challenging of my life. With my savings exhausted, I moved back to Los Angeles and found myself working long hours in a stressful position at a start-up company. Within two years, I had a complete breakdown, utterly exhausted and demoralised after years of illness, pain and an unsuccessful search for answers. I had seen world-renowned doctors, specialists in every field of alternative medicine, shamans, energy workers, psychotherapists and spiritual teachers. I'd taken multiple courses of antibiotics, steroids and anti-inflammatories. I'd tried every special diet under the sun; my 'supplement graveyard' had more than a hundred bottles of herbs, potions and pills I'd taken over the years. I was beginning to lose hope that I would ever regain my health.

Then one day I walked into a bookstore and saw a book called *Nourishing Traditions* on display. It advocated a 'real food, nutrient-dense approach' based on traditional diets. Something about this approach resonated deeply within me. Hey, I'd tried every other diet, why not give this one a shot? I started eating the foods the book recommended: bone broth soups, sauerkraut, fermented dairy products, slow-cooked meats, eggs and cold-water, oily fish. I felt better almost immediately; however, even with the extensive preparation methods suggested in the book (including soaking and fermentation), the whole grains and pulses recommended irritated my gut – so I eliminated them along with industrial seed oils (corn, soya, cotton, rapeseed, sunflower and safflower), sugar and all processed and refined foods. I didn't know it at the time, but I was on a Paleo diet.

I couldn't get over the dramatic change in my energy level and gut health. I felt like a different person: vibrant, energised, excited about my future and ready for a fresh start. I continued my meditation practice and added specific techniques for stress management to reduce the physical and psychological symptoms associated with chronic pain and illness, and I eventually formulated a supplement regime that further improved my health. I didn't have a name for it yet, but I'd discovered my own Personal Paleo Code – the individual prescription for my optimal health.

I felt a strong calling to use all of the knowledge and experience I had acquired in my own healing journey to help others with theirs, so I applied to the Acupuncture and Integrative Medicine College in Berkeley, California, to finish the degree in traditional Chinese medicine that I had started years before.

While there, I started a blog called The Healthy Skeptic (now ChrisKresser.com) – mainly as a 'journal' to keep track of my own research and study. My grandfather had died following complications after bypass surgery; I suspected he hadn't received the best treatment. The more I delved into the research about diet and cardiovascular disease, the more fascinated I became – why were my grandfather's doctors following a medical model that was half a century old? What other research was being overlooked?

I became deeply interested in the scientific evidence for various medical approaches to illness and began to blog on my website about my findings. I was quite surprised, then, the first time someone left a comment on one of my posts. I hadn't told anyone about the blog, and to this day I still don't know how people found it. Within a relatively short time, though, I had thousands of readers from all over the world. By the time I graduated and became licensed, I was fortunate to have a full and thriving private practice. Shortly thereafter, I was introduced to some members of the vibrant Paleo community. Now I had a name for the lifestyle I'd stumbled upon independently. I realised that I had found my tribe: a group of revolutionary individuals committed to helping people obtain optimal health.

Today, I'm blessed with excellent health, a loving family and a thriving private practice. It's incredibly rewarding to help patients discover their own Personal Paleo Diet and code for living, and recapture their health and vitality.

BEYOND DIET: 360-DEGREE GOOD HEALTH

The Personal Paleo Diet is not just a diet but also a way of life, a process for helping you discover your own ideal way of eating and living. The food we eat is perhaps the single most important influence on our health. But the ways we manage our stress, sleep, exercise, spend time outdoors, have fun and connect with other people really matter; I'd argue that they separate a life merely lived from a life worth living. Just as I'll help you customise the diet that works optimally just for you, I'll help you find the unique lifestyle 'code' that embraces every other part of your life so that you can live healthfully and joyfully. Diet and lifestyle, taken together, form 360-degree good health.

Everyone's path to health is unique. I can tell you from working with hundreds of patients in my practice, and guiding thousands of others through my blog, that it takes about 30 days of following the Reset Diet for you to experience dramatic relief from aggravating symptoms, lose your cravings for the foods that aren't good for you, see a pleasing weight loss and probably feel better than you ever have! After that, you'll feel powerfully motivated to follow the rest of my three-step plan to arrive at a recipe for living that works best for you. For some readers, it'll be a few more weeks. For others, I refuse to make an empty promise about what that timetable should be; that's for you to discover with my guidance. This is what makes this programme work: you!

You'll find some significant differences between the diet you develop and traditional Paleo/Primal diets, because my plan will be customised to your needs. What's 'forbidden' on those other diets may be a welcome addition to your table. Based on time-tested ancestral wisdom combined with the best of modern science, Your Personal Paleo Diet is firmly grounded in your personal experience, which means you'll find it easy to follow, its benefits will be sustainable and you'll thoroughly enjoy it.

Warning: conventional wisdom may be hazardous to your health

I'm going to challenge a lot of conventional wisdom in this book – not because I'm a contrarian or want to generate attention, but because I've spent years poring over original research and major studies. I don't believe a health claim simply because I've seen it repeated multiple times. I look at the evidence – the size of the original study samples, the length of the studies, the quality of the research design and other factors. I look for the difference between causation and correlation. If conventional wisdom holds that taking a certain medication will help us live longer or prevent a certain illness, I want to see the research that proves that. So that's what I do; I carefully investigate the evidence behind health claims.

And what I've found, based solely on the scientific evidence, is often very different from popular health claims; for example, I've found that saturated fat is not the evil nutrient we've been led to believe it is and that whole grains aren't nearly as healthy as we've been told they are. These ideas – and many similar ones – are so deeply ingrained in our collective psyche that few of us stop to question them. But the fact that a belief is widely accepted doesn't make it true.

There's often a significant time lag between gold-standard research, acceptance by the wider medical community and communication to the public. I'm no conspiracy theorist; I dislike those screaming headlines that shout, 'Doctors are withholding secrets that could SAVE YOUR LIFE!' The way I see it, part of the problem is that once something becomes accepted as medical dogma, and the more widely it gets reported, the fewer people invest themselves in studying alternative theories and those few researchers get less attention and funding.

Perhaps one of the best examples of dogma in medicine is the idea that eating cholesterol raises cholesterol levels in the blood. Early studies suggested this was true, but more recent and better-designed trials have shown that dietary cholesterol doesn't increase blood cholesterol levels in the majority of people. Today, few researchers working in the field believe that eating eggs has a significant effect on cholesterol levels in the blood. Yet the public, and much of the conventional medical establishment, still do. And millions of people in the US, UK and Australia continue to avoid nutrient-rich foods like eggs and red meat on the basis of this outdated science.

Admitting we don't have the all the answers is the key to progress in science and medicine. I would invite you to keep an open mind as you read this book, especially when you encounter sections that challenge your beliefs. If you have scientific training, or if you're just the adventurous type, you can also scour the detailed chapter notes and references for this book (listed on the website in the order they relate to each chapter) and read the original studies I cite throughout the book.

Our knowledge is constantly evolving. We look back on the people and theories of 100 years ago and think them ignorant. What do you imagine people living 100 years from now will think about us and our ideas?

THREE STEPS: RESET, REBUILD AND REVIVE

There are three steps to discovering your own Personal Paleo Diet: Reset, Rebuild and Revive.

In Step 1: Reset, you'll begin the 30-Day Reset Diet. This quick-start eating plan presses the reset button on your diet, targeting and eliminating the modern foods that we aren't genetically adapted to eat – the foods that are the leading culprits in weight gain and health issues. I designed this programme so that you'll feel better right away, and I think you'll be pleasantly surprised to discover how many of the foods you thought were 'off-limits' you can enjoy. You'll experience improved digestion, reduced inflammation (explained on page 66), fewer allergic reactions, more energy, and a smoothing out of your blood sugar and mood. You'll also burn fat and shed pounds. If you're like my patients, you'll feel better than you have in years!

In Step 2: Rebuild, you'll begin to customise Your Personal Paleo Diet by reintroducing some foods you eliminated during the 30-Day Reset to see how they work for your body. A lot of 'Paleo purists' believe we shouldn't eat anything that wasn't around at the time of our Palaeolithic ancestors. Therefore, they'd keep tomatoes, potatoes, peppers and other nightshade vegetables off your table for ever. They'd have you bid a permanent farewell to dairy products and all grains and pulses (called 'legumes' in the US). But the science doesn't support this stance, so neither do I. Why rule out dairy, for example, if you thrive on it? I'll show you my proven method for testing 'grey area' foods so that you can rebuild the repertoire of foods you love.

In Step 3: Revive, you'll take the final steps to creating your unique prescription for optimal health, tweaking Your Personal Paleo Diet until it's a perfect fit. What's the perfect balance of protein, carbohydrates and proteins for your unique needs? What makes you thrive the most? Three meals a day? Six? Intermittent fasting? We'll work all this out and more – including how to be flexible when you need to be (see 'The 80/20 rule' opposite), so that you can follow Your Personal Paleo Diet for life.

*

I'll help you get started on this exciting new way of eating with seven days of meal plans and delicious 'fan's favourite' recipes developed by a foodie/chef couple whose creations are big hits on my website as well as brand-new culinary delights created by a French chef trained at Paris's renowned Ecole de Cuisine La Varenne. You'll also find an additional three weeks of meal plans and recipes at the website.

Life is about so much more than what we eat. You'll also learn other ways to make your life more joyful, such as managing your stress, finding fun ways to move, sleeping more deeply, emphasising pleasure and play, and reconnecting with nature.

Do you have a specific health problem? I've got you covered. You'll learn even more specific diet and lifestyle tweaks to address conditions like weight gain, heart disease, high blood pressure, digestive problems, high or low blood sugar, anxiety and depression, thyroid disorders, brain fog and memory issues, and acne, psoriasis and other skin problems. These natural approaches are sometimes all it takes to halt, or even reverse, symptoms that have plagued you for years.

The 80/20 rule

Once you have worked through the 30-Day Reset in Step I and have fully customised Your Personal Paleo Diet, I recommend you follow it closely 80 per cent of the time, but then loosen up the other 20 per cent of the time and eat what you like. A truly healthy body is a resilient body, one that doesn't make you feel sick if you have foods outside Your Personal Paleo Diet.

In time, most people end up very happily eating more like 90/10 or 95/5, because they've lost the physical and psychological cravings for crisps or biscuits or a fizzy soft drink. Why?

Because after doing Step 1 they feel so much better without those foods, and they've filled out their diets with an array of new and delicious foods – as you will. They save their full-out 80/20 times for that special holiday abroad or a celebration.

I want you to nourish yourself at every level, including having the joy of eating foods outside Your Personal Paleo Diet: your mother's cherished Sunday dinners; the incredible buffet at the wedding; the chef's special at that fantastic new restaurant you and your friends are going to on Saturday. Enjoy yourself! (For more on how to follow the 80/20 rule for life, see Chapter 19.)

HOW TO USE THIS BOOK

Feel better right away If you're new to the Paleo approach and eager to get started because you're feeling lousy or you want to lose weight, start with Step 1. Once you're on the 30-Day Reset Diet, you'll experience the benefits of the Personal Paleo Diet right away and that will give you the motivation to continue with Steps 2 and 3. While you're going through your 30-Day Reset, read up on topics like nutrient density, minimising toxins in your diet and choosing the best possible foods – you'll realise why you feel so good. Continue with Step 2 (Rebuild Your Life) to find out how to improve your sleep, manage your stress, exercise more effectively, and more. Then move on to Step 3 (Revive Your Health) to help you customise your programme further for any particular health conditions or goals you might have and for tips on following Your Personal Paleo Diet for life.

Improve your results If you're already following a Paleo-style diet, but you're not getting the results you hoped for, you might want to start with Step 2, Rebuild, to focus on some of the important lifestyle factors you might have neglected until now. Then move on to Step 3, Revive, to learn how to personalise your diet and lifestyle according to your unique needs so that it is even more effective. (I do suggest you take a look at Step 1, Reset, to make sure that the diet you're currently following tracks with my recommendations.)

Doing the 30-Day Reset Diet is the essential first step in discovering Your Personal Paleo Diet, but in the same way that there's no one-size-fits-all approach to diet, there's no right or wrong way to read this book. Just choose what works best for you, depending on your background, needs and goals.

YOUR PERSONAL PALEO DIET – YOUR WAY

Throughout this book, I'm going to remind you to trust yourself. Of course, you should always partner with your health professional and learn all you can about health options from trusted resources like this one, but no one is more motivated than you to find out how to create your optimal health.

I'm not doctrinaire. I don't think that all medications and surgery are evil or even avoidable. I refer my patients to physicians when I think a drug or surgery may be necessary. We live in amazing times, when we can pick and choose from the best options available to us from many quarters. Stay curious, motivated and involved. Learn all you can. Let this book be one of many powerful tools at your disposal.

I've helped hundreds of my patients and thousands of blog readers and podcast listeners overcome chronic health problems using the knowledge and experience I have gained over my own ten-year healing journey, as well as my formal education as a practitioner of integrative medicine, but there's more work to be done. There are so many others out there still suffering from chronic illness or overweight who haven't been able to find help anywhere else. Perhaps you're one of them. If so, this book is for you. It will teach you how to heal yourself so that your health won't stand in the way of fulfilling your dreams. The methods I share in this book have changed my life and the lives of thousands of others. It is my deepest wish that they will also change yours.

So let's get started. In the next chapter, I'm going to give you a brief history lesson. (Don't worry; there's no pop quiz!) I'll lay out the scientific argument for why, if you want to live longer into the future, it makes sense to eat the way our ancestors did tens of thousands of years in the past.

CHAPTER 1

Why Paleo? From Cave
to Chronic Illness

Consider the following:

- Diabetes and obesity combined affect more than a billion people worldwide, including 100 million Americans.

- More than half of all Americans are overweight; a full third are clinically obese.

- Heart disease causes four out of every ten deaths in the US.

- One-third of Americans have high blood pressure, which contributes to almost 800,000 strokes every year – the leading cause of serious, long-term disability. There are 12.7 million strokes worldwide.

- One-quarter of the British population is obese, and two-thirds are overweight. Experts predict that by 2020 one-third of the population of the UK will be obese.

- Twenty-two per cent of Australians are obese, and 63 per cent are overweight.

Notes for this chapter may be found at ChrisKresser.com/ppcnotes/#ch1

- In England, approximately 30 per cent of the population has high blood pressure.

- In Australia, about 22 per cent of people have high blood pressure.

- More than 36 million people worldwide are now living with dementia.

- Depression is now the leading cause of disability, affecting more than 120 million people worldwide.

I could go on, but I think you get the point. We're getting fatter and sicker every year.

Now imagine, for a moment, a world where:

- Modern, chronic diseases, such as diabetes, obesity, some cancers, autoimmunity and heart disease, are rare or non-existent.

- We're naturally lean and fit.

- We age gracefully with strong bones, sharp vision and normal blood pressure.

Although this might sound like pure fantasy today, anthropological evidence suggests that this is exactly how human beings lived for the vast majority of our evolutionary history.

Today, most people accept diseases, such as obesity, diabetes and heart disease, as 'normal', but although these diseases may be common today, they're anything but normal. Humans evolved roughly 2 million years ago and for more than 66,000 generations we were free of the modern diseases that kill millions of people each year and make countless others miserable. In fact, the world I asked you to imagine above was the natural human state for our entire history on this planet up until the Agricultural Revolution occurred about 11,000 years (366 generations) ago – less than 0.5 per cent of the time we've been recognisably human. It's a tiny blip on the evolutionary time scale.

What happened to us? What transformed us from healthy and vital people free of modern, chronic diseases into a world of sick, fat and unhappy people?

In a word – mismatch.

AGRICULTURE: THE WORST MISTAKE IN HUMAN HISTORY?

Like it or not, humans are animals and, like all other animals, we are biologically adapted to a 'species-appropriate' diet and way of life.

When animals eat and live in accordance with the environment to which they're adapted, they thrive. Cats, with their sharp teeth and short intestinal tracts, evolved to be carnivores, so when we feed them grain-rich kibble, they develop kidney trouble and other woes. Cows naturally graze on grass. When they eat too much grain, harmful bacteria proliferate and make them sick. We humans face a similar mismatch. Our biology and genes adapted to a particular environment. Then that environment changed far faster than we could adapt – with a few important exceptions that I'll cover later in this chapter. The result? The modern epidemic of chronic disease.

For the vast majority of our existence, we humans lived as Palaeolithic hunter-gatherers, living off the meat we hunted, fish we caught and the vegetables, fruit and tubers we picked while on the move. The Agricultural Revolution dramatically altered our food supply and way of life. We learned to stay in one place, planting crops and domesticating animals such as cows, sheep, goats and pigs. Early farmers consumed foods that their hunter-gatherer predecessors didn't eat, such as cereal grains, milk and meat from domesticated animals, pulses (peas, beans and lentils, also called 'legumes') and other cultivated plants.

Although scientists have argued that these developments allowed us to flourish socially and intellectually, the consequences of this shift from a Palaeolithic to an agricultural diet and lifestyle were disastrous for human health. In evolutionary terms, 11,000 years is the blink of an eye, not nearly long enough for humans to completely adapt to this new way of eating. This is why the influential scientist and author Jared Diamond has called agriculture 'the worst mistake in human history'. He argued that hunter-gatherers 'practiced the most successful and longest lasting lifestyle in human history' and were all but guaranteed a healthy diet because of the diversity and nutrient density of the foods they consumed. Once we switched diets and became more sedentary, our naturally robust health began to decline.

How do we know that agriculture has been so harmful to humanity? There are three main lines of evidence:

1 A decline in health among hunter-gatherer populations that adopted agriculture.

2 The robust health of contemporary hunter-gatherers.

3 The poor health in people who rely heavily on grains as a staple.

Let's look at each of these in more detail.

WHAT HAPPENED WHEN HUNTER-GATHERERS BECAME FARMERS?

Studying bones gives us a window into the health of our distant ancestors and offers insight into what an optimal human diet might be. Some archaeologists and anthropologists today may have a better understanding of human nutrition than the average healthcare practitioner! So what have these scientists learned from examining the bones of humans that shifted from a Palaeolithic hunter-gatherer lifestyle to agriculture? The fossil record shows a rapid and clear decline in health in places where agriculture was adopted. Tooth decay and anaemia due to iron deficiency became widespread, average bone density decreased and infant mortality increased. These changes result in large part from the nutritional stress of eating a diet inappropriate for our species.

We also shrank in stature. Skeletal remains from Greece and Turkey indicate that the average height of hunter-gatherers at the end of the Ice Age was 5 feet 9 inches (1.75m) for men and 5 feet 5 inches (1.65m) for women. After agriculture was adopted in these areas, average height fell to a low of 5 feet 3 inches (1.6m) for men and 5 feet (1.5m) for women. Archaeologists have found similar shrinkage in skeletons all over the world when populations shifted to agriculture.

Early farmers didn't only lose inches from their skeletons – they lost years from their lives. Anthropologist Dr George Armelagos studied the American Indians living in the Ohio River Valley in approximately AD 1150. His team compared the skeletons of hunter-gatherers that lived in the same area with those of the early farmers who followed them. The farmers had 50 per cent more tooth enamel defects (suggestive of malnutrition), four times as much iron-deficiency anaemia, three times more bone lesions and an overall increase in degenerative conditions of the spine. Their life expectancy at birth also dropped from 26 years to 19 years.

In their book *The 10,000 Year Explosion*, anthropologists Gregory Cochran and Henry Harpending argue that these dramatic declines in health were brought on by a major shift in the human diet. When hunter-gatherers switched to farmers' diets, their average carbohydrate intake shot up, while the amount of protein plummeted. The quality of that protein also decreased, since almost any type of meat has a desirable amino-acid balance, whereas most plants do not. Vitamin shortages were common, because the new diet was based on a limited set of crops and was lower in more nutrient-dense animal products. Evidence suggests that these early farmers, who depended on one or two starchy crops, such as wheat or corn, may have developed vitamin-deficiency diseases such as beriberi, pellagra, rickets and scurvy. Their hunter-gatherer ancestors, who ate a wide variety of foods rich in vitamins and minerals, rarely suffered from these diseases.

Because of 'plentiful protein, vitamin D and sunlight in early childhood', our Paleo ancestors were 'extremely tall, had very good teeth and larger skulls and pelvises', according to one group of archaeologists. Their farming descendants, in contrast, suffered skull deformities because of iron-deficiency anaemia, had more tooth decay, were more prone to infectious disease and were much shorter, 'apparently because subsistence by this time is characterized by a heavy emphasis on a few starchy food crops'. Farming may have offered our ancestors a more stable and predictable food supply, but this stability came at a great price.

Didn't our Paleo ancestors die young?

A common question I hear from Paleo sceptics is something along the lines of 'Why should I eat Paleo? Didn't Stone Age people die before their thirtieth birthday?'

It's true that, on average, our Paleo ancestors died younger. However, these averages don't factor in challenges largely absent from our modern lives: high infant mortality, violence and accidents, infectious disease and lack of modern medical care.

Hunter-gatherers had infant mortality rates about 30 times higher than those in the US today – and early childhood mortality rates more than 100 times higher. These higher infant and childhood mortality rates were caused by accidents, trauma, exposure to the elements, violence, warfare and acute infectious disease – issues that, fortunately, few of us face today. These untimely deaths had the net effect of dragging down average life expectancy. If, out of ten people, three died in infancy, two died during childhood from exposure to the elements and two died as teenagers in warfare, even if the remaining three lived long, healthy lives, the average lifespan in this hypothetical group would still be short.

Recent research that has taken the high infant mortality rates of our Palaeolithic ancestors into account suggests that, if they survived childhood, they had average lifespans roughly equivalent to people living in industrialised societies, with a range from 68 to 78 years. Even more importantly, they reached these ages without any signs or symptoms of the chronic, inflammatory and degenerative diseases that we consider to be 'normal' in developed countries – including obesity, type-2 diabetes, gout, hypertension, cardiovascular disease and cancer. Of course, those of us living in modern, industrialised societies might live a little longer than acculturated hunter-gatherers on average. But most of our elderly people suffer from painful and debilitating diseases, take several medications a day and have a decreased quality of life.

Fortunately, we don't have to choose between eating like our ancestors or reaping the benefits of modern medicine. We can combine them to get the best of both worlds and enjoy long lifespans without the degenerative diseases that are so common in the industrialised world.

CONTEMPORARY HUNTER-GATHERERS: A STUDY IN GOOD HEALTH

Modern studies of contemporary hunter-gatherers – people who have had minimal exposure to industrial civilisation and still follow a traditional diet and lifestyle – suggest that they are largely free of the chronic, inflammatory diseases that have become epidemic in the industrialised world.

Anthropological and medical reports of these contemporary hunter-gatherers show that they have far fewer modern diseases such as metabolic syndrome, cardiovascular disease, obesity, cancer and autoimmune disease compared with Western populations. In their study, 'The Western Diet and Lifestyle and Diseases of Civilisation', nutrition researcher Pedro Carrera-Bastos and his colleagues compared traditional populations with people living in industrialised societies. The contemporary hunter-gatherers were superior in every measure of health and physical fitness, including:

- Lower blood pressure.

- Excellent insulin sensitivity and lower fasting insulin levels (meaning that they were less likely to develop diabetes).

- Lower fasting leptin levels (leptin is a hormone that regulates body fat).

- Lower body mass index (BMI) and waist-to-height ratio (one way of measuring optimal weight).

- Greater maximum oxygen consumption (a measure of physical fitness).

- Better vision.

- Stronger bones.

Let's look at some examples of contemporary populations around the world that (until recently) were still following their traditional diet and lifestyle.

The Kitavans

Kitava is a small island in the Trobriand Island chain in Papua New Guinea's archipelago. Although not technically hunter-gatherers (they are horticulturalists), when studied the Kitavans were one of the last populations on earth still following a traditional diet similar in composition to Palaeolithic diets. Residents of Kitava subsist 'exclusively on root vegetables (yam, sweet potato, taro, tapioca), fruits (banana, papaya, pineapple, mango, guava, watermelon, pumpkin), vegetables, fish and coconuts'.

A study of 2,300 Kitavans, conducted by Dr Staffan Lindeberg and detailed in his 1989 book *Food and Western Disease*, found that they enjoyed excellent health:

- None had ever experienced heart disease or stroke – particularly remarkable because most Kitavans smoke, and smoking is one of the strongest risk factors for heart disease.

- They were very lean, with an average body mass index (BMI) of 20 in men and 18 in women. (In contrast, the average BMI of Americans as of 2013 was 28.8, which is considered to be overweight and is only 2 points away from the obese category. In the UK average BMI is 27.)

- Kitavans had very low levels of leptin and insulin – the hormones that regulate food intake and energy balance – compared to Western populations. Low levels of each are associated with leanness and overall metabolic health.

Most significantly, most Kitavans didn't suffer the diseases of ageing that are so common in developed countries. Lindeberg noted:

The elderly residents of Kitava generally remain quite active up until the very end, when they begin to suffer fatigue for a few days and then die from what appears to be an infection or some type of rapid degeneration. Although this is seen in Western societies, it is relatively rare in elderly vital people. The quality of life among the oldest residents thus appeared to be good in the Trobriand Islands.

A long, healthy life followed by an easy, quick death. Don't we all want that?

The Inuit

The Inuit are a group of hunter-gatherers that live in the Arctic regions of Alaska, Canada and Greenland. They eat primarily fish, seals, whale, caribou, walrus, birds and eggs: a diet very high in fat and protein, with very few vegetables or fruits. They live in a harsh environment that is marginal at best for human habitation. Yet early explorers, physicians and other scientists unanimously reported that the Inuit they encountered enjoyed excellent health and vitality.

Dr John Simpson studied the Inuit in the mid-1850s. He noted that the Inuit were 'robust, muscular and active, inclining rather to spareness, rather than corpulence, presenting a markedly healthy appearance. The expression of the countenance is one of habitual good humour. The physical constitution of both sexes is strong.' This is especially remarkable considering the inhospitable environment the Inuit lived in and it's a testament to the nutrient density of the animal foods that comprised the majority of their diet.

Nearly 100 years later, an American dentist named Weston A. Price, noticing an alarming increase in tooth decay and other problems in his patients, set out to determine whether traditional peoples that had not adopted a Western diet suffered from the same problems. In 1933, he took a trip to the

Arctic to visit the Inuit, one of many cultures he studied, and he was deeply impressed by what he found. He praised the Inuit's 'magnificent dental development' and 'freedom from dental caries [cavities]'.

It's especially impressive that the Inuit enjoyed such robust good health considering that their diets were 80–85 per cent fat, a percentage that would surely horrify the American Medical Association and the NHS in the UK. Unfortunately, as modern Inuit people have moved away from their traditional diet, their health has suffered – as is the case with traditional populations around the world.

The Aboriginal Australians

Indigenous Australians – or Aboriginal Australians – were the original inhabitants of the Australian continent and surrounding islands. They traditionally lived as hunter-gatherers, consuming mostly animal products – including land mammals, birds, reptiles, seafood and insects – along with a variety of plants. The quality of their diet depended in large part upon where they lived: the subtropical, coastal areas were lush and provided abundant food, whereas the diversity and amount of food in the harsh desert interior was much lower.

Nevertheless, numerous studies suggest that even those Aboriginal Australians living in marginal environments were free from modern diseases like obesity, diabetes and heart disease. Weston Price described them as 'a living museum preserved from the dawn of animal life on the earth'.

Even today, contemporary Aboriginal Australians who live a traditional lifestyle are still lean and fit, with no evidence of obesity, insulin resistance, type-2 diabetes or cardiovascular disease. A study published in 1991 found that this population had optimal blood pressure, fasting glucose levels (an indicator of diabetes) and cholesterol levels, with an average BMI well below that of Australians living in urban environments.

In contrast, Aboriginal Australians develop unusually high rates of diabetes, cardiovascular disease and obesity when they make the transition from their traditional hunter-gatherer lifestyle to a Westernised lifestyle, according to the same study, and Westernised Aboriginal Australians experience a dramatic improvement in metabolic and cardiovascular health when they return to their traditional ways.

These three groups of hunter-gatherers have enjoyed good health with their traditional lifestyles into the 21st century, although each eats a very different diet. This may indicate that what we don't eat may be just as important as what we do eat.

ARE PEOPLE WHO EAT MORE GRAINS LESS HEALTHY?

Another way to consider whether traditional Palaeolithic diets are healthier is to look at cultures and groups that consume large amounts of grain. Are they more likely to have health problems? There's a great deal of research that says 'yes'. Whole grains, pulses, nuts and seeds contain the chemical phytate, which binds to minerals such as calcium, iron, zinc and manganese, making them more difficult to absorb. If a food contains nutrients that you can't absorb, you're not going to reap their benefits.

Studies show that children on vegetarian macrobiotic diets – 'healthy' diets composed of whole grains (especially brown rice), pulses, vegetables and some fruits – are deficient in vitamins and minerals and are more likely to develop rickets than their meat-eating peers. Breast-fed babies of macrobiotic mothers may be getting lower levels of vitamin B_{12}, calcium and magnesium, according to some research, resulting in delayed physical and cognitive growth.

Cultures that are heavily dependent upon grains often show

signs of severe vitamin A and protein deficiencies, which make them more susceptible to infectious disease. Dr Edward Mellanby, the discoverer of vitamin D, compared the agricultural Kikuyu tribe with the pastoralist Masai tribe, who consume primarily the milk, blood and flesh of the cows they raise. Dr Mellanby discovered that the Kikuyu, who lived mainly on cereals, had a far higher incidence of bronchitis, pneumonia, tropical ulcers and tuberculosis than the Masai.

We've been led to believe that 'healthy whole grains' are nutritional marvels, but cereal grains like corn, wheat and rice don't deserve that label. They're inferior to animal products as a source of protein, because they're considered 'incomplete', meaning that they're missing one or more essential amino acids. (Essential amino acids are the amino acids – the building blocks of protein – that our bodies can't synthesise themselves and must therefore get from our diets.) Grains are also lower in vitamins and minerals compared to meat and the variety of wild fruits and vegetables consumed by our ancestors.

The evidence suggests that when we eat grains at the expense of other more nutritious foods – especially when those grains are not properly prepared to reduce their phytate content and other toxins – our health suffers.

How meat made us human

Eating meat and cooking food is quite literally what made us human. The transition from a raw, exclusively plant-based diet to one that included meat and cooked food (along with starchy tubers) is what enabled the brains of our 'pre-human' ancestors to grow so rapidly.

Humans have exceptionally large, neuron-rich brains relative to our body size compared to non-human primates; for example, gorillas have bodies that are much larger than ours, but smaller brains with only about a third the number of neurons. So why is it that the largest primates don't also have the largest brains?

The answer is that the brain competes with other organs for resources in the body. Gorillas require a large, metabolically 'expensive' digestive tract to process the high-fibre, low-calorie plant matter they consume. This doesn't leave enough remaining resources for a larger, higher-performance brain (like ours). The human brain is an expensive metabolic tissue: it consumes 20 per cent of total body energy even though it represents only 2 per cent of body mass.

The larger you are, the more you need to eat. The more you need to eat, the more time you have to spend feeding yourself. Gorillas, who are vegetarians, already spend as much as 9.6 hours of a 12-hour day eating, in part because the fibrous plant matter they consume takes so long to break down and absorb. In order to provide enough energy for a human-like brain, they'd have to eat for an extra two hours a day! Likewise, early humans eating only raw vegetation would have needed to eat for more than nine hours a day to get enough calories to support their large brains.

Since gathering food was both dangerous and time-consuming, this makes a completely vegetarian, vegan, raw diet unlikely for our ancestors. When humans began cooking their meat, it became easier to chew and therefore to digest and absorb, increasing both the calorific content and nutritional density of the human diet.

As you'll see in Chapter 3 (which focuses on nutrient density), meat provides an ideal mix of amino acids, fats, vitamins and minerals for brain growth and maintenance. Vitamin B_{12} – available only in animal foods – is particularly important for developing brains.

It's possible to survive on vegan or vegetarian diets today, but they're far from optimal or normal for our species. People choose not to eat meat for many reasons, including concerns about the ethical treatment of animals, the amount of resources depleted in raising animals for consumption and religious observation. Those are complex issues beyond the scope of this book. My point is simply that we may not have become human as we know ourselves today without this nutritious food source.

THE INDUSTRIAL REVOLUTION: OUT OF THE FRYING PAN INTO THE FIRE

The Agricultural Revolution began the transition out of 66,000 generations of good health. But this shift didn't really hit full stride until about six generations ago, when we reached another milestone in human development: the Industrial Revolution ushered in a new age of industry, mass production, transportation, urbanisation and economic development.

Although the Industrial Revolution dates to the 18th century, its dietary effects didn't become evident until the late 1800s. Improved transportation meant greater access to food for more people. Mass-production methods meant that foods like white flour, table sugar, vegetable oil and dairy could become fixtures at every table. White flour, for example, became widespread in the US after 1850, but didn't reach 'saturation point' until the 1890s. Mid-Victorians living in England between 1850 and 1890 generally enjoyed great health and still ate a fairly 'pre-industrial' diet. With falling prices and improved transportation, however, by around 1900 these modern foods comprised 70 per cent of total calories consumed each day – a remarkable change when you consider that none of them was available for the vast majority of human history.

Another significant change that came with the Industrial Revolution was a decrease in the diversity of the diet on a global scale. Palaeolithic hunter-gatherers consumed a large variety of plant species, primarily fruits, tubers and vegetables, as do their contemporaries; for example, the Alyawara tribe in central Australia consumed 92 plant species and the Tlokwa tribe in Botswana ate 126. Thanks to improved railways, roads and canals in the 19th and 20th centuries, a limited number of crops could be grown cheaply and shipped to every corner of the planet. Today, 80 per cent of the world's population lives on only four principal staple plants: wheat, rice, corn and potatoes.

The food introduced on a large scale by the Industrial Revolution (and grown with newly invented pesticides containing toxins) may be cheaper for us, but it isn't better. A 100g piece of sweet potato (about half a potato) contains only about 90 calories and 100g (one small serving) of wild-game meat contains about 150 calories, but both of these foods contain a wide spectrum of beneficial micronutrients. On the other hand, 100g (less than a cup) of refined wheat flour or sugar contains 361 or 387 calories respectively and virtually no beneficial nutrients at all. The same quantity of corn oil (about 7 tablespoons), a staple of modern diets, contains a whopping 881 calories and has essentially no nutritional value.

Even worse, industrialisation completely changed the way we lived. In 1800, 90–95 per cent of Americans still lived in rural areas, farming or living in small villages and towns. In 1900, about half the population remained in a non-urban environment. Today, less than 16 per cent of all Americans live in rural areas; in the UK it is less than 10 per cent, Australia is less than 11 per cent. With more people working in cities, we became more sedentary. Longer working hours meant less time in the sun and less sleep. Stress – chronic, unrelenting – became a fixture in everyday life. Although the Industrial Revolution undoubtedly improved our health in many ways (for example, greater protection against infectious disease, better emergency medical care, and so on) these benefits did not come without a significant cost. We have the Industrial Revolution to thank for new 'diseases of civilisation' that were rare or virtually non-existent in pre-industrial cultures:

- In the early 1950s in Uganda, only 0.7 per cent of people above the age of 40 showed any evidence of a previous heart attack, according to an autopsy study. Today, in a country where the Western-style diet has taken hold, heart disease is the fourth leading cause of death.

- In Papua New Guinea, heart attacks were unknown prior to urbanisation. Today, those rates are sky-rocketing, with upwards of 400,000 heart attacks a year in a population of 5.4 million people.

- Among the Pima Indians in Arizona, the first confirmed case of diabetes was in 1908. Thirty years later, 21 cases were reported, but by 1967 the number had risen to 500. Today, half of all adult Pima Indians have diabetes.

- When the South Pacific people of Tokelau migrated to nearby New Zealand and switched to a Western diet, they developed three times the rate of diabetes as those who remained in Tokelau.

As study after study shows, the more 'Westernised' a traditional culture becomes, the more disease it experiences. Today, obesity, diabetes, heart disease and other chronic, degenerative conditions collectively affect well over a billion people worldwide and kill millions of people each year. It may be nearly impossible for you to imagine life without them. Yet they've been common only for the last 150–200 years, a tiny fraction of human existence on the planet.

WE'RE STILL EVOLVING

So far I've argued that humans are 'mismatched' with an agricultural diet, because our environment changed faster than our genes and biology could adapt. But this doesn't mean that we haven't developed any adaptations to agriculture, or that human evolution stopped in the Palaeolithic era.

In fact, the pace of genetic change in humans has actually increased during the last few thousand years. Evolutionary biologist, Scott Williamson, suggests that evolution is occurring 100 times faster than its long-term average over the 6 million years of hominid evolution and that as much as 10 per cent of the genome shows evidence of recent evolution in European-Americans, African-Americans and Chinese.

This rapid increase in genetic change has been primarily driven by two factors, say anthropologists Gregory Cochran and Henry Harpending in their book *The 10,000 Year Explosion*:

- A significant change in our environment, which increased the selective pressure to adapt to it.

- A dramatic increase in our population, which increases the likelihood that adaptive mutations will arise by chance.

If there's a new source of slightly indigestible food available to a population that previously lacked abundant food sources, there would be a lot of selective pressure for those people to adapt to be able to consume that food. That's exactly what happened with milk. For most of our history, we stopped producing lactase, the enzyme that helps digest the milk sugar, some time in childhood. Since mother's milk was the only lactose-containing food in the human diet at that time, there was simply no need for children to continue making lactase after they stopped breastfeeding, which was at about age four for most hunter-gatherers.

This all changed, however, with the dawn of the Agricultural Revolution and the domestication of cattle, which made cow's milk a readily available food source. Early farmers who relied heavily on grains were prone to mineral deficiencies – especially calcium. Their skeletons, shorter than those of their hunter-gatherer predecessors, indicated that they also probably lacked vitamin D, which plays a role in skeletal development. Milk is rich in calcium, contains some vitamin D, is a complete protein and may promote growth during childhood. It also provided hydration and sustenance during periods of drought. Individuals who carried a genetic mutation allowing them to digest milk beyond their breastfeeding years would have been favoured by natural selection, and their genes would have spread rapidly through farming populations.

In fact, archaeological evidence and gene mapping studies suggest that a genetic mutation that continued the production of lactase into adulthood originated about 8,000 years ago somewhere in Europe and spread rapidly thereafter. Today, approximately one-third of the global population produces lactase into adulthood. In cattle-herding tribes in East Africa, like the Tutsi, the rate is up to 90 per cent. In some Northern European countries, like Denmark and Sweden, the genes are present in up to 95 per cent of people.

There are several other relatively recent changes – genetic and otherwise – that have influenced our response to modern foods. For example:

- Populations with historically high starch intake produce more amylase in their saliva. Amylase is an enzyme in the saliva that helps to digest starch and glucose, which are both forms of carbohydrate.

- New versions of genes that affect insulin and blood sugar regulation have also arisen in the relatively recent past. These mutations appear to increase carbohydrate tolerance and reduce the likelihood that a higher carbohydrate diet will lead to problems like diabetes.

• Changes in the expression of certain genes (which can happen much faster than changes to the underlying genes themselves) may help some populations that rely on grains as staples to process them more effectively.

• Finally, changes in the gut microbiota – the beneficial microorganisms that live in our digestive tract – can also directly affect our ability to assimilate certain nutrients. Researchers have identified a bacterium in the colon of Japanese people that produces an enzyme that helps them to digest seaweed (nori in particular). And some studies suggest that lactose intolerance can be eliminated simply by eating increasing amounts of yoghurt containing lactose and live bacteria – all of which can naturally metabolise lactose.

Our bodies, therefore, have adapted in some ways to offset the challenges of an agricultural diet. Human innovation has also helped us. As I mentioned in the previous section, cereal grains and pulses contain phytate, which bonds with calcium, iron, zinc and other minerals. The human gut is unable to break these bonds, which means that it's difficult for us to absorb the minerals from grains. But traditional cultures soaked grains and grain flours in an acid medium (such as whey or lemon juice), fermented them, germinated (sprouted) them, or leavened them (for example, baking bread with a natural sourdough starter), which significantly reduced their phytate content and thus made the minerals they contain more bioavailable (that is, easier to absorb).

WILL EVOLUTION CATCH UP
WITH WESTERN DIETS?

Humans, it would seem, are well adapted to Palaeolithic foods such as meat, vegetables, fruits and tubers, because we've been eating them for millennia, and the evidence shows our health declined with the introduction of agricultural foods; however, the fact that a food wasn't available during the Palaeolithic era doesn't necessarily mean we should avoid it entirely. The genetic and cultural changes I've described above occurred (at least in part) to help us adapt to an agricultural diet, and they do influence how each of us tolerates 'Neolithic' foods. This explains why some people are able to include moderate amounts of dairy, grains and/or pulses in their diet – especially when they are 'pre-digested' by fermentation, soaking, sprouting or leavening – without ill effect. (I'll have more to say on this topic later in the book.)

These genetic changes don't mean we can eat a diet high in cereal grains and low in animal protein without adverse health consequences, however. These adaptations are often simple mutations of single genes. They're also relatively crude; for example, the mutation that enables us to digest milk beyond childhood simply 'breaks' the genetic switch that turns off lactase production after infancy. This rather haphazard fix reflects the short time frame in which it took place – it's much easier for the body to break something that already exists than to create something new.

If we waited for long enough, it's at least possible that humans could evolve a more complex adaptation (involving the coordinated action of several different genes) to a grain-heavy diet. This might include changes in our gastrointestinal tract that would allow us to better assimilate nutrients from grains. But even if such an adaptation were to occur, it wouldn't change the fact that grains are far less nutrient dense than meats, fish and vegetables – the staple foods of our

Palaeolithic ancestors. This is especially true when you take into account the bioavailability of nutrients, which is high in animal products and low in grains.

For these reasons, the best approach is to make the 'Palaeolithic' foods we're adapted to eat the foundation of your diet and then to personalise it depending on your own unique combination of genetics, health status, activity level, life circumstances and goals. That's exactly what I'm going to show you how to do, starting in the next chapter.

Obviously, a lot has changed since our Palaeolithic ancestors roamed the earth, and most of us aren't living like the contemporary hunter-gatherer populations I've mentioned in this chapter. How do we know their lifestyle is our best option today? Beyond the considerable anthropological record, there are several lines of modern, clinical evidence supporting the health benefits of a 'Paleo template' diet and lifestyle. These include:

- The high nutrient density of Paleo foods.

- The minimal presence of toxins and anti-nutrients in Paleo foods.

- The superior balance of fats in a Paleo diet.

- The importance of the gut microbiota to human health and the beneficial effects of the Paleo diet on gut bacteria.

- The benefits of integrating physical activity throughout the day and minimising sedentary time, as our Paleo ancestors did.

- The importance of sleeping at least seven to eight hours a night and minimising exposure to artificial light, something our Paleo ancestors never had to contend with.

- The benefits of sun exposure (which go beyond vitamin D) and spending time outdoors.

- The importance of pleasure, play and social connection.

I'll cover each of these – and much more – in Steps 1 and 2 of the book. Again, the good news is that we don't have to live in caves or roam the earth for food to enjoy the benefit of a Paleo-style diet. And there's no need to run to a geneticist to see if you have the right alleles (variations of genes) to digest milk or wheat. Your Personal Paleo Diet will lead you to the perfect diet. For now, I hope I've convinced you that a Paleo template is the right place to start.

Ready? Let's get started!

STEP 1

Reset Your Diet

CHAPTER 2

Reset to Feel Better – Fast

When your computer starts running slowly, applications are crashing left and right and you can't even move the cursor anymore, what do you do?

You press the reset buttons – control-alt-delete (or whichever combination works on your system). Sometimes we need to do the same thing with our bodies. They're under constant assault in the modern world. Refined, processed food, environmental toxins, stress, sleep deprivation and chronic infections can all wreak havoc with our health.

We're simply not adapted to live this way. With a few exceptions (which I'll cover later), we're still hard-wired to eat the foods our hunter-gatherer ancestors ate. When we follow that 2-million-year-old genetic template, as we did for thousands of generations, we're naturally healthy and vital. But when we stray from it, as we have in the recent past, we suffer. If you want to feel better fast, the best thing to do is to get back to basics.

How do you hit reset?

Notes for this chapter may be found at ChrisKresser.com/ppcnotes/#ch2

With Step 1's 30-Day Reset Diet. You commit to a 30-day period where you eliminate the modern foods that contribute to disease, as well as the foods people are most often allergic to or intolerant of, and focus on the safe, nourishing foods our ancestors have thrived on for more than 66,000 generations.

Then, after you've 'hit reset' and returned to that basic template, you can customise it to find the approach that works best for you over the long term (as you'll see later in Steps 2 and 3).

THE 30-DAY RESET DIET

The Reset Diet is designed to reduce inflammation, improve digestion, burn fat, identify food sensitivities, reduce allergic reactions, boost energy, regulate blood sugar and stabilise your mood.

It almost seems too good to be true, but I've not only done this myself I've also guided thousands of people through it. And I can tell you this: it works! No other therapy – natural or otherwise – can come even remotely close to accomplishing all these goals in such a short period.

Why 30 days? Because that's how long, on average, it takes my patients to experience the full benefits of the reset. It's absolutely essential that you commit to making these changes for at least 30 days – without cheating. Later on in the pro-gramme, you'll have more leeway to go off the rails every now and then. After all, there's more to life than food! But the Reset phase is not one of those times. This is where you gather your strength and buckle down. I know you can do it, because thousands of other people just like you already have.

In Step 2 of the programme, you'll be able to reintroduce some of the foods you eliminated during the 30-Day Reset Diet to see if you tolerate them. In Step 3, you'll learn how to make them part of a flexible lifestyle. But for now, the only way to find out if these foods are causing problems is to avoid them entirely.

As with any new diet or exercise programme, check with your healthcare professional before you begin.

WHAT FOODS CAN YOU EAT?

I've broken down the foods you can and can't eat into three categories to make it as easy as possible:

Eat liberally You can enjoy as much of these foods as you like. No counting calories or calculating ratios of protein, fat or carbohydrate. This isn't a 'cleanse' or a fast. If a food is on this list, you're free to eat it.

Eat in moderation You can eat these foods, but don't go wild. I've indicated how often or how much of them I think is safe, but in general you want to limit consumption of these foods compared to those in the 'eat liberally' category.

Avoid completely Yes, completely. The success (or failure) of the programme hinges on your ability to steer clear of these foods during the 30-day Reset.

As you'll see in later chapters, there are convincing reasons for choosing or avoiding specific foods in each of these categories. For now, however, let's look at what's on – or off – the list during the Reset.

Eat liberally

Meat and poultry Emphasise beef and lamb or mutton, but also pork, chicken, turkey, duck, goat and wild game such as venison, ostrich, and so on. Organic and free-range is always preferable, but it is especially important during this programme, when you're trying to minimise all toxins; however, if that option is not available, don't let that get in the way of your Reset.

Organ meats (especially liver) Liver is the most nutrient-dense food on the planet, rich in vitamin A, iron and all the essential amino acids. If you don't like its taste, chop fresh liver into 1cm cubes and freeze them in an ice-cube tray, then pop them out, transfer them to a freezer bag and store in the freezer. When you're making any meat dish, defrost a cube, chop it finely and mix it in. You won't notice the taste, but you'll get all the nutrients. If you're adventurous, try heart, kidneys, spleen, tongue and brains. (**Note** If you have iron overload, a condition of excess iron storage in the body, you should not eat organ meats. See page 176 for more information.)

Bone broth soups It's essential to balance your intake of muscle meats and organ meats with home-made bone broths. Bone broths differ from stocks in that they're simmered for a long time – up to 48 hours – to get the maximum nutrition from the bones. They're not only delicious but they're also rich in glycine, an amino acid found in collagen, which is a protein important in maintaining a healthy gut lining. (See the recipe on page 448 and the website for instructions on making your own bone broth.)

Fish, especially oily fish such as salmon, sardines, mackerel, anchovies and herring. Wild is preferable. It's best to eat three 175g servings of oily fish per week to meet your needs for the omega-3 fats, EPA and DHA, as I'll discuss in Chapter 5.

Eggs, preferably free-range and organic. And yes, yolks are allowed, if you've believed in the past that they are unhealthy – I even encourage them, because they're an excellent source of vitamin D, selenium and other important nutrients.

Starchy plants Yams, sweet potatoes, tapioca, yuca (also sold as cassava or manioc), taro, lotus root, plantains (ripe and unripe), breadfruit, celeriac and parsnip. (Boil the peeled yuca for 30 minutes, then roast or mash it before eating to remove toxic goitrogens – compounds that can impair thyroid function in susceptible individuals.) No white potatoes are allowed during the Reset, but don't worry, you can see whether they belong back on your plate during Step 2.

Non-starchy vegetables, either cooked or raw. These include artichoke, asparagus, aubergine, beetroot, broccoli, Brussels sprouts, cabbage, carrots, cauliflower, celery, chillies, courgette, cucumber, garlic, leaves (beetroot, spring, dandelion, mustard), kale, leeks, lettuce (endive, iceberg, leafy varieties, radicchio, cos), mushrooms, okra, onions, parsley, peppers, pumpkin, radishes, spring onions, spinach, swede, Swiss chard, tomato, turnips.

Fermented vegetables and fruit Sauerkraut, kimchi, beetroot kvaas, coconut kefir, and so on. Loaded with 'good' bacteria, fermented foods are excellent for gut health.

Traditional fats Coconut oil, red palm oil, palm kernel oil, macadamia oil, lard (rendered from free-range pigs, if possible), duck fat, beef tallow (from free-range cattle if possible) and olive oil (preferably extra virgin).

Olives, avocados and coconuts (including coconut milk).

Sea salt and spices Avoid sugar or artificial flavourings.

Eat in moderation

Processed meat Sausages, bacon, salami, pepperoni and jerky. Make sure they're gluten-, sugar- and soya free, and organic/free-range meat is preferable. Two to four servings a week is fine.

Whole fruit Up to four servings per day, depending on your blood sugar balance (see below) and the type of fruit. Choose a wide variety of colours: green, red, orange and yellow. All fruit is permitted, but favour low-sugar fruits such as berries, grapefruit, oranges and peaches over tropical fruits, apples, grapes and pears. Watch out for dried fruit – it's easy to consume a lot of sugar with a single handful. (See NutritionData.com to find the amount of sugar in fruits, as well as nutrient values for other foods.)

Nuts and seeds Allowed nuts include almonds, Brazil nuts, cashew nuts, hazelnuts, macadamia nuts, pecan nuts, pine nuts, pistachio nuts and walnuts. (**Note** Peanuts are actually legumes, not nuts, and they're not allowed during the 30-Day Reset Diet.) Favour nuts lower in omega-6, such as hazelnuts and macadamia nuts, and minimise nuts high in omega-6, such as Brazil nuts and almonds. Allowed seeds include chia, flax, pumpkin, sesame, sunflower, and so on. It is easy to overeat nuts and seeds, so limit yourself to a handful per day. (See page 82 for important information on how to prepare nuts to make them easier to digest and more nutritious.) Sesame oil should be used only sparingly, because it contains relatively high levels of omega-6 linoleic acid, which is not good. I'll explain more in Chapter 5.

Green beans, sugar snap peas and mangetout Although technically legumes, they are usually well tolerated. You may eat four to six servings of these per week.

Coffee and black tea All teas and coffee are permitted – black, or with coconut milk. Limit caffeinated coffee and tea to one 225ml cup (not one triple espresso, but one cup of brewed coffee) and only before noon; however, if you experience fatigue, insomnia, anxiety, hypoglycaemia, mood swings or depression, you should eliminate all caffeine entirely. (Check labels; you'll find caffeine lurking in many headache and cold preparations.) Caffeine stimulates the adrenal glands and can worsen all of these conditions. Once your adrenal issues have been addressed – see Chapter 20 – you may be able to add caffeine back in moderation.

Vinegar Cider, balsamic, red wine and other varieties. Cider vinegar is especially well tolerated. Vinegar may be used in small amounts every day as part of a salad dressing or sauce.

Restaurant food Restaurants cook with industrial seed and vegetable oils (on the 'avoid' list, below), which can wreak havoc with your health. Also, it's hard to escape grains hidden in breaded coatings, salads and other dishes, as well as some of the other foods on the 'avoid' list. For these reasons, limit restaurant food as much as possible during the 30-Day Reset. I'd suggest eating out no more than twice a week (lunch included). I'll offer tips on how to order in restaurants in Chapter 19.

Avoid completely

Dairy, including ghee, butter, cheese, yoghurt, milk, cream and any dairy product that comes from a cow, goat, sheep or other mammal.

Grains, including wheat, rice, cereal, oats or any pseudo grains and non-gluten grains, such as sorghum, teff, quinoa, amaranth, buckwheat, spelt, rye, barley, couscous, malt, matzoh, tabbouleh, udon, gram flour, and so on. In other words: no bread, pasta, cereal or pizza. And for now, don't go shopping for 'gluten-free' substitutes, which can cause inflammation.

Pulses, including beans of all kinds (soya, kidney, cannellini, haricot, black, pinto, and so on), peas, lentils and peanuts.

(Read labels: soya is present in miso, tofu, bean curd, natto, tamari, tempeh, texturised vegetable protein (TVP) and other vegetarian versions of meat, edamame and elsewhere.)

Sweeteners, whether real or artificial, including sugar, high-fructose corn syrup (HFCS), dextrose, coconut sugar, molasses, maple syrup, honey, agave, brown rice syrup, Splenda, Equal, Nutrasweet, xylitol, mannitol, stevia, and so on.

Chocolate Milk chocolate contains both dairy and sugar and should be avoided for that reason. There's nothing wrong with dark chocolate (more than 75 per cent cocoa); in fact, it's one of the most nutrient-dense foods available, as you'll learn in Chapter 3; however, many people who are intolerant to gluten are (unfortunately!) also intolerant to the proteins in chocolate, so it should be avoided during the Step 1 Reset. You can reintroduce it during Step 2.

Processed or refined foods As a general rule, if it comes in a bag or a box, don't eat it. This also includes highly processed 'health foods' such as protein powder, energy bars, dairy-free creamers, and so on.

Industrial seed and vegetable oils Soya, corn, safflower, sunflower, rapeseed, peanut, cottonseed, and so on. Read labels – seed oils are in almost all processed, packaged and refined foods (which you should be mostly avoiding during this phase anyway).

Fizzy drinks, including diet drinks, as well as fruit juice, in all forms, including 'natural' brands. Avoid fruit juice during the Reset, because it's high in sugar and easy to over-consume. Coconut water is fine, but limit to 125ml a day – it's quite sweet. Plain soda water or mineral water is fine.

Alcohol – in any form. (Don't freak out – you'll be adding this back in Step 2.)

Processed sauces and seasonings Soy sauce, tamari and other processed seasonings and sauces (which often contain sugar, soya, gluten, or all of the above).

Visit the website for a version of the list above that you can print out and post on your fridge and take with you to the shops or supermarket.

Does red meat cause heart disease?

You might be surprised that red meat is included in the 'eat liberally' category. After all, haven't we been told for years that red meat contributes to heart disease? It's true that some studies do show an association between red meat consumption and heart disease. Yet others – especially those that separate fresh red meat consumption from processed meat consumption – have found none. This includes a large review of studies in 2010 covering more than 1.2 million participants, which found that consumption of fresh, unprocessed red meat was not associated with increased risk of coronary heart disease (CHD), stroke or diabetes. In addition, it's hard to draw conclusions from observational studies on red meat and disease, because of something known as the 'healthy user bias': because red meat has been viewed as unhealthy for so long, those who eat more of it are also more likely to engage in other behaviours perceived (correctly, in these cases) as unhealthy, such as smoking, eating processed and refined food and not getting enough exercise.

If eating red meat did cause heart disease, we'd expect to see lower rates of heart disease in vegetarians and vegans.

Again, early studies suggested this was true, but they suffered from the same 'healthy user bias' as the red meat studies (that is, vegetarians tend to be more health-conscious on average than the general population, so there could be other factors explaining their lower incidence of heart disease, such as more exercise, less smoking, and so on). Newer, higher-quality studies that have attempted to control for these confounding factors haven't found any difference in rates of heart disease between omnivores and vegetarians; for example, one study compared the risk of death from heart disease of people who shopped in health-food shops (both vegetarians and omnivores) to people in the general population. They found that both vegetarians and omnivores in the health-food shop group had a lower risk of death from heart disease than people in the general population, but there was no difference between the health-food shop omnivores and the vegetarians.

So there's no reason to feel guilty or frightened about digging into that juicy steak or beef stew!

HOW TO BE A FOOD DETECTIVE

Before you begin your 30-Day Reset, police your pantry and get rid of food that's off-limits. (You can donate it to your local food bank, if you like.) Dairy, sugar and fat lurk in many products, so read the ingredients labels – you might be surprised where culprits are hiding!

Where dairy hides Anything containing casein, whey, malt, or with the prefix 'lacto-' is off-limits during the Reset, as are foods with 'curds', 'pudding', and 'custard' on the packaging. Many artificial flavours and colourings also have dairy in them.

Where sugar hides You'd expect to find sugar in cereals and drinks, but did you know it's frequently in salad dressing, canned soup, peanut butter, beef jerky, or tomato sauce, in 'healthy' granola bars and yoghurt? Dried fruit may also contain added sugar. 'Fat-free' is often code for 'We added a lot of sugar to this so that you won't miss the fat.' You'll also find sugar 'hidden' inside other words commonly found on food labels. Watch out for fruit juice concentrate, corn sweetener, malt syrup, maltodextrin, evaporated cane juice or syrup, or any word ending in '-ose', such as sucrose, dextrose, galactose or maltose. Sugar is sugar, no matter whether it comes from beetroot or other healthy-sounding sources, or if it arrives in a special form, like confectioner's, muscovado or 'raw' sugar.

Where industrial seed oils hide Read the labels to make sure that your healthy nuts aren't roasted in unhealthy fats. Also, if a product has been processed to be 'shelf stable', it probably has industrial seed oils and artificial trans-fats (watch for the words 'partially hydrogenated') – another reason to avoid boxes and bags, especially during the Reset phase.

CAVEATS AND TWEAKS FOR SPECIAL CONDITIONS

If you've been diagnosed with certain health conditions, you'll need to modify the 30-Day Reset Diet. If you're not sure, take the Reset Diet Symptoms Questionnaire on pages 56–57. Add up the total number of points in each section for the symptoms you experience. Then use the answer key to determine which diet you should follow.

Questionnaire: Reset Diet Symptoms

1 Blood sugar and weight regulation

	Points
Diagnosed with diabetes, impaired glucose tolerance or hypoglycaemia	50
Feel fatigued directly after meals	5
Crave sweets during the day	5
Eating sweets doesn't relieve cravings for sugar	5
Must have sweets after meals	5
Feel agitated if you don't eat frequently	5
Irritable or light-headed between meals	5
Eating relieves fatigue	5
Feel shaky or jittery, especially between meals	5
Need caffeine to get yourself started in the morning	5
Easily upset or nervous	5
Poor memory or forgetful	5
Waist circumference equal to or larger than hip circumference	5
Difficulty losing weight	5
Increased thirst or appetite	5
Frequent urination	5
Blurred vision	5
TOTAL	

Answer key:

Score	Blood sugar and weight regulation
0–49	Follow the normal 30-Day Reset
More than 50	Follow the 30-Day Reset with blood sugar and weight regulation modifications (listed on page 58)

2 Autoimmune problems

	Points
Diagnosed with autoimmune disease	50
High C-reactive protein and other inflammatory markers on lab tests	5
Muscle or joint aches and pains	5
Persistent fever	5
Extreme fatigue	5
Swollen glands	5
Abdominal pain, digestive problems, constipation or diarrhoea	5
Itchy skin or skin rashes	5
Tingling in hands and/or feet	5
Sudden, unexplained weight loss or weight gain	5
Changes in skin colour	5
Food allergies or multiple food sensitivities	5
TOTAL	

Answer key:

Score	Autoimmune problems
0–49	Follow the normal 30-Day Reset
More than 50	Follow the 30-Day Reset with autoimmune modifications (listed on page 58)

If you scored over 50 on both parts of the questionnaire, you should follow the modifications for blood sugar *and* autoimmune problems during the 30-Day Reset, and consult with your physician or healthcare provider.

Tweaks for problems with blood sugar or weight regulation

If you scored 50 points or more in this category and/or you're trying to lose weight, you should limit fruit and starchy vegetables during your 30-Day Reset. Eat all the non-starchy vegetables you want, but limit your fruit and starchy vegetables to roughly 10–15 per cent of calories from carbohydrate. This amounts to roughly 65–100g daily for a moderately active male and 50–75g daily for a moderately active female. To give you a general idea of what this looks like in terms of food, 50g of carbohydrate is equal to one large sweet potato and ½ cup of blueberries; 100g of carbohydrate is equal to ½ cup of blueberries, ½ cup of strawberries and two large sweet potatoes. You can search online databases like the ones from the USDA to determine the carbohydrate content of foods (http://ndb.nal.usda.gov/).

Tweaks for autoimmune problems

If you scored 50 points or more in this category, please follow the 30-Day Reset, but also avoid the following:

- Eggs (both whites and yolks). Eggs contain proteins that are common allergens, particularly in susceptible people.

- Nightshades (potatoes, tomatoes, peppers, chillies, aubergine, tomatillos, pimentos, paprika and cayenne pepper). Nightshades have compounds called alkaloids that can cause inflammation and worsen joint pain in susceptible people.

Not everyone with an autoimmune condition needs to be on the protocol for ever – you'll experiment with adding these foods back in Step 2.

FREQUENTLY ASKED QUESTIONS ABOUT STEP 1: THE 30-DAY RESET DIET

If you're completely new to this way of eating, you might be feeling pretty overwhelmed right now. 'I thought saturated fats were bad,' you say. 'Aren't whole grains healthy?' I'll take up all these questions in the chapters that follow. For now, let's tackle some of the more immediate questions you may have.

How do I do it?

I recognise this will be a dramatic change for many of you. The best way to do it is to just dive right in. Begin right now. If you procrastinate or delay, it just gets harder.

Use the meal plans and recipes in Chapter 21 to plan what you're going to eat for the first week. (You can find additional recipes and cheat sheets, sample menus, worksheets and shopping lists on the website.) Then set off for the supermarket, farmers' market, butcher's, fishmonger, greengrocer, or wherever you shop, and stock up for the next week. All you have to do is think about what to eat and what not to eat. There are no calories to count. Just eat the foods that are allowed and don't eat the ones that aren't.

When will I get results?

The first few days can be hard. Your body will be going through withdrawal from 'everyday' substances such as sugar and wheat. You may notice symptoms like mood swings, strong cravings, irritability and fatigue, as your body adjusts to life without them. If you've been drinking four cups of coffee every day for 20 years, cutting back to one cup will be tough. Does that mean you shouldn't do it? That it wouldn't benefit your health in the long run? No. It just means you're probably going to need some support along the way.

If you've been eating a poor diet with a lot of processed food, smoking, drinking too much alcohol and leading a sedentary life filled with chronic stress, I truly understand that the transition to a healthy diet will be a big challenge. But at some point you will recover and start feeling better than you did before you began the programme.

Most of my patients say that the first four to seven days are the hardest. After that, you'll start having a lot more energy. Those familiar dips in energy in the afternoon may well disappear completely – without the 'hit' of that afternoon coffee and chocolate bar. In fact, your cravings may disappear altogether. You'll find yourself eyeing that pizza or pasta dish and thinking, 'No thanks.' Your skin will clear up, the outbreaks and redness disappearing. Your digestion will smooth out. You'll sleep more deeply and wake feeling more rested. Those up-and-down mood swings will stabilise. You'll start shedding some pounds (only if you need to, usually). Even if the scale doesn't budge, you may find that muffin top melting. Aches, pains and the mysterious symptoms you've had for ages will – seemingly miraculously – begin to improve.

This programme has the potential to change your life. I realise that it's difficult; I know how much work it is, and I remember what it was like to cut out all these foods. I've been there myself, although I can hardly remember why I used to love some of that junk food so much (cold cereal was a particular weakness). But I also know from my own experience, and from supervising many people through this transition, that the results are worth the effort.

I thought fat was bad for me, but some of the foods on the 'OK' list seem fatty

The biggest mistake people make on this programme is not eating enough fat. You're eliminating a lot of foods from your diet (bread, grains, beans, and so on) and you have to replace those calories with something. Healthy fat is that something. If you're concerned about your weight, take comfort in the knowledge that the vast majority of my patients and readers shed pounds on the 30-Day Reset. Fat is the preferred fuel source of the body and should constitute about 40–70 per cent of your calories, depending on individual needs. (My only caveat is chicken fat, which is delicious, but often comes from chickens that have been fed on grains, so the ratio of healthy omega-3 fat to not-so-healthy omega-6 fat isn't great. In a later chapter, you'll see why that ratio matters. If you can find chicken fat from pastured chickens, that's fine and healthy to eat.) You can exchange that dry, boneless, skinless chicken breast for a luscious pork chop or a nice juicy steak.

A little cheat here and there can't hurt, can it?

Once you've worked out your ideal diet, I'd agree that a little cheat occasionally is fine but, as I said above, this isn't the time to cheat. Don't do it. It's not worth it.

By removing the foods that most commonly cause problems, you allow your body to rest and recover from whatever symptoms those foods have been provoking. Just one cheat could trigger a whole new cascade of reactions. A single piece of bread or one glass of milk could restart the inflammatory process and throw your body back into the chaos that led you to the Personal Paleo Diet programme in the first place. Some of the greatest benefits of the Reset Diet don't kick in until the third week – right when the finish line is in sight.

At some point you won't even miss those foods you think you can't live without. So don't cheat. It could set you back. If you go for the full 30 days, it will get easier. I promise.

Shouldn't I be counting calories and calculating the percentage of fat, protein and carbohydrate I eat?

Relax – no calculators. (The only exceptions here are people with specific health conditions; see below.) In the next chapter, I'll discuss why the concentration of nutrients in the food we eat (that is, nutrient density) is often a more important consideration than the absolute quantity of food (or calories) we eat. And in Step 3, I'll discuss how to determine the optimal amount of fat, carbohydrate and protein (macronutrients) to eat based on your individual circumstances. For now, we're focusing more on the quality of macronutrients than the quantity. That said, you can use the following ranges as a starting point during the Reset (keep in mind that these measurements refer to the amount of each macronutrient in the food, not the total weight in the food):

- **Fat** 40–70 per cent of total calories (that is, 115–200g for a moderately active male eating 2,600 calories per day, or 100–155g for a moderately active female eating 2,000 calories per day).

- **Carbohydrate** 15–30 per cent (that is, 100–200g for a moderately active male eating 2,600 calories per day, or 75–150g for a moderately active female eating 2,000 calories per day).

- **Protein** 10–20 per cent (that is, 65–130g for a moderately active male eating 2,600 calories per day, or 50–100g for a moderately active female eating 2,000 calories per day).

Don't overanalyse what you're eating. Enjoy your food. Make cooking fun and leave time to savour your creations. You'll find recipes and meal plans in Chapter 21. There are also more recipes on the website. You've got real, delicious, nutrient-dense foods to choose from.

Can I juice?

If you juice with whole fruits or veggies or make into smoothies with water, unsweetened nut milk, or 125ml coconut water with no sugar added, you should be fine, although some of my patients say that they tend to feel hungrier when they 'drink their meals'. Focus on the veggies and the lower-sugar fruit like berries. And avoid prepared juices or smoothies, which often contain large amounts of natural sugar or processed sugars, such as high-fructose corn syrup, which you should avoid completely on the Reset.

This is too hard.
How can I make it easier?

No man (or woman) is an island. Change is hard and the more support you have in doing this, the easier it will be. Try enlisting your spouse, significant other, or a good friend to do this with you. (They may not be eager, but they'll thank you later when they realise that it might have benefits for them too.) Invite friends over to cook with you – focusing on the Personal Paleo Diet foods. Connect with others online who are following this approach. Be sure to look on the online forum where you can discuss your dietary changes with fellow adventurers. Ask questions. Get help.

Focus on what you're getting out of the 30-Day Reset Diet instead of what you can't have: not just that juicy steak or delicious omelette, but that looser waistband; not feeling exhausted in the middle of the afternoon; seeing a clearer complexion in the mirror; your knees not feeling so achy anymore; feeling sharper, less moody; your digestion running more smoothly; knowing that you're on your way to feeling better than you have felt for years – or perhaps ever before!

I'm really physically active.
Should I eat more?

If you're an athlete or very physically active, you will generally need more calories and a higher carbohydrate intake, especially after working out. As a general idea, you should aim for 25–60 per cent of calories from carbohydrate if you're seeking to maintain your current weight or to gain muscle, or 7–20 per cent of calories from carbohydrate if you're trying to lose fat. For protein, most athletes should aim for 0.8–1.0g of protein per pound of bodyweight per day if you're trying to lose fat or maintain weight, or 1.0–1.25g per pound of bodyweight per day if you're trying to gain muscle or increase performance. See Chapter 18 for detailed recommendations for those with high activity levels.

I'm going out to eat/I've got a trip planned.
What should I do?

If you're dining out, choose a place that can accommodate your needs. Call ahead and ask if they have gluten-free items on the menu. Pick a restaurant offering meat and vegetable dishes and order a side salad. (Skip the dressing, since it may have sugar, and ask for vinegar and olive oil to add yourself instead.) Don't put yourself in a situation where you're starving because you haven't planned in advance and then eat a big plate of pasta because that's all that's available. If you're travelling, stock up on Personal Paleo Diet-friendly snacks, such as nuts and veggies. See Chapter 19 for more tips and tricks for sticking to your 30-Day Reset Diet when eating out or on the road. Advance planning makes it possible!

I'm taking a lot of medication/supplements. Should I continue taking them during Step 1?

This one's a little harder to answer. Always check with your healthcare provider before starting or stopping any prescription medication or supplement. If you know the supplement helps you, or you're taking it for a specific goal or purpose (for example, iodine for thyroid function), by all means continue. If you can't even remember why you're taking a certain supplement, or you're uncertain about whether it's helping you, I suggest stopping it during Step 1. Not all supplements are beneficial, and some may even cause harm. (I'll discuss which supplements are most likely to help and cause harm in more detail in Chapter 18.)

How can I stay organised and motivated? Will your website help?

Go to ChrisKresser.com/PPC to register for the free Personal Paleo Diet resources I mention throughout the book, including cheat sheets with the most important information in bite-sized format; reference guides on bone broth, fermented foods and other topics; additional recipes; shopping lists; a Paleo Troubleshooting Guide; and other resources to take all of the guesswork out of it for you. Take a look around the website and familiarise yourself with what's available. Print out charts or whatever you need, put them up on your fridge and take them with you to the shops if you get stuck. Don't forget to get involved with the forum, where you can get support from other Personal Paleo Diet users who may be dealing with similar issues and who may have helpful recommendations to get you through each phase of the programme.

If you're having some difficulty beyond the usual adjustment period, don't be alarmed. It doesn't mean the Personal Paleo Diet won't work or isn't a good choice for you. Not all damage done to the body is immediately reversible; sometimes the 30-Day Reset Diet isn't enough to reverse that damage without additional help. You may need to tweak things a bit and add a few things to your programme.

Inflammation: why Your Personal Paleo Diet will protect you

Throughout this book, I'll be discussing foods and nutrients which may have inflammatory or anti-inflammatory properties. It's important to note which of these can trigger inflammation or alleviate it, as this condition is the cause of so many modern, chronic diseases.

When healthcare professionals and scientists talk about 'inflammation', you may automatically think of conditions like joint pain, most notably arthritis, which can involve swelling that you can often actually see; however, although swelling can be a symptom of inflammation, inflammation itself is actually the body's response to infection or other threats, through the production of white blood cells and other substances.

In many cases this inflammation is invisible, because it's occurring inside the body – but that doesn't mean it's any less harmful. In fact, just about all of the modern diseases that plague us today are caused at least in part by inflammation, including bowel diseases like Crohn's and ulcerative colitis, autoimmune diseases like Hashimoto's thyroiditis and rheumatoid arthritis, cardiovascular disease, obesity, type-2 diabetes, Alzheimer's and even depression. The good news is that when you follow a diet that aligns with Your Personal Paleo Diet, you naturally reduce the risk of inflammation and protect yourself from related illness.

'I'm so glad I stuck with it'

The 30-Day Reset Diet can be a big adjustment, but it offers big rewards! I hope you'll be inspired by these reports from people who took the plunge:

- 'My acid reflux went away after one week and my knee stopped swelling after two weeks. Imagine jumping into a time machine and travelling back in time 20 years! Imagine fitting into the clothes you wore when you were 25 years old! Imagine shocking your doctor and watching his double take when he reviews your new cholesterol levels! I am 51 years old and I feel as if I was 30 years old again.'

- 'No more haemorrhoids, no more pimples, no more dry skin, no more acidity in my mouth, no more farting – more energy. No post-lunch fatigue – better sleep, less sugar cravings.'

- 'After about a week, I started noticing moles that had been raised were now flat as a pancake and starting to disappear. I stayed with it for 45 days just because I was feeling so much better. I also dropped 12 pounds [5.4kg] with no effort. What a difference. Leg cramping, that "heavy" feeling, lethargic issues are all gone. Fingernails started to grow faster and stronger.'

- 'On the fifth night, I started sleeping deeply for the first time in my life. I lost weight for the first time since being diagnosed with hypothyroidism three years ago and have maintained a 2 stone 2lb [13.6kg] weight loss. I have more energy than I have ever had before. Also my digestion is solid.

   'Energy levels more even, tennis elbow inflammation disappeared, asthma improved, waistline shrunk. Definitely glad I stuck with it.'

- 'There were a couple of days with the flu-ish feeling as my body adjusted to the lack of sugar and salt. Within days, though, my digestion was improved. Dropped 25 points on both sides of my blood pressure and dropped cholesterol from a starting 7.25mmol/l to 3.8mmol/l about six months later. I avoided statins and dropped my blood pressure prescription that I'd been on for five years.'

- 'I feel the best ever. No insulin anymore and no more of the three big drugs for blood pressure.'
- 'My blood chemistry has improved greatly, especially my triglyceride count, from 4.3 to 0.5 in 30 days. I lost about 1 stone 1lb [6.8kg] in the first month. I got my health back and my family's health back. Once you learn the truth about anything, diet included, you can never go back.'
- 'After 30 days, my IBS was gone and my acne had cleared up. I had tons of energy at the gym and slept really well.'
- 'I kept wondering when the magic was going to happen, then digestion, sleep, energy, hunger, skin tone and weight all seemed to improve as quickly as if I had passed through a doorway. I am so glad I stuck with it. My mental and physical health have improved tenfold. It is amazing how much your body can heal in only 30 days.'

HOW DO I KNOW WHEN TO MOVE ON TO STEP 2?

Follow the Step 1 Reset Diet for a minimum of 30 days – even if you're feeling significantly better, or if most of your symptoms have improved, in less time. As mentioned, I've found that 30 days is the minimum amount of time it takes to establish a new pattern in the body. If you move on too quickly, you risk sabotaging your hard-won improvement.

If you feel you're still making progress and want to give

yourself more time to reap the benefits of the Reset, then continue for as long as you like. The Reset Diet is completely safe to follow for a lifetime. (Remember, though, as mentioned at the beginning of this chapter it is essential to check with your healthcare professional before you start the programme.) When you're ready to reintroduce some foods, or if you begin to feel like your improvements are levelling off, that's an indication that you're ready for Step 2.

If you stay on the Reset Diet for more than 30 days and your progress plateaus for more than two weeks, it's unlikely you will see further improvement by continuing with Step 1, so I recommend moving on to Step 2. In many cases, adding foods back during Step 2 can kick-start the improvement again.

Feeling better fast is a powerful motivation to move on to Step 2. In the following chapters, I'm going to explain the core principles behind the Personal Paleo Diet, which will give you even more motivation while you are doing the Reset.

CHAPTER 3

Nutrient Know-How: Maximising Nutrient Density in Every Bite

Ruth, aged 65, came to see me complaining of numbness, tingling and weakness in her legs, reduced mobility and decreased balance and coordination. She also had brain fog – difficulty focusing, solving problems, and even spelling common words – and her memory sometimes failed her. 'I have suffered for years from these symptoms,' she said, 'but I always thought they were just a normal part of getting older.' When her symptoms worsened, she sought help. Two doctors she visited both suspected multiple sclerosis, but Ruth was sceptical of this diagnosis and came to see me for another opinion.

In discussing her medical history and asking about her diet, I learned that Ruth had been a vegetarian for the last 25 years but had never had her B_{12} levels tested. Vitamin B_{12} deficiency can mimic many of the symptoms of multiple sclerosis (MS) – including peripheral neuropathy (numbness and tingling in the arms and legs), cognitive decline and poor coordination and

Notes for this chapter may be found at ChrisKresser.com/ppcnotes/#ch3

balance – and is extremely common among long-term vegetarians. Sure enough, after I ran a full range of blood tests for her I found that her B_{12} levels were dangerously low. I immediately started her on intensive B_{12} supplementation, and within a matter of weeks her symptoms had vastly improved. Unfortunately, her recovery was not complete, because some damage caused by B_{12} deficiency is irreversible. This highlights the importance of this essential vitamin.

'I can't believe something so simple to diagnose and treat could cause so many problems,' she told me, upon learning of her B_{12} deficiency. 'I only wish I could have known this sooner.' Although she'd been a vegetarian for more than two decades, Ruth decided to start incorporating meat and fish back into her diet to give her body the B_{12} it so desperately needed.

There are many reasons why people choose to eat a vegetarian diet, and I respect individual choice. However, Ruth's story is a good example of what happens when we don't choose a nutrient-dense diet, and it highlights one of the greatest benefits of the Personal Paleo Diet approach: it contains the full spectrum of nutrients that humans require for optimal health.

WHY NUTRIENT DENSITY MATTERS

There are two types of nutrients in food: macronutrients, which include protein, carbohydrate and fat; and micronutrients, which are made up of vitamins, minerals and other compounds required in small amounts for normal metabolic function.

The 'nutrient density' of foods refers primarily to micronutrients and amino acids – the building blocks of protein. Carbohydrates and fats are important to health, but with the exception of two fatty acids – which we'll discuss in Chapter 5 – they can be synthesised by the human body if dietary intake is insufficient. The same cannot be said for micronutrients and the essential amino acids found in protein, which must be obtained from the diet.

Your body needs about 40 different micronutrients for proper physiological function; sub-optimal intake of any of them will contribute to disease and shorten lifespan. Unfortunately, nutrient deficiency is widespread in people following an industrialised diet that is energy- but not nutrient-dense. 'Energy density' is defined as the number of calories per a given weight of food, whereas nutrient density is defined as the concentration of nutrients in a given weight of food. With that in mind, you can understand why a large sugary fizzy drink has high energy density (lots of calories) but virtually no nutritional density.

Vegetable oils and sugar contribute about 36 per cent of calories in a typical US diet, yet are essentially devoid of micronutrients. Not surprisingly, studies have shown that the more energy-dense, nutrient-poor foods someone consumes, the more likely they are to have nutrient deficiencies. More than half of Americans are deficient in zinc, calcium, magnesium, vitamin A, vitamin B_6 and vitamin E, according to a 1997 survey. Approximately one-third are also deficient in riboflavin, thiamin, folate, vitamin C and iron. In many cases, these aren't mild nutrient deficiencies. Up to 50 per cent of Americans consume less than half the recommended daily allowance (RDA) for several micronutrients.

This is especially alarming when you consider the fact that the RDA is based on the amount of a nutrient required to avoid acute deficiency symptoms. It does not reflect the amount required to avoid deficiency symptoms over an extended period of time. This amount is not known for most micronutrients, but it is almost certainly higher than the RDA, which means that an even larger percentage of Americans than listed above is not getting enough of these vitamins and minerals (and the same is likely regarding people in the UK and Australia). Ruth, my patient with the B_{12} deficiency, is hardly alone!

THE CONSEQUENCES OF
NUTRIENT DEFICIENCY

You've already read about the precipitous decline in health among ancient hunter-gatherers when they adopted agriculture; those effects were in large part due to nutrient deficiencies caused by their new grain-based diet. Unfortunately, 366 generations later, we're still witnessing an inadequate intake of micronutrients and the widespread problems that causes.

It starts at a subcellular level in the body, where nutrient deficiency can mimic the effect of radiation and chemicals on DNA, causing single- and double-strand breaks, oxidative lesions or both. Simply put, nutrient deficiency threatens your body's ability to function normally and can shorten your lifespan. Here are just some of the conditions triggered by nutrient deficiency:

Immune function is adversely affected by poor intakes of nearly every essential vitamin and mineral, which compromises our ability to fight infections. And antioxidant vitamins, carotenoids and minerals are required to prevent premature ageing and protect against cellular damage.

Cardiovascular disease affects more than 65 million Americans and is the leading cause of deaths each year (responsible for almost four out of ten deaths). Sixty-five per cent of US adults are overweight and 34 per cent meet the criteria for metabolic syndrome: a constellation of medical disorders including high triglycerides, low HDL cholesterol, high fasting blood sugar, high blood pressure and abdominal obesity. Diabesity – a term coined by Dr Mark Hyman, which refers to the continuum of metabolic disorders from mild blood sugar imbalance to full-blown type-2 diabetes – affects one in two Americans. And the UK and Australia are not far behind the Americans for all of the above.

Micronutrient deficiency may contribute in part to all of these conditions; for example, magnesium deficiency is associated with an increased risk of metabolic syndrome and cardiovascular disease. Vitamin K_2 deficiency is associated with heart disease and coronary calcification. Deficiency of folate leads to increased levels of a compound that damages the fragile lining of blood vessels and is thought to contribute to heart disease. Folate deficiency also impairs a process called methylation, which in turn can lead to altered expression and suppression of genes and increase the risk of cancer.

WHOLE FOODS VS SUPPLEMENTS

You might be thinking that a multivitamin can prevent nutrient deficiency, but supplemental nutrients do not have the same effect on the body as nutrients from food. Humans are adapted to getting nutrients from whole foods – not supplements. Most nutrients require specific enzymes and other substances to be properly absorbed. Although these are naturally present in foods, they are often not included in synthetic vitamins with isolated nutrients. This may explain why several trials have shown that adding antioxidant supplements to a typical American diet not only doesn't prevent heart disease and cancer but it may increase the risk. Although supplements can (and should) be used for therapeutic effect in certain health conditions, or to replace certain nutrients that are difficult to obtain from food, they should never replace nutrients that could otherwise be found in a nutrient-dense diet.

Are vegetarian and vegan diets healthier than omnivorous diets?

Many vegetarians and vegans choose not to eat meat or animal products for ethical reasons, and I respect that choice. That said, from a nutritional perspective, it is difficult to justify a diet that causes deficiencies of several nutrients critical to human function. Although it may be possible to address these shortcomings through targeted supplementation (an issue that is still debated), it makes far more sense to meet nutritional needs from food. Humans are adapted to obtaining nutrients from food, and some evidence suggests that supplemental nutrients don't have the same effect on the body that nutrients in whole foods do. For more on my thoughts regarding vegetarianism versus omnivorous eating, as well as detailed information on B_{12} deficiency and other nutritional challenges posed by following a plant-based diet, please see the notes for this chapter on my website.

YOU ARE WHAT YOU ABSORB: THE IMPORTANCE OF BIOAVAILABILITY

Now you understand the importance of eating nutrient-dense food, but the most nutrient-dense food on the planet is worthless to us unless the nutrients it contains are bioavailable. Bioavailability refers to the portion of a nutrient that is absorbed from the diet and used for normal body functions. The level of bioavailable nutrients in a food is almost always lower than the absolute level of nutrients it contains.

The grass on your front lawn is a perfect example. Grass contains several vitamins and minerals, but they are largely inaccessible to humans because of its cellulose content. Cellulose is a fibre that forms the walls of cells in most green plants. Cows and sheep that eat grass are known as ruminant animals, because they have a specialised organ in their stomachs, called a rumen, which produces an enzyme that breaks down cellulose so that the nutrients in the grass can be absorbed. Ruminants also have three other chambers in their stomach to help them assimilate the nutrients from grass.

Humans have neither a rumen nor the other special chambers or enzymes, so we can't extract any nutrients from grass if we eat it. Fortunately, there is a solution to this problem: rather than eating the grass, humans can let animals do the hard work of assimilating the nutrients from grass, and then we can eat the animals.

There are three primary factors that affect the bioavailability of a given food.

First, minerals and other nutrients exist in different chemical forms in food. The classic example of this is iron, which exists in two forms: heme and non-heme. Heme iron is found only in animal products such as meat, fish, poultry and egg yolks, whereas non-heme iron is found in both plant and animal foods. Only about 2–20 per cent of non-heme iron is absorbed, compared to 15–35 per cent of heme iron. In addition, non-heme iron (but not heme iron) absorption is reduced by several different food components, such as the antioxidant compound known as phytate (found in whole grains and other foods), tannins (found in tea and coffee) and oxalates (found in spinach, sweet potatoes and Swiss chard).

Second, the absorption of most nutrients is dependent upon or influenced by the presence of other nutrients. Nutrient enhancers can keep a nutrient soluble or protect it from interaction with nutrient inhibitors; for example, beta-carotene, lutein and lycopene are fat-soluble, which means that these nutrients require fat for optimal assimilation. Adding avocado to a green salad (which increases its fat content by 47 per cent) can increase the absorption of lutein sevenfold and beta-carotene 18-fold. Another example is heme iron. Not only is heme iron better absorbed than non-heme iron (the form found in plant foods), but heme iron actually improves non-heme iron absorption. Vitamin C also has been shown to increase iron absorption as much as threefold.

Third, nutrient inhibitors and 'anti-nutrients' can decrease nutrient bioavailability. They can do this in several different ways: by binding the nutrient into a form not recognised by the digestive tract's uptake systems; by rendering the nutrient insoluble and so unavailable for absorption; and by competing for the same uptake system used by that nutrient. Phytate is an example of an anti-nutrient that we've already discussed; it binds to minerals such as calcium, iron and zinc and makes new compounds that the body can't absorb. Most cereal grains and pulses contain significant amounts of phytate, which is one of the reasons early farmers developed nutritional deficiencies after adopting agriculture.

Even beneficial nutrients can inhibit the absorption of other nutrients; for example, both calcium and non-heme iron bind to a transporter in the intestines, but whereas non-heme iron is absorbed this way, calcium basically stays in that doorway and blocks the entry of iron into the bloodstream. This is why calcium supplements are sometimes used in patients with haemochromatosis, a genetic disorder that causes dangerously high iron levels, to impair iron absorption.

Focusing on the nutrient density of foods alone is not enough. Instead, our goal should be to maximise the intake of foods that are high in bioavailable nutrients and substances that improve nutrient absorption, and minimise intake of foods that are poor in nutrients and substances that impair nutrient absorption. The Personal Paleo Diet allows you to do just that.

MEASURING NUTRIENT DENSITY

There are several issues involved in measuring the nutrient density of foods, including:

Deciding which nutrients to measure Experts don't entirely agree on which nutrients are most essential to human health and which are detrimental; however, there are several nutrients that are universally accepted to be beneficial, and these should be included in any nutrient-density scale. Likewise, nutrients that have not yet been conclusively shown to be important should not take the place of these essential nutrients.

Outdated science Many nutrient scales penalise saturated fat and cholesterol content, although recent long-term studies show that eating saturated fat and cholesterol does not raise cholesterol in the blood for most people. The same is true of sodium. Early studies suggested that sodium raises blood pressure, but later studies have shown that this is only true in a small group of sodium 'hyper-responders'. On the other hand, many scales don't include nutrients now known to be important for human health, such as the omega-3 fats EPA and DHA, and vitamin K_2.

Bioavailability As I explained in the previous section, it doesn't matter how many nutrients a food contains; what matters is what we absorb when we eat that food. If bioavailability were taken into consideration on nutrient-density scales, foods such as cereal grains, pulses, and nuts and seeds (which are high in phytate) would score even lower compared to foods like meat and dairy with highly absorbable forms of nutrients.

Distribution of nutrients in the food supply Some nutrients, such as vitamin D, vitamin A (retinol) and magnesium are difficult to find in food in bioavailable forms, whereas other nutrients used in density rankings such as protein and many minerals are relatively easy to obtain. Ideally, the difficult-to-obtain nutrients should be weighted more heavily and vice versa.

Combining calorie density with energy density Many nutrient-density scales penalise foods for higher calorie content. Although it's true that some calorifically dense foods (for example, processed and refined foods) promote overeating and weight gain, the same is not always true for unprocessed high-calorie foods such as dairy products and animal fats. Nutrient density and calorie density should be considered separately.

In order to address these shortcomings of existing nutrient-density scales, Harvard University chemist Dr Mat Lalonde created a new scale that he presented at the Ancestral Health Symposium in August 2012. Using the USDA Nutrient Database for Standard Reference, Dr Lalonde ranked foods according to the following qualifying nutrients:

Qualifying nutrients for characterising nutrient density (adapted from Lalonde)

Vitamin A (RAE)	Choline	Thiamin (B_1)
Riboflavin (B_2)	Niacin (B_3)	Pantothenic acid (B_5)
Pyridoxine (B_6)	Folate (B_9)	Vitamin B_{12}
Vitamin C	Vitamin D	Vitamin E
Calcium	Copper	Iron
Magnesium	Manganese	Phosphorus
Potassium	Selenium	Vitamin K
Zinc	Sodium*	

*Although sodium is an essential nutrient, it was excluded from the calculation to prevent foods high in sodium from being penalised.

The results of Dr Lalonde's analysis are shown below:

Average nutrient-density score of selected food categories (adapted from Lalonde)

Category	Average nutrient-density score
Organ meats	21.3
Herbs and spices	12.3
Nuts and seeds	7.5
Cacao	6.4
Fish and shellfish	6.0
Beef	4.3
Lamb, veal and wild game	4.0
Vegetables (raw)	3.8
Pork	3.7
Eggs and dairy	3.1
Poultry	3.1
Processed meat	2.8
Legumes (pulses)	2.3
Vegetables (cooked or canned)	2.0
Fruit	1.5
Plant fats and oils	1.4
Grains and pseudo-cereals	1.2
Animal fats and oils	1.0
Canned grains	0.8

On the Lalonde scale organ meats were the most nutrient-dense foods by far. Seafood, red meat and wild game were more nutrient dense than raw vegetables; all forms of meat, fish, fruit and vegetables (raw and cooked) were more nutrient dense than grains and pseudo-cereals.

Unfortunately, the USDA Nutrient Reference Database does not have data on bioavailability, so Dr Lalonde was not able to take it into account in his analysis; however, given what we know about the anti-nutrients in pulses and grains, these foods would have been even lower on the scale when compared to organ meats, other meats, dairy products and fruits and vegetables had bioavailability been considered.

With this in mind, let's look at each category in more detail, using Dr Lalonde's scale as the reference.

Organ meats

Calorie for calorie, organ meats are one of the most nutrient-dense foods on the planet. This is even more true when bioavailability is taken into account, since the amino acids, iron, zinc and other vitamins and minerals organ meats contain are in a highly absorbable form. Even without that consideration, organ meats were nearly 18 times more nutrient dense than whole grains and almost 11 times more nutrient dense than cooked vegetables. (This isn't a criticism of cooked vegetables as much as it is praise for organ meats!)

Herbs and spices

Second only to organ meats on the nutrient-density scale, herbs and spices have approximately half the score. But while it makes sense to consume a variety of herbs and spices for their nutrient value, they are unlikely to make a significant contribution to overall nutrient intake because of how little of them we eat in comparison to other foods.

Nuts and seeds

Third on the nutrient-density scale are nuts and seeds with about one-third the score of organ meats; however, most nuts and seeds contain phytate, the anti-nutrient which reduces the bioavailability of some of the minerals they contain. Fortunately, soaking nuts overnight and either dehydrating them (with a food dehydrator) or roasting them at a low temperature (65–75°C) in an oven for four to eight hours breaks down much of the phytate and improves bioavailability. These methods also make nuts easier to digest, which is of particular benefit for those with sensitive digestive systems.

Cacao

Chocolate lovers will be happy to see cacao, the raw form of cocoa, listed as the fourth most nutrient-dense food that was analysed. Like nuts and seeds, cacao contains high levels of phytate; however, cacao is fermented in the process of making chocolate, which is likely to break down some of the phytate and make it more bioavailable.

Fish and shellfish

Shellfish and oily fish were the most nutrient-dense animal foods apart from organ meats. Shellfish and oily fish are indeed rich in several vitamins and minerals, but they're also the only significant source of DHA in the diet. As you'll learn in Chapter 5, DHA is crucial to human health and most people from the US, UK and Australia do not get enough.

Red meat

Beef, lamb and wild game came just after seafood on the scale. This may surprise many of you, because red meat has been demonised for decades by the mainstream media and medical establishment. (See page 53 in Chapter 2, on red meat and heart disease, as well as the box on page 88.) Yet 100g (about one serving) of beef typically contains more B_{12}, niacin, vitamin

E, vitamin D, retinol, zinc, iron, potassium, phosphorus, and EPA and DHA than the same amount of blueberries or kale, which are two of the most nutrient-dense fruits and vegetables. In addition, as is the case with organ meats, the nutrients in red meat are highly bioavailable when compared to foods such as cereal grains, nuts and seeds and pulses. Studies have shown, for example, that the bioavailability of zinc in meat is four times higher than it is in grains.

Vegetables (raw)

The placement of vegetables (both raw and cooked) on the ranking scale will likely come as the biggest surprise to most of you. Vegetables are a good source of many of the vitamins and minerals that were measured on this scale. They're also rich in some nutrients that weren't included in this nutrient-density scale but that an increasing number of studies suggest are beneficial, such as bioflavonoids and polyphenols. They are an important part of the diet for this reason. Note that raw vegetables would likely have scored lower if bioavailability had been considered, because a portion of their nutrients are bound to fibres that are either difficult or impossible for humans to digest.

Pork

Pork is another meat that we are often told to avoid because of its high fat content. Yet it was more nutrient dense on this scale than pulses, cooked vegetables, fruit and grains.

Eggs and dairy

One egg provides 13 essential nutrients, all in the yolk (contrary to popular belief, the yolk is far higher in nutrients than the white). Eggs are an excellent source of B vitamins, which are needed for vital functions in the body, and also provide good quantities of vitamin A, essential for normal growth and development. The vitamin E in eggs protects against heart disease and some cancers. Eggs from pasture-raised (but not conventionally raised) chickens also contain significant amounts of vitamin D, which promotes mineral absorption and good bone health. (There are a few outlets in the UK that sell pasture-raised poultry, although eggs from truly free-range hens are rare.) Finally, eggs are one of the few significant dietary sources of choline, which helps maintain healthy cell membranes, nervous system function, immune balance and cognitive function.

Many people unnecessarily limit egg consumption because of concerns about cholesterol and heart disease, a misconception I will address in the bonus chapter on High Cholesterol and Heart Disease available on my website.

The dairy category included yoghurt, cheese and milk. Dairy is one of the few good sources of retinol and calcium, which are difficult to obtain elsewhere in the diet. Dairy protein is also highly absorbable, as I'll explain in Chapter 7.

Poultry

The scale shows that poultry is less nutrient dense than organ meat, red meat or any type of seafood. That said, it's still a good source of bioavailable protein and other nutrients, especially niacin and selenium.

Processed meat

Sausages, hams, meats made from reconstituted meat products (such as most cooked, sliced ham and chicken from supermarkets), supermarket bacon, all come under the heading of processed meats, which contain preservatives. Processed meats were more nutrient dense than legumes, cooked vegetables, fruits and grains. This is in large part because processed meats are made from red meat and pork, both of which scored highly on the nutrient-density scale. Some studies have shown an association between processed red meat consumption and both cardiovascular disease and premature death, but people who eat more processed meat are also more likely to engage in other unhealthy behaviours that could increase their risks. Moderate consumption of processed meats within the context of a nutrient-dense, whole-foods diet is unlikely to cause problems.

Legumes (pulses)

Legumes, which include pulses such as chickpeas, red kidney beans and lentils as well as peanuts, scored higher than cooked vegetables and fruit, but lower than most animal foods. Like grains, nuts and seeds, legumes contain significant amounts of phytate. This means that many of the minerals found in legumes will not be absorbed unless they are soaked, sprouted or fermented prior to consumption. Most traditional societies that included legumes in their diet did this, but people living in Western, industrialised societies rarely do. If you go to a Mexican restaurant and eat a bean burrito, for example, it's almost certain that the beans were not prepared in such a way that would reduce the phytate.

Vegetables (cooked)

Cooked vegetables scored lower than raw vegetables for three reasons. First, some of the cooked vegetables contained more water, which would dilute the nutrient concentration. Second, the water used to boil vegetables washes away nutrients. Third, heat destroys some of the nutrients that were included in the analysis. On the other hand, the nutrients in cooked vegetables are more bioavailable than those in raw vegetables because cooking breaks down some of the tough fibres in raw vegetables that limit nutrient absorption. This makes up for at least some of the nutrients lost in the process of cooking.

Fruit

Although fruit is placed below all forms of meat and fish, eggs, dairy, legumes and vegetables in terms of nutrient density, it remains a nutritious addition to the diet and an especially important source of vitamin C.

Plant fats and oils

This category includes oils from olives, nuts, seeds, avocados and coconut. In general, fats – whether from animals or plants – are not significant sources of micronutrients; however, it's important to note that many nutrients in vegetables are fat-soluble, which means that they require the presence of fat for optimal assimilation. Eating steamed vegetables with butter, or salad leaves with olive oil, and avocado will markedly improve your absorption of the nutrients in those vegetables.

The suitability of fats for human nutrition depends more on the specific fatty acids they contain; for example, many plant oils are high in omega-6 linoleic acid, which can promote inflammation when consumed in excess. I'll discuss this in more detail in Chapters 4 and 5.

Cooked grains and pseudo-cereals

Cooked grains and pseudo-cereals were close to the bottom of the list, ahead of only animal fats and canned grains. Since most grains and pseudo-grains contain phytate, they would have scored even lower had bioavailability been taken into account. Although Dr Lalonde didn't test whole and refined grains separately, refined grains would certainly have a lower score than whole grains. This is significant because 85 per cent of grain consumed in the US is in the highly refined form, and refined flour accounts for approximately 20 per cent of calories consumed by the average American and all other industrialised, urban populations.

Animal fats and oils

As I mentioned above, fats and oils aren't significant sources of micronutrients, but they are required to absorb fat-soluble vitamins, which are crucial to health and, along with glucose, are the main source of energy for the body. In addition, some animal fats do contain modest amounts of uncommon nutrients like retinol and vitamin K_2 (in butter from pastured cows) and vitamin D (in lard).

Canned grains

The canned grains category primarily includes cooked and creamed corn. As I explained above, even fresh, cooked whole grains and pseudo-cereals are low in nutrient density, so it's not surprising that canned grains are even lower on the scale.

Dr Lalonde's scale, which encompasses a wide-ranging and exhaustive amount of nutritional data and science, suggests that a diet centred around fish, meat, eggs, dairy, vegetables, nuts and seeds, fruit, and herbs and spices provides all the essential nutrients we require in sufficient quantities – an approach that is consistent with the Personal Paleo Diet. Despite claims by some nutrition 'experts' to the contrary, there is absolutely no need for grains or pulses in the human diet – foods that have only been part of our diet for a tiny fraction of our evolutionary history.

Does red meat cause cancer?

Some studies suggest that red meat increases the risk of cancer, especially colon cancer. Is that true?

One of the fundamental principles of scientific research is: 'correlation is not causation'. In other words, just because two things are correlated – that is, they appear together – it doesn't mean that one caused the other. In some observational studies, people who ate more red meat tended to die earlier than people who ate less. But it's possible that it's not red meat itself that's causing the increased mortality or cancer, but some other lifestyle factor.

In most of the red meat studies, people who eat the most red meat are also the least physically active, the most likely to smoke and the least likely to take a multivitamin (the health effects of which are unknown, although it is a proxy marker in our culture of how health-conscious someone is). They also have a higher body mass and higher alcohol intake, are more likely to eat more processed food, sugar and other less healthy foods, and have higher rates of diabetes. Perhaps it's not the hamburger that's increasing cancer and mortality risk, but the highly refined-flour bun or sugary chocolate milkshake that goes with it?

When all of this is taken into account, the case against red meat falls apart. In 2011, a research group published a study in the prestigious journal *Obesity Reviews* criticising the epidemiological studies linking red meat and colorectal cancer. They performed a critical analysis of 35 studies that claimed to associate red meat with cancer and concluded that 'the currently available epidemiological evidence is not sufficient to support an independent positive association between red meat consumption and colorectal cancer.'

So rest easy. You can safely return steaks and hamburgers to your plate.

Summary: maximising nutrients

- Build your diet around foods that are highest on the nutrient-density scale, such as organ meats, meat, fish, poultry, dairy, eggs, nuts and seeds, vegetables, fruits, and herbs and spices. (And don't forget dark chocolate!)
- Avoid or significantly reduce your intake of foods that are lowest on the nutrient-density scale, like grains, pseudo-cereals and pulses.

CHAPTER 4

Three Foods to Avoid: Minimising Toxicity in Your Daily Diet

If exchanging the standard Western diet for a full-scale Paleo diet still feels overwhelming, you can nevertheless take a major step towards hitting the reset button by eliminating three toxins that contribute significantly to modern disease. Here they are:

1 Gluten (grains aren't 'super-foods')

2 Industrial seed oils (they are anything but 'heart-healthy')

3 Refined sugars (in a word, they're 'toxic')

At the simplest level, a toxin is something capable of causing disease or damaging tissue when it enters the body. When most people hear the word 'toxin' they think of chemicals such as pesticides, heavy metals or other industrial pollutants. But even beneficial nutrients like water, which are necessary to sustain life, are toxic at high doses.

Notes for this chapter may be found at ChrisKresser.com/ppcnotes/#ch4

The body has a built-in detoxification system that was designed to process and excrete toxins in small amounts; however, the detox system evolved over millions of years in an environment that was relatively pristine in relation to the modern environment; we've simply never been exposed to the range or volume of toxins we face today.

This is important to understand as we examine the role of dietary toxins in contributing to modern disease. Most of us won't get sick from eating a small amount of the foods I discuss in this section, but if we eat them in excessive quantities, our risk of developing modern diseases rises significantly.

That's exactly what's happening today. These three food toxins – gluten-containing grains, industrial seed oils and excess sugar – comprise the bulk of the modern diet. Bread, pastries, cakes, biscuits, fizzy drinks, fruit juice, fast food and other convenience foods are all loaded with these toxins. In the US, vegetable oils, grain flour and table sugar (along with dairy and alcohol) now comprise 70 per cent of total calories consumed each day. When the majority of what most people eat on a daily basis is toxic, it's not hard to understand why our health is failing.

Let's look at each of these food toxins in more detail.

GLUTEN

Plants, like animals, have an imperative to survive and reproduce. But, unlike animals, plants can't run away from predators (like us). They had to evolve other mechanisms for protecting themselves. These include:

- Producing toxins that damage the lining of the gut.

- Producing toxins that bind essential minerals, making them unavailable to the body.

- Producing toxins that inhibit the digestion and absorption of other essential nutrients, including protein.

One of these toxic compounds is the protein gluten, which comprises 80 per cent of the protein found in wheat, barley and rye. Due to modern food-processing techniques, gluten can also often be found in trace amounts in other grains such as oats and corn – unless they are specifically marked as gluten-free.

Coeliac disease (CD) was initially described in the first century AD by a Greek physician named Aretaeus of Cappadocia. But neither Aretaeus nor anyone else knew that CD is caused by an autoimmune reaction to gluten: a protein in wheat. That didn't become clear until 1950 – several centuries later – when Dr Willem Dicke, a Dutch paediatrician, conclusively proved that gluten was the culprit. Dicke's discovery saved millions of children and adults from the perils of untreated coeliac disease, including malnutrition, stunted growth, cancer, severe neurological and psychiatric illness and even death.

Since then, the mainstream view of gluten intolerance has been relatively black or white: either you have coeliac disease, in which case even a small amount of gluten will send you running to the bathroom in three seconds flat, or you don't and you can chug down beer and munch bread without fear. This 'all-or-nothing' view has led to some doctors telling patients who suspect they're sensitive to gluten, but test negative for CD, that they're simply imagining an affliction that doesn't exist.

It turns out those doctors are wrong. We now know that it's possible to have gluten intolerance without having coeliac disease – a condition known as 'non-coeliac gluten sensitivity' (NCGS) – and that gluten intolerance is more of a spectrum of conditions than a single condition, with full-blown CD on one end, complete tolerance on the other and NCGS in the middle. Let's discuss each of these three possible reactions to gluten in more detail.

1 Coeliac disease

CD is an autoimmune disease characterised by an inflammatory response to gluten and damage to the tissue in the small intestine. Signs and symptoms typically include diarrhoea, bloating, abdominal pain, fatigue, lethargy and malnutrition. But CD can also manifest with atypical signs and symptoms, ranging from chronic headache to dermatitis to joint pain to insomnia.

Coeliac disease has become dramatically more common over the past half-century. According to a study comparing blood samples from Air Force recruits 60 years ago to more recent samples, CD has increased by 400 per cent during that period. Today, official statistics indicate that CD affects between 0.7 per cent and 1 per cent of the US population, but many experts in the field of gluten intolerance believe the actual prevalence is higher. Why the spike in CD? We don't know for certain, but many scientists believe that changes in our gut microbiota as well as changes in the way wheat is cultivated play a role.

Contrary to popular belief, coeliac disease is not simply a digestive disorder. One in two new patients diagnosed with CD do not have gut symptoms. For every one case of CD that is diagnosed, there are 6.4 cases that remain undiagnosed – the majority of which are atypical or 'silent' forms with no damage to the gut. This 'silent' form of CD is far from harmless, however: it is associated with a nearly fourfold increased risk of death from all causes.

These findings surprised many researchers and physicians, because it was long believed that the damage done by CD was limited to the gastrointestinal tract. But research over the past few decades has revealed that gluten intolerance can affect almost every other tissue and system in the body, including (but not limited to) the brain, endocrine system, stomach, liver, blood vessels, smooth muscle and even the nuclei of cells.

This explains why CD is associated with numerous diseases.

The following is only a partial list:

Type-1 diabetes

Multiple sclerosis

Dermatitis herpetiformis

Autoimmune thyroid disease

Osteoporosis

Heart failure

Depression

ADHD

Arthritis

Migraine

Allergies

Asthma

Obesity

How could a single condition be associated with such an astonishing array of diseases? CD causes the gut barrier to become permeable. As I explain in Chapter 10, when this happens large proteins and gut microbes 'leak' across the gut barrier and provoke a chronic, low-grade inflammatory response. But this response isn't limited to the gut; it can affect nearly every tissue in the body, as the list of conditions above suggests.

'Removing gluten put my Hashimoto's into remission'

Elise, aged 29, came to me complaining of Hashimoto's disease, an autoimmune condition that attacks the thyroid gland and eventually causes hypothyroidism. Elise had several symptoms related to poor thyroid function, including brain fog, constipation, hair loss, cold hands and feet and crushing fatigue. Hashimoto's is diagnosed by measuring levels of antibodies to thyroperoxidase (TPO), an enzyme required to make thyroid hormone and thyroglobulin (TG), a protein in the thyroid gland. 'I have high levels of thyroid antibodies,' she said, 'but the doctors told me there's nothing I can do about it.'

I explained to Elise that the key to treating her thyroid condition was to balance and regulate her immune system. I also explained that there's a strong association between both coeliac disease and non-coeliac gluten sensitivity and Hashimoto's. I suggested she remove gluten (and all grains) from her diet for a period of 90 days. 'I couldn't believe what happened,' she said. 'I felt so much better that I was able to go off Synthroid [prescription thyroid medication] completely. But if I ever fall off the wagon and eat gluten, my thyroid symptoms come back almost immediately.' Gluten was aggravating Elise's immune system, which in turn exacerbated her Hashimoto's disease. When she removed gluten from her diet, her immune system settled down – and so did the attacks against her thyroid gland, which is what enabled her to get off her medication.

2 Non-coeliac gluten sensitivity

There's no consensus definition of NCGS yet, but the most common understanding is that it's a reaction to gluten that is not autoimmune (like CD) or allergic (like wheat allergy). Another way of defining it is a reaction to gluten that resolves when gluten is removed from the diet, and CD and allergy have been ruled out. It's difficult to estimate the prevalence of NCGS, because there is no definitive diagnostic test for it (see the box 'Testing for coeliac disease and gluten intolerance' on page 97 for more on this). Another problem is that the range of symptoms associated with NCGS are so broad and 'non-specific' (meaning that they could be attributed to any number of causes) that many patients and doctors don't suspect it and thus don't order the necessary testing or perform a gluten challenge to find out.

Even with these limitations, some estimates suggest NCGS may occur in as many as one in ten people.

While some mainstream medical professionals continue to insist that NCGS doesn't exist, scientists have validated it as a distinct clinical condition. In one major study, researchers reviewed the charts of all 276 patients with irritable bowel syndrome (IBS) who had been diagnosed with NCGS using a double-blind, placebo-controlled wheat challenge, where patients go on a gluten-free diet and are then given capsules containing either wheat or an inert substance. As a whole, the NCGS group had higher frequency of anaemia, weight loss, self-reported wheat intolerance and food allergy in infancy than those with IBS without NCGS. The authors concluded that their data 'confirm the existence of non-coeliac wheat sensitivity as a distinct clinical condition'.

As with coeliac disease, NCGS can affect almost every cell/tissue/system in the body. The list of documented signs and symptoms is diverse (and far too long to present in its entirety here), but primarily includes:

IBS-like symptoms, including abdominal pain, bloating, changes in stool frequency

Brain fog

Headache

Fatigue

Joint and muscle pain

Numbness and tingling in the arms and legs

Dermatitis (eczema or skin rash)

Depression

Anaemia

There is a particularly strong connection between NCGS and neurological and psychiatric disease, including schizophrenia, autism and even depression; for example, studies suggest up to 40 per cent of patients with ataxia (a nerve disorder affecting balance and coordination) and 25 per cent of schizophrenic patients produce antibodies to gluten. And while the relationship to autism is less clear in the scientific literature, anecdotal evidence from the autism community indicates that gluten-free diets are very effective in some cases.

Testing for coeliac disease and gluten intolerance

Dr Alessio Fasano, a pioneer in the field of gluten intolerance, has proposed that a positive diagnosis for CD can be made if any four of the five factors below are present:

1 You have typical symptoms of CD (diarrhoea, bloating, abdominal pain, fatigue, lethargy and malnutrition).
2 You have elevated antibodies to alpha-gliadin (a type of gluten protein) or tissue transglutaminase-2 (an enzyme found in the gut and other organs).
3 You improve on a gluten-free diet.
4 You have a positive small intestine biopsy (indicating intestinal damage).
5 You have the genes that predispose you to CD (known as HLA-DQ2 and HLA-DQ8).

What about diagnosing NCGS? This turns out to be far more complicated, because of the limitations with current laboratory testing; many people can react to parts of the wheat compound that are not screened for during most gluten intolerance testing. That's why most experts on gluten sensitivity agree that the only reliable test for NCGS is a 'gluten challenge'. This involves removing gluten from the diet completely for a period of at least 30 days (although preferably three months) and then adding it back after that. If symptoms improve during the elimination period and return when gluten is reintroduced, a diagnosis of NCGS can be made.

For many people, however, a gluten-free diet isn't enough. Some grains that don't contain gluten, such as corn, oats and rice, contain proteins that are similar enough in structure to gluten to elicit an immune response in people with CD or NCGS. Moreover, about 50 per cent of patients with CD show signs of intolerance to casein (the protein in milk) and up to 30 per cent of CD patients continue to have symptoms or clinical signs after adopting a gluten-free diet. This is one reason why the Step 1 Reset forbids all grains and dairy in addition to gluten.

3 Tolerance

The final category of response to gluten is tolerance. Dr Weston Price, the American dentist who studied the health of traditional peoples (see page 28), documented cultures that maintained excellent health consuming gluten-containing grains, such as the people of the Loetschental valley in Switzerland. Why did they remain so healthy, if gluten can make so many ill? We don't currently understand all the factors that contribute to gluten sensitivity, but genetics certainly play a strong role in CD and probably in NCGS as well. Researchers estimate that patients who test negative for the two main genetic patterns associated with coeliac disease – HLA-DQ2 and HLA-DQ8 – are significantly less likely to have the disease. Diet, the gut flora, immune status and other factors we don't yet understand are also likely to influence susceptibility to NCGS and CD.

The problem is that it's difficult to know what category of gluten response you're in. Fewer than one in six people with CD are aware that they have it, and the percentage is almost certainly lower in the case of NCGS. The testing is flawed and the symptoms are so broad and non-specific that many doctors and patients with symptoms not typically associated with gluten sensitivity will overlook it. Another issue is that we don't currently understand what moves someone from tolerance to intolerance or sensitivity.

Considering the seriousness of the conditions that gluten sensitivity can cause, the complete lack of requirement for gluten in the diet and the low nutrient density and bioavailability of gluten-containing grains, I recommend that everyone perform a gluten challenge to determine whether they are intolerant. If you have a reaction to gluten when you add it back into your diet after the three-month challenge period, it's crucial that you strictly avoid gluten indefinitely. If you do not react to gluten, I still recommend avoiding it for the most part because of its potential to cause harm and our uncertain understanding of what shifts people from tolerance to intolerance. That said, if you don't have an obvious reaction to gluten, an occasional piece of bread or gluten-containing food when you're out with friends or travelling is unlikely to cause problems.

The myth of 'healthy whole grains'

At this point you may be asking yourself, 'If the nutrient-density scores for grains are so low, even without taking bioavailability into account, and gluten is so potentially toxic, why are they constantly referred to as healthy?' That's a great question and not easy to answer quickly. There are many reasons for the emphasis on grains in the standard Western diet, including their low price and ease of storage, a widespread lack of understanding of the nutrient inhibitors they contain and the misguided fear of animal foods that has swept over the US, UK, parts of Europe and Australia over the past 50–60 years.

But the low nutrient scores of grains and their potential toxicity should cast serious doubt on the recommendation of groups like the American Heart Association, which says you should consume six to eight servings of grains a day. Following this recommendation will almost certainly lead to a less nutrient-dense diet, especially if the grains are eaten in refined form (which is by far the most common way they are consumed in the industrialised world).

In addition to their generally low nutrient density, grains have significant nutritional shortcomings; for example, they contain no retinol (active vitamin A) at all and, with the exception of yellow corn, no grains contain its precursor (beta-carotene) either. (A precursor means that the substance in question, in this case beta-carotene, will eventually result in the formation of a new substance.) Nor do grains contain vitamin C or vitamin B_{12}. In the context of a mixed diet containing fish, meat, and fruit and vegetables, these shortcomings aren't particularly problematic, but in people following grain-heavy vegetarian and vegan diets, they can be serious problems.

Poor nutrient content is not the only thing to be concerned with when it comes to grains. As I've explained in this chapter, many grains contain proteins capable of provoking an immune response or allergic reaction. Gluten, which, as we have seen, is found in wheat, barley, rye and (sometimes) oats, is the best example of this.

When taken together, the evidence indicates that grains are a sub-optimal food source when compared to meat, fish, vegetables, fruit and nuts. Does that mean you should strictly avoid them 100 per cent of the time? Not necessarily. In my clinical practice, I've found that most people feel better without any grains or pulses in their diet at all; however, if you're fundamentally healthy and you're following a nutrient-dense diet, you may be able to tolerate them in moderation. If you do choose to include grains and pulses in your diet, they should be prepared properly (soaked, sprouted or fermented) to improve nutrient bioavailability and inactivate food toxins, and they should never replace more nutrient-dense foods like animal products, vegetables and fruits. See my website for links to resources on how to properly prepare grains and pulses.

INDUSTRIAL SEED OILS

Industrial seed oils are oils made from the seeds of plants such as corn, soya, cotton, sunflower and safflower. Historically, they've been used in a variety of applications, ranging from manufactured products (for example, soaps, candles, perfumes, cosmetic products, insulators) to lubricants, to pet food additives, to fuel (such as biodiesel). (Their use in the preparation and manufacturing of so many products is why they're referred to as 'industrial' seed oils.) But today they're marketed primarily as 'heart-healthy' oils and used in just about all processed, packaged and refined foods, as well as by most restaurants. This has led to a dramatic increase in the consumption of these oils; for example, intake of soya oil has increased more than 1,000-fold since the early 1900s, and consumption of linoleic acid, the primary fatty acid in seed oils, has risen more than threefold during that period.

We're only beginning to understand the consequences of such a dramatic increase in seed oil consumption, but based on current evidence I believe they should be minimised in the diet for three reasons:

1 They contain high amounts of linoleic acid (LA), which some research suggests is harmful when consumed in excess.

2 They are easily oxidised (damaged), and oxidative damage is associated with numerous modern, inflammatory diseases.

3 There's no strong evidence that they protect against heart disease in humans, and some evidence that they may increase the risk.

Let's look at each of these reasons in more detail.

Excess linoleic acid

Linoleic acid (LA) is an essential fatty acid, which means the body requires it for proper function, but must obtain it from the diet. However, the actual requirement for LA is very small: as little as 0.1 per cent of total calories consumed per day. Studies show that intake of LA in the modern diet averages between 4 and 10 per cent of total calories per day (mostly from highly processed seed oils), which means that we're getting up to 100 times the amount that we require for proper function.

In contrast, most traditional cultures had very low intakes of LA, which came exclusively from whole foods such as vegetables, nuts and seeds, and meat. As you'll see below, LA from industrial seed oils has a different effect on the body than LA from whole foods, because it is more likely to oxidise.

Oxidative damage

Linoleic acid is highly vulnerable to oxidation when exposed to heat (during food processing or cooking). It promotes the formation of compounds called OXLAMs, which are by-products of LA associated with a variety of diseases ranging from Alzheimer's to fibromyalgia to non-alcoholic fatty liver disease

(NAFLD). OXLAMs are a major component of oxidised LDL and atherosclerotic plaques, and they play a central role in the development of heart disease. Oxidised linoleic acid causes atherosclerosis in animal studies, and at least one human study has shown that higher intake of LA in the presence of risk factors for oxidative damage (such as smoking) increases the risk of heart disease. Reducing linoleic acid intake has been shown to decrease circulating OXLAM levels.

High intakes of linoleic acid are particularly problematic when the long-chain omega-3 fat DHA, found exclusively in seafood, is absent from the diet. This creates a pro-inflammatory environment in the body and may interfere with neurological function, because of the important role DHA plays in the brain and nervous system. Unfortunately, the combination of high LA intake and low DHA consumption is common in the modern diet, which is rich in processed and refined foods and low in cold-water, fatty fish.

Heart disease

For years we've been taught that saturated fats found in foods such as red meat and butter will clog our arteries and give us a heart attack, and that vegetable oils are a 'heart-healthy' alternative. As of 2013 the American Heart Association still recommended using liquid vegetable oils (such as corn, rapeseed, safflower, sunflower and soya) or non-fat sprays for cooking and drastically limiting use of coconut oil, butter, palm oil and other saturated fats.

Yet these recommendations are based on evidence that is decades old. Although it's true that some early studies suggested that vegetable oils were heart-healthy, those studies did not distinguish between the effects of omega-3 and omega-6 polyunsaturated fats (which I'll cover in the next chapter) found in these oils. More recent research that studied the effects of omega-3s and omega-6s separately has found that vegetable oils high in omega-6 linoleic acid not only do not prevent heart disease but they may increase the risk. Patients in one study who increased their intake of linoleic acid and reduced their saturated fat intake had a higher risk of death from cardiovascular disease and all other causes. This occurred despite a reduction in LDL and total cholesterol in these patients. An analysis of other randomised, controlled trials – considered the gold-standard of medical evidence – also found that higher intakes of linoleic acid increase the risk of heart disease and death.

Finally, it's important to note that industrial seed oil has almost no nutritional value: it is calorie-dense but nutrient-poor. Given the serious health problems it can contribute to, and the fact that it was entirely absent from the diets of healthy, traditional cultures, I think it's wise to avoid industrial seed oils as much as possible.

REFINED SUGAR

Studies going back more than 40 years have shown that naturally occurring sugars in fruits and vegetables are beneficial to health and do not promote weight gain. Traditional cultures such as the Hadza of north-central Tanzania and the Kuna of Panama obtain a high percentage of total calories from foods that are high in natural sugars, such as fruit, starchy tubers and honey. Yet they are remarkably lean, fit and free of modern disease.

Excess refined sugar, however, in the form of table sugar and high-fructose corn syrup, is a different story. Added sugars are harmful primarily because they promote overeating and weight gain. When people add fat to their diet, they tend to eat less of something else (usually carbohydrate) and if they eat more carbs they'll usually eat less fat; however, the same kind of swap is not true for sugar – especially in liquid form (for example, soft drinks and other sugar-sweetened beverages). Most people fail to compensate for extra sugar in their diet by reducing intake of calories from other sources; for example, a study of 323 adults found that the calories from sugar-sweetened beverages didn't displace calories from other foods and thus led to greater calorie intake overall. Another study showed that total calorie intake among 16 patients was greater on the day that a sugar-sweetened beverage was given at lunch than on the preceding day. Added sugar causes weight gain to the same degree, whether it's eaten as glucose or fructose, but, contrary to popular belief, excess fructose is no more fattening than excess glucose.

Excess weight isn't just a cosmetic problem; it contributes directly to metabolic and cardiovascular disease. Studies consistently show that overfeeding and fat gain cause insulin resistance. Insulin resistance, in turn, is associated with diseases ranging from diabetes to heart disease to Alzheimer's.

Added sugar can also cause problems in the digestive tract, where it promotes bacterial overgrowth in the small intestine and may cause gas, bloating and constipation or diarrhoea. Excess fructose may be particularly harmful for the gut; it's poorly absorbed and leads to bacterial fermentation and excess gas production, particularly in people with digestive problems.

In fact, there's almost no end to the list of problems too much refined sugar in the diet can cause. About 20 years ago, Nancy Appleton, Ph.D., began researching all the ways in which sugar destroys our health. Over the years the list has continuously expanded and now includes 141 points. Here's just a small sampling (the entire list can be found on her blog). Excess sugar:

- Suppresses the immune system

- Causes imbalances of essential minerals like copper and zinc

- Decreases tissue elasticity and function

- Interferes with nutrient absorption

- Causes tooth decay

- Decreases growth-hormone levels

- Contributes to depression and other mood disorders

- Increases the risk of breast cancer

There's a lot more to the Paleo diet than removing these food toxins from your diet. That said, if everyone on a standard Western diet stopped eating cereal grains, industrial seed oils and excess sugar tomorrow, I'm willing to bet that the rates of obesity, diabetes, heart disease and just about every other chronic, inflammatory disease would plummet over the next decade.

As I said at the start of this chapter, if starting a full-scale Personal Paleo Diet seems overwhelming after reading this book, or you're not prepared to begin for whatever reason, start with eliminating (or at least greatly reducing) these toxins from your diet. If you're like most of the people I've worked with, you'll feel like a different person. And that will give you the motivation and energy you need to take the next steps towards feeling even better.

Summary: minimising toxins

- Avoid gluten completely during the Step 1 Reset and for at least two months afterwards (for a total of 90 days). Then reintroduce it and see how your body reacts.
- If you feel better without gluten and worse when you reintroduce it, you are gluten intolerant and should strictly avoid it. If you don't react adversely, I still recommend avoiding or minimising gluten, but you may choose to have it occasionally

as part of your 80/20 rule (like a slice of birthday cake, Mum's lasagne, or a piece of bread when you're dining out).

- Avoid industrial seed oils and refined sugar. They are high in calories, low in nutrients and may contribute to inflammation and other health problems. As with gluten (assuming you're not gluten intolerant), you may choose to have small amounts of them infrequently as part of your 80/20 rule.

CHAPTER 5

Fats as Fuel: Give Yourself an Oil Change

Fats are a primary energy source (along with glucose) for the body. They also play a role in maintaining healthy skin and hair, regulating body temperature, supporting immune function, insulating internal organs and aiding in the absorption of the fat-soluble vitamins (A, D, E and K).

Fats, in general, though, get a bad rap in our 'heart-healthy' and fat-obsessed diet culture, partly because we're trained to put fat in the 'foods to avoid' category. A food that is described as 'high-fat' sets off alarm bells for most of us. But, as you're about to see, not all fats affect the body in the same way and, while some are harmful, many have beneficial, life-extending properties. When you follow Your Personal Paleo Diet, you'll find that it's easy to select the right variety and combination of fats.

Notes for this chapter may be found at ChrisKresser.com/ppcnotes/#ch5

THE FACTS ON FAT

Petrol and diesel are both fuel that cars can run on. If you put petrol in a diesel engine, or vice versa, the engine may run but it won't run well – or for very long. In a similar way, the human body can run on the entire range of fats (combined with carbohydrates and proteins), but it runs much better on the types it was designed to run on, and if you eat too much of the others, the body will eventually break down.

With this classification in mind, let's begin by examining the different types of fat to determine which ones are the preferred 'fuel' for the human body. The main fats we encounter in foods are:

- Saturated fats (long- and medium-chain)

- Monounsaturated fats

- Trans-fats (natural and artificial)

- Polyunsaturated fats

During the Step 1 Reset, it's best not to worry too much about macronutrient ratios. That said, as a starting place the best approach is to choose a rough target for carbohydrate intake based on your individual circumstances (see Chapter 18 for more on this) and eat that amount. Your remaining calories will come from protein and fat, and since most people naturally eat the amount of protein their body needs, you also won't have to think about how much fat to eat – that will fall into place without any calculations on your part. For example, say you decide to go for 30 per cent of calories from carbohydrate. In the US, most people eat about 15 per cent of calories from protein. That means your fat intake would be about 55 per cent of calories. This may be much more fat than you're accustomed to eating, especially if you've been following a low-fat, high-carbohydrate diet. But remember that the *quality* of fat you eat is often more important than the *quantity* when it comes to health and even weight regulation.

With this in mind, let's take a closer look at the various types of fat and their effects in the body.

SATURATED FAT

All fats are made up of molecular 'chains' of carbon, hydrogen and oxygen atoms. They are classified as short, medium or long based on the length of the molecular chain.

Long-chain, saturated fats (myristic, palmitic and stearic acid) are found mostly in the milk and meat of ruminant animals such as cattle and sheep. They form the core structural fats in the human body, comprising 75–80 per cent of fatty acids in most cells and they're our primary storage form of energy. In other words, when the body stores excess energy from food for later use, it stores it primarily as long-chain saturated fat.

Unlike polyunsaturated fats and carbohydrates such as glucose and fructose, saturated fats have no known toxicity – even at very high doses – presuming insulin levels are in a normal range. Long-chain saturated fats are more easily burned as energy than polyunsaturated fats, and the process of converting saturated fat into energy leaves no toxic by-products. In fact, it leaves nothing but carbon dioxide and water.

Saturated fats have many other benefits. They:

- Play an important role in bone health by helping to incorporate calcium into the skeletal system.

- Protect the liver from alcohol, damage from medications such as acetaminophen (paracetamol) and other toxins.

- Have beneficial effects on cardiovascular function, including reducing levels of Lp(a), an inflammatory substance in the blood that promotes heart disease, thereby reducing mortality caused by stroke; and improving lipid profiles by increasing HDL (which you probably know as the 'good' cholesterol, as opposed to LDL), decreasing triglycerides and making LDL particles larger and more buoyant, which makes them less likely to cause harm.

- Support healthy immune function.

- Deliver the fat-soluble vitamins A, D, K and E to the cells and tissues of the body.

- Regulate the availability of beneficial polyunsaturated fatty acids such as DHA.

Main dietary sources Fattier cuts of beef, lamb and pork; cream, whole milk, butter, ghee; in smaller amounts in coconut products and egg yolks.

Foods and oils rich in saturated fat

Food	Saturated fat, %
Coconut oil	87
Dairy products	64
Tallow (beef)	50
Palm oil	49
Beef, chuck steak	40
Lard*	39
Beef, brisket	39
Beef, minced (20% fat)	38
Duck fat	33
Chicken fat	30
Egg yolks	30

*Lard from conventional, grain-fed pigs is also very high in omega-6 linoleic acid, which is harmful in excess quantities. Look for lard from pastured pigs.

Verdict: eat liberally Along with monounsaturated fat (which we'll discuss shortly), saturated fat should comprise the bulk of your fat intake.

If you're worried about saturated fat causing heart disease, it's true there are certain situations where saturated fat intake should be moderated, and I'll explain those in later chapters; however, for most healthy people, the evidence that saturated fat leads to heart disease is weak at best. For decades we've been told that eating saturated fat increases cholesterol levels in our blood and that high cholesterol levels clog our arteries and cause heart disease. But does the research actually support that theory?

It's true that some studies show that saturated fat intake raises blood cholesterol levels. But these studies are almost always short term, lasting only a few weeks. Longer-term studies have not shown an association between saturated fat intake and blood cholesterol levels. In fact, of all the long-term studies examining this issue, only one of them showed a clear association between saturated fat intake and cholesterol levels, and even that association was weak.

Perhaps saturated fat contributes to heart disease by some mechanism other than raising cholesterol? Not according to the research. A large review of 21 studies covering almost 350,000 participants found no association between saturated fat intake and cardiovascular disease. Moreover, studies on low-carbohydrate diets (which tend to be high in saturated fat) suggest that they not only don't raise blood cholesterol but have several beneficial impacts on cardiovascular disease risk markers. (For detailed information on these studies and other findings, please see the notes for this chapter on my website.)

Medium-chain saturated fats (often called medium-chain triglycerides) are found in coconut milk and breast milk and they have unusual properties. They're metabolised differently from long-chain saturated fats: they don't require bile acids for digestion and they pass directly to the liver via the portal vein. This makes medium-chain triglycerides a great source of easily digestible energy. They're so easy to digest, in fact, that they're used in the liquid hospital formulas fed to patients who have had sections of their intestine removed and are unable to digest solid food.

In addition to being a good energy source, medium-chain triglycerides have therapeutic properties:

- They're high in lauric acid, a fat found in mother's milk that has anti-bacterial, anti-viral and antioxidant properties.

- They promote weight loss. They have a lower calorie content than other fats; they are not stored in fat deposits as much as other fats and they enhance fat burning (thermogenesis).

- They promote the development of ketones, one of two substances (along with glucose) that the brain can use as fuel. Ketones and ketone-generating diets have been shown to benefit several neurological conditions, including seizure disorders, Parkinson's and Alzheimer's.

Main dietary sources Coconut: its flesh, oil, milk and butter.

Verdict Eat liberally. Coconut oil is an especially good cooking fat, because it is not vulnerable to the oxidative damage that occurs with high-heat cooking using other fats.

How traditional fats helped Kara get pregnant

Kara was 36 years old and had been trying to get pregnant for the previous two years when she came to see me. When I reviewed her diet I noticed that she was drinking skimmed milk and severely limiting other traditional, saturated fats like butter, ghee, lard and coconut oil.

This isn't unusual, of course. Most of us have been told for decades that saturated fat will clog our arteries and cause heart disease. Yet many traditional cultures emphasise the importance of these fats in promoting optimal health, and this is especially true during the pre-conception period; for example, the Masai tribe in Africa allowed couples to marry and become pregnant only after spending several months drinking full-fat milk in the wet season when the grass is lush and the nutrient content of the milk is especially high.

Modern research has confirmed that saturated fats may promote fertility. A study at the Harvard School of Public Health found that women who ate two or more servings of low-fat dairy foods per day, particularly skimmed milk and yoghurt, increased their risk of infertility by more than 85 per cent compared with women who ate less than one serving of low-fat dairy food per week.

I instructed Kara to re-incorporate traditional saturated fats into her diet and switch from non-fat to full-fat dairy products. After just three months on this new dietary regime, Kara emailed me with the news: she was pregnant! Kara continued eating this way throughout her pregnancy (gaining a normal amount of pregnancy-related weight) and delivered a healthy, 8lb 2oz (3.7kg) baby girl.

MONOUNSATURATED FAT

Also known as oleic acid, monounsaturated fat is found primarily in olives, avocados, some meat and certain nuts such as macadamia nuts. Like saturated fats, monounsaturated fats form the core structural fats of the body and are non-toxic even at high doses. Interestingly, monounsaturated fats seem to be the only fats that typically fat-phobic groups like the

American Heart Association and the British Heart Foundation, and fat-friendly groups such as Atkins and other low-carbers, can agree are completely healthy.

Monounsaturated fats are also known for their beneficial effects on cardiovascular disease risk markers. They reduce LDL and triglycerides and increase HDL; decrease oxidised LDL, reduce oxidation and inflammation; lower blood pressure; decrease thrombosis (blood clotting); and may reduce the incidence of heart disease. Some studies also suggest that monounsaturated fats promote healthy immune function.

Main dietary sources Olives, olive oil, avocados, lard (pork fat), duck, chicken, egg yolk, macadamia nuts, almonds.

Dietary sources of monounsaturated fat

Food	Monounsaturated fat, %
Macadamia nuts	77
Olives and olive oil	74
Avocado	64
Almonds	62
Duck fat	49
Egg yolks	46
Lard	45
Chicken fat	45
Tallow (beef)	42
Butter	26

Verdict Eat liberally, but be aware that certain foods that are high in monounsaturated fats, such as nuts and avocados, can contain significant amounts of linoleic acid, an omega-6 polyunsaturated fat. As I'll explain below, linoleic acid is pro-inflammatory if consumed in high amounts when intake of EPA and DHA are low.

TRANS-FATS

There are two types of trans-fats: natural and artificial.

Naturally occurring trans-fats are formed when bacteria in the stomachs of grazing animals such as cows or sheep digest the grass the animal has eaten. Conjugated linoleic acid (CLA) is a natural trans-fat found in moderate amounts (between 2 and 9 per cent of total fat) in grass-fed meat and dairy products, and to a lesser degree in grain-fed products. It is also produced in our bodies from the conversion of other naturally occurring trans-fats in those same animal products.

Research over the last two decades suggests that CLA may protect against several different diseases. For example:

- CLA is inversely associated with heart disease. In other words, those who ate higher amounts of CLA had a lower risk of heart disease, and vice versa.

- CLA may help prevent and manage type-2 diabetes by improving glucose tolerance and insulin sensitivity, and observational studies show an inverse association between CLA levels in fat tissue and diabetes risk.

- CLA has been shown to reduce the risk of cancer, primarily by blocking the growth and metastatic spread of tumours, controlling the cell cycle and reducing inflammation.

- Some research suggests that CLA can help reduce body fat and promote weight loss in those who are overweight and obese.

Grass-fed vs intensively reared meat

Cattle that are grazed on pasture provide healthier meat and dairy products than those that are intensively reared in barns. In the UK most dairy is pastured for most of the year, and you can also buy pastured beef, but it's important to check first, because cheaper meat will be intensively reared and fed on maize (corn) and a mixture of other feed. You are more likely to be able to buy grass-fed meat from a butcher than a super-market, as many butchers use meat from their own farms or from farms producing meat in the traditional way; however, some supermarkets are now stating that their beef is grass fed for most of the year and fed on silage (grass cut in the summer and stored) during the winter months when the cattle are kept in barns. It might not be clearly stated on the packs, so check their websites. Farmers' markets are another good source. Always ask your butcher or farmers' market vendor whether the meat they are selling is grass fed. You can also buy grass-fed meat and dairy products online – a number of farms are specialising in selling quality meat through their websites.

Artificial trans-fats have slightly different chemical structures than natural trans-fats found in beef and butter. But these minor differences in structure lead to dramatically different effects in the body. Whereas natural trans-fats may reduce the risk of cancer, heart disease, obesity and other inflammatory conditions, artificial trans-fats have been shown to *increase* the risk of those diseases – even at relatively low doses.

Their effects on cardiovascular health are particularly harm-ful. They promote inflammation, damage the fragile lining of the blood vessels, increase the number of LDL particles, reduce HDL cholesterol and reduce the conversion of shorter-chain omega-3 fats into DHA. Artificial trans-fats are the quintessential junk food, because they provide no benefit and have no role in human physiology, yet they cause significant harm.

Main dietary sources – natural trans-fats Pastured dairy and meat are the best sources of CLA and other natural trans-fats. In fact, 100 per cent grass-fed animal products contain from three to five times more CLA than products from animals fed grain. And since CLA is in the fat, the best sources will be fattier cuts of meat, bone marrow, high-fat dairy products like butter, whole milk and full-fat cheeses.

Main dietary sources – artificial trans-fats Highly processed, refined and fried foods (doughnuts, margarine, fast food, frozen food, crisps, biscuits, crackers, chocolate bars, and so on); packaged foods (instant soups, cake mixes, microwave popcorn, flavoured rice and pasta mixes, and so on).

Foods high in naturally occurring CLA

Food	CLA, mg per g fat*
Cow's milk	3.4–23.6
Beef	3.7–17
Lamb	5.6–14.9
Butter	4.7–14.1
Goat's milk	5.8–10.5
Yoghurt (cow's milk)	2.8–10.5
Cheese (cow's milk)	2.9–9.8
Cheese (goat's milk)	2.7–6.3

*Milligrams of CLA per gram of fat. The large range of values displayed depends largely on whether the animals were grass-fed (higher values) or grain-fed (lower values), although altitude, the status of the bacteria in the grazing animal's stomach and other factors may play smaller roles.

Foods high in artificial trans-fat Artificial trans-fat is found exclusively in processed foods, such as biscuits, bars, cakes, cake mixes, margarines, crisps and ready-made convenience foods. Note that food manufacturers are not required to list 'trans-fats' on nutrition labels if the per-serving portion contains less than 0.5g; however, if you eat more than one serving of a food such as crisps (many brands list 0 trans-fats), you may be getting several grams of trans-fat.

Verdict – conjugated linoleic acid (CLA) Eat pastured meat and dairy products (if you tolerate them) to obtain CLA. Note that CLA supplements do not have the same benefits as naturally occurring CLA. Most CLA supplements are derived from linoleic acid in safflower oil, and some studies have shown that CLA supplementation in humans can cause fatty liver disease, inflammation, unfavourable changes in lipid profiles (high LDL cholesterol and triglycerides, and low HDL cholesterol) and insulin resistance. Furthermore, CLA supplements have not demonstrated the beneficial effects seen from dietary intake of CLA in human trials.

Verdict – artificial trans-fats (ATF) Avoid like the plague.

POLYUNSATURATED FATS

Polyunsaturated fats can be divided into two categories: omega-6 and omega-3. Omega-3 fats are present in green leaves and algae (and the animals that eat them) and omega-6 fats are found primarily in seeds (as well as the animals that eat them).

Polyunsaturated fats play both a structural and regulatory role in the body. They comprise cell membranes, regulate gene expression and help to control cell function. Omega-3 and omega-6 fatty acids have specific effects on the cells close to where they are formed, including both pro-inflammatory and anti-inflammatory effects. In general, both too much omega-6 and too little omega-3 cause inflammation, whereas restricting omega-6 and getting adequate omega-3 will prevent inflammation.

Polyunsaturated fats are a complex subject involving a lot of biochemistry. I'm going to spare you the unnecessary details, but there are a few basic concepts you'll need to understand about them before we proceed.

- Like all fats, polyunsaturated fats are chains of carbon, hydrogen and oxygen atoms.

- There are six different omega-6 fats and six different omega-3 fats. They are classified by the length of the chain (that is, the number of atoms in it) and the number of double bonds.

- Essential fatty acids are the shortest-chain polyunsaturated fats. They are called 'essential fatty acids' because they're required for proper function but can't be produced in the body and thus must be obtained from the diet. There is one essential omega-6 fat (linoleic acid) and one essential omega-3 fat (alpha-linolenic acid).

- Linoleic acid (LA) and alpha-linolenic acid (ALA) are converted into longer-chain derivatives in our bodies. The most important long-chain omega-6 fat is called arachidonic acid (ARA) and the most important long-chain omega-3 fats are called EPA and DHA.

- Although LA and ALA are considered essential, because they can't be manufactured in the body, the longer-chain derivatives (ARA, EPA and DHA) are primarily responsible for the health benefits we get from polyunsaturated fats.

With that in mind, let's take a closer look at omega-6 and omega-3 fats.

Omega-6

Linoleic acid (LA) is the essential omega-6 fatty acid. It is found in small or moderate amounts in a wide variety of foods, including fruits, vegetables, cereal grains and meat. But it is present in large amounts in industrial processed and refined oils, such as soya, cottonseed, corn, safflower and sunflower. These oils are ubiquitous in the modern diet, present in everything from salad dressing to crisps and crackers to restaurant food. LA is also relatively high in most nuts and in all poultry, especially in the dark meat with skin.

The evidence suggests that a moderate intake of linoleic acid from whole foods such as poultry, vegetables, and nuts and seeds is unlikely to cause problems in the context of a diet containing sufficient amounts of long-chain omega-3 fats like EPA and DHA. But when consumed in excess amounts – especially in the form of industrial seed oils (which have a tendency to oxidise) – and when intake of EPA and DHA is low, linoleic acid has a pro-inflammatory effect and may contribute to modern, chronic disease.

Arachidonic acid (ARA) is a longer-chain omega-6 fat that can be produced in our bodies by converting the LA we eat. It is also found in animal foods like chicken, eggs, beef and pork, because animals are also capable of making this conversion. ARA is present in cell membranes, involved in cellular signalling (aiding cells in exchanging information) and can also act as a vasodilator (relaxing the blood vessels). It is necessary for the growth and repair of skeletal muscle tissue and, along with DHA, is one of the most abundant fatty acids in the brain.

You may have seen stories in the media claiming that eating meat and other animal products causes inflammation in the body. This is based on the idea that the ARA leads to the production of inflammatory compounds. Animal products are high in ARA, so it stands to reason that eating animal products would increase inflammation. Right?

Not so fast. Although it's true that the compounds derived from ARA can be pro-inflammatory, recent evidence suggests that they may have important anti-inflammatory actions as well. Moreover, it's now clear that ARA serves as a precursor for a potent group of compounds that help reduce and resolve inflammation. ARA is needed to make a class of molecules called lipoxins, which trigger the release of anti-inflammatory compounds synthesised from EPA and DHA. In epidemiological studies, higher plasma levels of both ARA and EPA and DHA were associated with the lowest levels of inflammatory markers. And clinical studies have found that adding up to 1,700mg of ARA per day to the diet has no discernible effect on the production of inflammatory cytokines – a type of protein manufactured by cells that promotes inflammation.

Main dietary sources – omega-6 linoleic acid In whole foods, such as nuts, seeds, poultry and avocado; also present (in large amounts) in industrial seed oils like corn, soya, cottonseed, safflower and sunflower. These oils are ubiquitous in processed and refined foods, and most restaurants cook with them (because they're so cheap).

Main dietary sources – omega-6 arachidonic acid Primarily in animal foods such as meat, poultry and eggs.

Verdict – omega-6 linoleic acid (LA) Limit LA intake to moderate consumption of whole foods such as nuts, avocados and poultry. Avoid industrial seed oils as much as possible.

Verdict – omega-6 arachidonic acid (ARA) Eat liberally in animal foods such as meat, poultry and eggs. Intakes of more than five times the average have been shown to be safe.

Industrial seed oils with high omega-6 content

Oil	Omega-6, %
Safflower oil	72
Sunflower oil	63
Wheat germ oil	53
Corn oil	52
Cottonseed oil	50
Soya oil	49
Groundnut (peanut) oil	31
Rapeseed oil	18

Foods with high omega-6 content

Oil	Omega-6, %
Chicken leg	19
Chicken breast with skin	18
Chicken breast without skin	17
Ham	13
Duck, roasted	12
Tilapia	11
Eggs*	11
Bacon	10

*Eggs are low in total fat, so the relatively high percentage of omega-6 is not a concern. Also, eggs from pastured chickens that are not grain fed are likely to have a lower percentage of omega-6 than conventional eggs. See Chapter 8 for more on this.

Omega-3

Alpha-linolenic acid (ALA), the essential omega-3 fat, is found in plant foods such as walnut and flaxseed. Eicosapentaenoic acid (EPA) and docosahexaenoic acid (DHA) are the most important long-chain omega-3 fats (and now you know why it's easier to refer to them as EPA and DHA!). They are found in seafood and, to a lesser extent, the meat and fat of ruminant animals.

Although ALA is considered 'essential', it's really EPA and DHA that are responsible for the benefits we get from eating omega-3 fats. (Some researchers have even proposed that DHA be considered an essential fatty acid, because like ALA and LA, it's essential for human health and must be obtained from the diet to ensure adequate levels.)

A common misconception is that we can meet our omega-3 needs by taking flaxseed oil or eating plant foods containing ALA. It's true that the body can convert some ALA to EPA and DHA. But that conversion is extremely inefficient in most people. On average, less than 5 per cent of ALA gets converted into EPA, and less than 0.5 per cent of ALA gets converted into DHA. Since this conversion depends on adequate levels of nutrients such as B_6, zinc and iron, these numbers are likely to be even lower in those who are likely to be deficient in these vitamins and minerals, such as vegetarians, the elderly or the chronically ill.

During the Palaeolithic era, daily consumption of EPA and DHA averaged between 450–500mg per day – a figure that greatly exceeds current intakes, which average around 90–160mg per day for most Americans. This finding, along with the studies indicating extremely poor conversion of ALA to DHA, suggests that we evolved to eat pre-formed EPA and DHA – in other words, readily available EPA and DHA that does not have to be converted from ALA. Research suggests that the ALA-to-EPA/DHA conversion pathway may not have been used at all by our ancestors.

The complete absence of pre-formed, ready-to-eat DHA in plant foods (other than marine algae, which isn't exactly a staple in Western cuisine) is one of the primary reasons I believe vegetarian and vegan diets are not optimal for health.

How too much omega-6 and not enough omega-3 is making us sick

One of the most profound differences between traditional, ancestral diets and the modern, industrialised diet is in the balance of essential fatty acids consumed. Anthropological research suggests that our intake of omega-6 and omega-3 fats was relatively low throughout most of human history (around 4 per cent of total calories), with a ratio of omega-6 to omega-3 of between 1:1 and 2:1.

Today, people in the US, UK, Australia and other countries that are following the standard Western diet have an intake of omega-6 fat that is far higher than the evolutionary norm, primarily due to increased consumption of industrial seed oils: corn, cottonseed, soya, sunflower, safflower and rapeseed. On the other hand, we're eating much less omega-3 than we used to. Despite a slight increase in fish consumption in recent years (fish being a primary dietary source for omega-3), intake is still far below historical levels. These changes have shifted the ratio of omega-6 to omega-3 in the modern diet to between 10:1 and 20:1, with a ratio as high as 30:1 in some individuals! This is between five and 30 times higher than the ratio has been for most of our history. Many scientists believe that this increase in total polyunsaturated fat intake, as well as the dramatic rise in omega-6 consumption relative to omega-3, is at least in part to blame for the rise of chronic, inflammatory conditions such as obesity, type-2 diabetes, metabolic syndrome, autoimmune disease and cardiovascular disease.

Why EPA and DHA are so important

A large body of evidence indicates that EPA and DHA are essential to health and that deficiency of EPA and DHA has played a significant role in the epidemic of modern, inflammatory disease. In general, inadequate intakes of EPA and DHA cause systemic inflammation. Systemic inflammation – the body's response to infection or other threats, through the production of white blood cells and other substances – is associated with nearly every modern, chronic disease, from arthritis to Alzheimer's, to autoimmunity, to gastrointestinal disease; for example:

- Even modest consumption of EPA and DHA (200–500mg per day) reduces deaths from heart disease by 35 per cent – an effect much greater than that observed with statin drug therapy.

- DHA is essential for the proper development of the brain and preservation of brain function as we age. Low levels of DHA in pregnant women are associated with lower scores in learning and memory tasks in their offspring, and low DHA levels in the elderly are associated with multiple markers of impaired brain function.

- Regular consumption of fish or fish oil reduces the overall risk of death (described as 'total mortality') by 17 per cent. Statin drugs reduce total mortality by only 15 per cent – and even then, only in populations at very high risk of heart disease, specifically middle-aged men with pre-existing heart disease – but keep in mind that's a relative-risk statistic, so the absolute risk goes from something like 3 per cent to 2.55 per cent.

How eating more fish and less vegetable oil helped Mark

Mark, aged 62, was an avid golfer his entire life. He played 18 holes at least three times a week for more than 20 years and he always walked the course. A few years before he came to see me, however, he began experiencing pain in his shoulders and knees. It had become so bad that he had to start using the golf buggy and, more recently, stop playing altogether because he couldn't swing a club without pain.

I looked at Mark's diet and noticed that he was eating a lot of omega-6 fat. He ate at restaurants every day during the week (he went out to lunch near his office and bought a take-away for dinner at least twice a week at home), and often on the weekend too, and his main cooking oil was rapeseed (because he was trying to avoid saturated fat). At the same time, Mark wasn't eating much omega-3 at all. The only fish he ate was an occasional can of tuna – which is low in EPA and DHA.

I asked Mark to start taking a lunch to work and to cut back on takeaways at home. Restaurants primarily use industrial seed oils rich in omega-6 linoleic acid, because they're so cheap. I also alleviated his fears about saturated fat and instructed him to cook with ghee, coconut oil, butter, tallow and lard instead of rapeseed oil. Finally, I told Mark to eat at least four 140g servings of cold-water, oily fish such as salmon, mackerel, herring and sardines each week.

After six weeks on this programme, Mark came back to the office beaming. He was able to walk without pain for the first time in three years and he was back out on the golf course – on foot, instead of in the buggy.

Don't underestimate the power of simple dietary changes!

How to raise your EPA and DHA levels

There are two ways to increase your levels of EPA and DHA:

1　Significantly reduce the amount of LA consumed.

2　Eat sufficient amounts of pre-formed EPA and DHA.

Of these two steps, the second is the most important, because, even at relatively low levels of LA intake, the conversion of ALA to EPA and DHA is negligible and, as you've read, eating too much LA may be harmful. Excess LA has been shown to cause vitamin E depletion, intestinal dysbiosis, oxidative damage and inflammation as well as contributing to weight gain, liver disease, cancer, autoimmune disease, inflammatory bowel disease and premature ageing.

Main dietary sources – omega-3 ALA In fruits, vegetables, nuts and seeds, especially walnuts and flax.

Main dietary sources – omega-3 EPA and DHA EPA and DHA are found primarily in cold-water, oily fish such as salmon, mackerel, herring, sardines, anchovies and sea bass, as well as shellfish such as oysters and mussels, and to a much lesser extent in grass-fed meat and wild game. It's important to note that freshwater fish and other species of ocean fish and farmed fish are generally lower in EPA and DHA and there-fore not as beneficial.

Verdict – omega-3 alpha-linolenic acid (ALA) Consume in moderation in whole foods such as fruits, vegetables and seeds. Avoid large amounts of flaxseed oil and flaxseed, which unnecessarily increase total polyunsaturated fat intake with-out significantly increasing EPA and DHA.

Foods highest in EPA and DHA

Food	EPA + DHA, g per 85g
Caviar (fish eggs)	5.5
Herring	1.8
Salmon, farmed	1.8
Anchovy	1.7
Mackerel	1.5
Salmon, wild	1.5
Bluefin tuna	1.3
Oyster	1.1

Verdict – omega-3 EPA and DHA Eat liberally. How much fish should you eat to get the benefits of EPA and DHA? Death from heart disease can be significantly reduced by 25 per cent or more by consuming about 3.5g of EPA plus DHA per week, according to some studies. This is equivalent to about 280g a week of wild salmon; however, studies of Western populations without substantial levels of EPA and DHA in their diet (and with higher levels of LA in their diet) suggest a continued reduction of cardiovascular disease when they consume up to 7g of EPA and DHA per week, which is about 550g of wild salmon. With this in mind, I recommend the following:

- If you're healthy and free of heart disease, and your intake of LA is relatively low, aim for the lower-end target of 3.5g of EPA/DHA, or 280g of fish a week. This equates to two 140g servings per week.

- If you're at risk of heart disease, or you're unable to significantly reduce your intake of LA (perhaps you eat out a lot), aim for the upper end of the range at 7g of EPA/DHA or 550g per week. This equates to four approximately 140g servings per week.

Be aware that, depending on the dose of EPA and DHA, it takes about three to six months to re-establish a healthy long-chain omega-3 polyunsaturated fat balance in the tissues.

Why not just take 20g of fish oil per day to change your tissue levels of EPA and DHA as quickly as possible? The answer is that all polyunsaturated fats are highly vulnerable to oxidative damage – a process associated with cancer, heart disease and other inflammatory conditions – and EPA and DHA are no exception. In fact, they are the most vulnerable of all fats. A randomised trial showed that 6g per day of fish oil increased oxidative damage in healthy men, regardless of whether they were supplemented with 900iu of vitamin E (an antioxidant).

This argues for getting the majority of EPA and DHA from cold-water, oily fish in the diet, rather than fish oil. Supplementing with fish oil should be reserved for therapeutic purposes and should usually be short term and limited to 2–3g per day, depending upon background fish intake. The exception would be cod liver oil, which tends to have relatively low levels of EPA and DHA compared to other fish oils but is rich in important fat-soluble vitamins such as A and D. (I'll discuss cod liver oil and therapeutic supplementation with fish oil in later chapters.)

FATS AT A GLANCE: WHAT TO EAT, WHAT TO AVOID

Saturated fat and monounsaturated fat should form the bulk of your fat intake. The omega-3 fats EPA and DHA and omega-6 fat arachidonic acid (ARA) should be consumed regularly, while omega-6 linoleic acid should be consumed only in whole food form (nuts, seeds, avocados) in moderate amounts. See my website for a printable version of this chart that you can put on your fridge.

Fats to eat and to avoid

Eat liberally	Eat in moderation	Avoid
Coconut oil	Sesame oil	Soya oil
Palm oil	Walnut oil	Groundnut (peanut) oil
Olive oil	Pecan oil	Corn oil
Ghee	Almond oil	Safflower oil
Butter	Flaxseed oil	Wheat germ oil
Lard*	Avocado oil	Rapeseed oil
Tallow (beef and lamb)	Nuts and seeds	Sunflower oil
Duck fat*	Nut butters	Cottonseed oil
Dairy fat		Grapeseed oil
Macadamia oil		Rice bran oil
Eggs, meat and seafood		

*Choose pasture-raised lard and duck fat. Conventional alternatives are significantly higher in omega-6 LA, which should be limited.

When choosing fats for cooking, it's important to be aware of their smoke point. The smoke point is the temperature at which the flavour and nutritional integrity of the fat or oil begins to break down. Once an oil exceeds its smoke point, it will usually produce bluish and pungent smoke that is irritating to the eyes. Oils that have passed their smoke point are likely to contain oxidised fats, which have been shown to damage cells and contribute to numerous diseases.

I've listed the approximate smoke point of various fats and

oils below. For high-heat cooking, choose fats with the highest smoke points, such as ghee, extra light (not extra virgin) olive oil, palm oil, expeller-pressed (refined) coconut oil, macadamia oil and beef tallow. Butter, extra virgin olive oil and extra virgin coconut oil have relatively low smoke points and are best for uncooked uses (that is, putting them on cooked or raw foods).

Smoke points of fats

Fat	Smoke point (°C)
Ghee	252
Olive oil (extra light)	242
Palm oil	235
Coconut oil (expeller-pressed)*	232
Macadamia oil	212
Beef tallow	204
Duck fat	190
Lard	188
Coconut oil (extra virgin)	176
Olive oil (extra virgin)	160
Butter	120–149

*Expeller-pressed coconut oil is nearly odourless and tasteless, which is advantageous for those who do not like the taste of coconut.

Summary: fats

- Saturated and monounsaturated fats from meat, poultry, animal fats, nuts and seeds, avocados, coconut, olives and dairy products should form the foundation of your fat intake.
- Eat pastured meat and dairy products (if you tolerate them) to obtain conjugated linoleic acid, a healthy form of trans-fat.
- Avoid industrial seed oils as much as possible. They are almost completely devoid of nutrients and associated with numerous health problems.
- Eat between 280g and 550g of cold-water, oily fish such as salmon, mackerel, herring, anchovies or sardines each week. The higher end of the range is for those still eating a significant amount of industrial seed oil and/or those with cardiovascular disease or other inflammatory conditions.
- Avoid high doses (greater than 3g per day) of fish oil, which can promote oxidative damage.

CHAPTER 6

Choosing Carbs for Energy: Glucose, Fructose and Fibre

Carbohydrates are one of the two main energy sources (along with fats) for humans. They are found in many foods, including refined grains and sugars that have contributed to so much modern disease. But there are many excellent (and often overlooked) dietary sources of healthy carbohydrates, which you'll learn about in this chapter, as you continue to construct Your Personal Paleo Diet.

First, however, let's look at how carbs work. In our bodies, all carbohydrates in food are ultimately broken down or converted into simple sugars (that is, glucose and fructose) or indigestible fibre. But whereas glucose, fructose and fibre are all technically carbohydrates, they each have different effects on the body. Let's look at each of them in more detail.

Notes for this chapter may be found at ChrisKresser.com/ppcnotes/#ch6

GLUCOSE

Glucose is a simple sugar (or monosaccharide) found mostly in plant foods such as fruits, vegetables, starches and grains. It can be broken down from sweeteners like table sugar (sucrose) and honey. Glucose has three main uses in the body:

1 It forms structural molecules called glycoproteins.

2 Like fat, it is a source of energy for cells (especially in the brain).

3 It's a precursor to compounds that play an important role in the immune system.

Glucose preceded fatty acids as a fuel source for living organisms by a very long time and it is the building block of foods that have the longest evolutionary history of use by mammals like us. The fact that glucose can be produced in the body from protein is often used as an argument that we don't need to eat glucose. But rather than viewing this as evidence that glucose isn't important, we might view it as evidence that glucose is so metabolically essential that we evolved a mechanism to produce it even in its absence in the diet.

One of the few differences between our digestive tract and that of a true carnivore, like a lion, is that we produce an enzyme called amylase. Amylase allows us to digest starch – a long chain of glucose molecules we can't absorb – into single molecules of glucose that easily pass through the gut wall into the bloodstream.

Although glucose from fruits, vegetables and starches is generally well tolerated, too much of it – in the form of sucrose-sweetened beverages or concentrated sweeteners, for example – can cause weight gain and metabolic problems.

FRUCTOSE

Fructose is another simple sugar found primarily in fruits and vegetables. Although it has the same chemical formula and calorific content as glucose, it is processed differently. Rather than being absorbed by the cells directly, it is shunted directly to the liver for conversion into glucose or fats. About 50 per cent of fructose ends up as glucose, 25 per cent becomes lactate (a chemical produced during normal metabolism and exercise) and 15 per cent or more becomes glycogen, the principal storage form of glucose. The remainder is burned directly for energy and a small portion – as low as 2–3 per cent – is converted to fat.

There's little question that excess fructose from high-fructose corn syrup-sweetened beverages such as fizzy drinks contributes to weight gain. One of the main reasons for this is that most people don't cut calories somewhere else to compensate for the additional calories that come from drinking a couple of fizzy drinks each day. They simply end up taking in more calories overall. It's also true that excess fructose has distinctly harmful metabolic effects when compared to glucose.

Despite some claims to the contrary, however, there's no evidence that we should avoid whole fruit simply because it contains fructose. There's nothing fattening or toxic about fructose when it's consumed in moderate amounts from whole fruits and vegetables. And since whole fruit contains fibre and other nutrients, it's difficult to eat a lot of fruit without simultaneously reducing intake of other foods. Fruit has been part of the human diet for longer than we've been recognisably human. We're well adapted to eating it and capable of processing the fructose it contains. Studies overall suggest that eating whole, fresh fruit might actually decrease the risk of obesity and diabetes, and that limiting fruit intake has no effect on blood sugar, weight loss or waist circumference.

Although fructose in whole fruits and veggies is unlikely to cause metabolic problems, it can be an issue for some people with digestive problems. When glucose is present in equal or greater amounts than fructose in a food – such as bananas, berries and cantaloupe melon – the fructose will be well absorbed (because glucose helps with fructose absorption); however, when there's more fructose than glucose in a food – as with apples, peaches and papaya – that additional fructose will linger in the gut where it is rapidly fermented by bacteria. If you have digestive issues, you may wish to limit foods with more fructose than glucose. Please see Chapter 20 for more information on this.

FIBRE

Fibre is plant matter that is indigestible to humans. There are two types of fibre: soluble fibre and insoluble fibre. Soluble fibre dissolves in water. It is fermented by bacteria in the colon and creates a viscous, gel-like substance in the digestive tract. Insoluble fibre does not dissolve in water. It is not fermented in the colon (with some exceptions) and it adds bulk to the stool. Soluble and insoluble fibre are often lumped together in discussions about the merits of fibre, but their effects on the body are quite different. This has caused confusion and led to dangerous dietary and supplement recommendations.

Many studies suggest that soluble fibre is important for human health. Although we can't digest it, some of the 100 trillion bacteria that live in our gut can. Intestinal bacteria 'eat' soluble fibre by fermenting it. In the process of fermenting the fibre, the bacteria produce short-chain fats such as butyrate, propionate and acetate. These short-chain fats are the primary energy source for intestinal cells in the colon, and butyrate in particular has been associated with several health benefits: it has anti-inflammatory effects; increases insulin sensitivity; delays the development of neurodegenerative diseases; and has shown promise in the treatment of diseases of the colon such as Crohn's, IBS or ulcerative colitis. Butyrate may also play a role in healthy metabolic function, stress resistance and the immune response. In fact, the benefits observed in epidemiological studies of a diet high in naturally occurring fibre are likely due to the higher butyrate production from these diets.

Soluble fibre may also protect against heart disease. Research shows a strong inverse association between dietary fibre intake and heart disease, heart attack and peripheral artery disease. In one major study, subjects followed for more than 19 years with the highest dietary soluble fibre intake had a 15 per cent lower risk of heart disease and had a 10 per cent lower risk of cardiovascular events. Soluble fibre binds cholesterol, increases the activity of LDL receptors in the liver (which helps clear LDL from the bloodstream), improves insulin sensitivity, and increases satiety (the feeling of fullness) with lower overall calorie consumption.

On the other hand, most insoluble fibres (with the exception of resistant starch, which I'll discuss below) have only partial or low fermentability. Insoluble fibres provide a bulking action and tend to increase stool regularity, but they do not generate short-chain fatty acids like butyrate and thus don't have the same health benefits as soluble fibres. Whereas soluble fibre has been shown to protect against heart disease, insoluble fibre has not. What's more, excess insoluble fibre can bind to minerals such as zinc, magnesium, calcium and iron, preventing the absorption of these vital nutrients.

The effects of whole-grain fibre (which is mostly insoluble) may be especially harmful. In one study involving men who had previously suffered a heart attack, there were 22 per cent more deaths in the high-fibre group (who doubled their grain fibre intake from 9g to 17g per day) than in the control group.

Resistant starch is an insoluble fibre with unique properties. Starch exists as a large chain of glucose molecules in plants. Since humans produce amylase, the enzyme that breaks down starch, most forms of starch are easily absorbed in our digestive tract; however, resistant starch is unique among starches in that it cannot be broken down in the small intestine and digested by humans. But unlike other types of insoluble fibre, resistant starch can be fermented by gut microbiota in the large intestine to produce beneficial short-chain fatty acids like butyrate. Resistant starch has several other benefits, including increasing our uptake of minerals such as calcium, boosting levels of bifidobacteria (a healthy species of bacteria in our large intestine) and reducing harmful pathogens, improving motility and reducing blood sugar and insulin levels. On a Personal Paleo Diet, resistant starch is found in unripe bananas, potatoes that have been cooked and cooled, potato starch, plantain flour, tapioca flour and some pulses (for those who tolerate them). It can also be used as a supplement for those with digestive and/or blood sugar problems, which I'll discuss in later chapters.

As with most nutrients, there's a sweet spot with fibre; both too little and too much fibre can cause problems. The best approach is to obtain fibre in the context of a whole-foods diet. Although soluble fibre is probably more beneficial than insoluble fibre, many foods in the Personal Paleo Diet – such as yams and sweet potatoes, green leafy vegetables, carrots and other root vegetables, fruits with an edible peel (such as apples and pears), berries, seeds and nuts – contain both. There's no need to restrict insoluble fibre when it naturally occurs in these foods (unless you have digestive problems, which I'll discuss further in Chapter 10); however, grains are high in insoluble fibre and low in bioavailable nutrients and are best avoided.

Does a high-fibre diet prevent colorectal cancer?

The US Institute of Medicine recommends a daily fibre intake of 38g for men and 25g for women, from dietary fibres (both soluble or insoluble) or the addition of 'functional fibres' (that is, fibre added to cereals, breads and other foods) to the diet. The British recommendations are more sensible; they suggest 18g per day. But is there any evidence to support these recommendations?

Although initial studies seemed to support the theory that high-fibre diets protect against colorectal disease, later studies have not. Newer, better-designed epidemiological studies covering as many as 38 countries worldwide found that increased dietary fibre was not associated with a reduction in colon cancer. Long-term longitudinal studies (observational research that studies a particular variable, like fibre intake, over a long period of time) including more than 725,000 participants have also failed to find an association, as have interventional studies (where they give one group a higher-fibre diet and the other group a lower- or normal-fibre diet). Finally, an analysis of five randomised, clinical trials with almost 4,500 total participants found that increased fibre does not reduce the incidence of polyps in the colon. (Colorectal cancer usually begins as a polyp.)

There is little evidence supporting current recommendations for a very high-fibre diet, or for taking fibre supplements to prevent colorectal disease. In the vast majority of cases, you can get all the fibre you need from a whole-foods diet that includes vegetables, fruits, starchy tubers, nuts and seeds.

WHICH DIETARY SOURCES OF CARBOHYDRATE ARE BEST?

Now that you have a better understanding of the different types of carbohydrate and how they are processed in the body, let's look at the best dietary sources of carbohydrate from a Paleo perspective. These should form the foundation of your carbohydrate intake during the Step 1 Reset. In Step 2, you may choose to reintroduce moderate amounts of other sources of carbohydrate, such as dairy products, certain grains like white rice and buckwheat, and concentrated sweeteners.

In Step 3, you'll explore how much carbohydrate is optimal for you, based on your activity level, health status, digestive function and other factors. During Step 1, the focus is on carbohydrate quality: replacing refined grains and sugars with the more nutrient-dense, whole-food carbohydrates listed below.

During the Step 1 Reset you can aim for approximately 15–30 per cent of calories from carbohydrate. For a moderately active male eating 2,600 calories a day that works out at 100–200g of carbohydrate per day. As a point of reference, a large sweet potato (37g), a large potato (64g), one medium banana (27g) and one medium apple (27g) amount to about 125 grams of carbohydrate. For a moderately active female eating 2,000 calories a day, 15–30 per cent works out at 75–150g of carbohydrate per day. Those with blood sugar issues or who wish to lose significant amounts of weight should aim for 10–15 per cent of calories from carbohydrate, which works out at 65–100g on a 2,600 calorie diet or 50–75g on a 2,000 calorie diet.

Non-starchy vegetables

Non-starchy vegetables include cruciferous vegetables such as broccoli and cauliflower, as well as lettuces, cabbages and greens, summer squashes, onion, tomato, asparagus and more.

Non-starchy vegetables are excellent sources of micronutrients and fibre, but overall they are quite low in carbohydrate. Most have less than 80 calories of carbohydrate per 450g, typically in the form of glucose and fructose. What's more, some evidence suggests that the human body expends up to 40 calories for every 450g of non-starchy vegetables consumed. This suggests a net gain of a mere 40 calories per 450g of vegetables eaten.

Carbohydrate content of selected non-starchy vegetables*

Vegetable	Quantity	Carbohydrate, g
Artichokes	1 medium	14
Swede	140g	12
Spring greens	35g	11
Romaine/cos lettuce (raw)	½ head	10
Green (French) beans	100g	10
Red pepper	90g	9
Onion	1 medium	9
Mushrooms, button	70g	8
Turnip	130g	8
Beetroot	70g	8
Kale	65g	7
Peas	35g	7
Broccoli	90g	6
Carrots (raw)	1 medium	6
Courgette	115g	5
Cauliflower	100g	5
Asparagus	4 spears	2

*Cooked unless otherwise indicated.

Verdict Eat liberally. I recommend consuming as many non-starchy vegetables during the day as you like, but not counting them towards your total carbohydrate intake. Your optimal intake of non-starchy vegetables will depend on digestive function (some of them are high in insoluble fibre, which can be hard on an inflamed gut) and personal preference, but approximately 450g per day is a good target for most people.

Fruit

Fruit contains a mixture of glucose and fructose. It also contains a wide range of micronutrients and is a good source of fibre (mostly soluble). Along with starchy plants (see the next section), fruit should be a primary source of carbohydrate in your diet.

Carbohydrate content of selected fruits

Fruit	Quantity	Carbohydrate, g
Banana	1 medium	27
Pear	1 medium	27
Pomegranate	½ × 10cm fruit	27
Mango	165g (about ½ fruit)	25
Apple	1 medium	25
Pineapple	165g	22
Orange	1 medium	18
Grapes	150g	16
Papaya	145g	16
Peach	1 medium	14
Cantaloupe melon	160g	13
Strawberries	150g	12
Watermelon	150g	12
Blueberries	75g	11
Raspberries	60g	8
Plum	1 × 5cm fruit	8
Tomato	180g	7

Verdict Three to four servings of fruit a day is fine for most people. Those with insulin resistance, diabetes or metabolic syndrome may see improvements by restricting fruit intake to one to two servings a day and by choosing fruits that are lower in sugar, such as berries and melon. See Chapter 18 for more on how to determine your optimal carbohydrate intake.

Starchy plants

Starchy plants include tubers such as potatoes and sweet potatoes, roots like taro and yuca (cassava/manioc) and fruits like plantain and breadfruit. They are primarily broken down into glucose and are thus well absorbed by most people. There are a few caveats to this, however:

- Although all humans produce amylase, some produce less than others and may not tolerate starch as well, as a result.

- The intestinal bacteria feed on starch. This is generally a good thing; however, when there's an overgrowth of bacteria in the small intestine (as is often the case with digestive conditions like GERD – gastro-oesophageal reflux disease – and IBS), starch may worsen the problem and cause gas, bloating and changes in stool frequency.

- Those with diabetes, impaired glucose tolerance or other problems with blood sugar regulation may find that starch aggravates their condition.

The key, as always, is to experiment. I have patients with digestive and blood sugar issues that are able to tolerate moderate amounts of starch without a problem.

How starchy plants made Ron regular again

Ron, aged 46, came to see me complaining of constipation. He averaged only two to three bowel movements per week and even those were not complete evacuations. His abdomen was bloated and tense most of the time and his wife constantly complained about his bad breath.

While reviewing Ron's case history, I noticed that he had been on a very low-carb diet for several years. He told me that he wasn't constipated before going low-carb, but he had lost 1 stone 11lb (11.3kg) on the diet so he had stuck with it over the years. I asked Ron to add some starchy plants such as potatoes, sweet potatoes, taro, plantain and yuca (cassava/manioc) back into his diet. I explained that these foods were high in fermentable fibres that feed healthy gut bacteria and that constipation is often caused by an imbalance of good and bad bacteria in the gut.

Ron was concerned about adding these foods back into his diet because of their carbohydrate content. He told me he'd been on a low-fat, high-carb diet prior to switching to low-carb and he felt the high-carb intake had contributed to his weight gain; however, the carbs Ron was eating prior to going low-carb were almost all processed and refined. I explained to Ron that starchy plants are not only lower in carbohydrate than grain flours and sugar but they are also higher in nutrients and less likely to promote overeating.

Within a few weeks of adding starch back into his diet, Ron began having a complete, daily bowel movement. His energy and sleep also improved and despite his concern about gaining weight, he actually lost a few pounds.

I've listed several different starchy plants in the table on page 146. If you can't find some of these at your local supermarket, check out ethnic markets in your area. You can often find taro and lotus root at Asian markets, for example, and yuca and plantains at markets or some supermarkets. You can make great chips with yuca and crisps with taro, especially if you roast them in duck fat or lard.

Carbohydrate content of selected starchy plants

Starchy plant	Quantity	Carbohydrate, g
Potato (floury, e.g. King Edward)	1 large	64
Tapioca	½ cup	63
Plantain	150g	48
Taro	100g	46
Yuca (cassava/manioc)*	100g	39
Sweet potato	1 large	37
Yam	140g	37
Breadfruit	110g	30
Acorn squash	200g	30
Butternut squash	200g	22
Lotus root	10 slices	14

*Yuca should never be consumed raw because it contains harmful toxins. Putting it in cold water, bringing it to the boil, boiling for 30 minutes and discarding the water is sufficient to reduce its toxicity to safe levels.

Verdict Starchy plants should be the foundation of your carbohydrate intake along with fruit. Your optimal intake of starchy plants will depend on several factors, which we'll explore in more detail in Chapter 18. As a starting place, I'd recommend about 450g per day. That comes to roughly two to four servings of starchy plants per day.

Summary: carbohydrates

- Most people should aim for between 15–30 per cent of total calories from carbohydrate per day. If you have blood sugar issues or are trying to lose significant amounts of weight, aim for between 10–15 per cent of total calories.
- Eat as many non-starchy vegetables as you'd like throughout the day. How much you eat depends largely on personal preference and how well you digest them, because they don't make a significant contribution to total carbohydrate intake.
- Eat approximately two to five servings of fruit per day. If you have a blood sugar issue or are trying to lose weight, aim for the lower end of the scale and choose low-sugar fruits such as berries and melon. If you're lean, active and have no blood sugar issues, aim for the higher end of the scale.
- Eat approximately two to four servings of starchy plants per day. If you're restricting carbs, eat fewer servings and smaller amounts at each serving.
- Avoid grains, concentrated sweeteners and dairy products as carbohydrate sources during the Step 1 Reset. You'll have a chance to reintroduce some of these, if you choose, during Step 2.
- Avoid fortified fibre products and most fibre supplements. Soluble fibre or prebiotic supplements may be useful in some situations, which we'll discuss in later chapters.

CHAPTER 7

Proteins for Life: Optimise Protein Quality

The great thing about protein, an essential nutrient for humans, is that most of us naturally eat the right amount of it without paying it much attention. Our brains strongly influence our desire to consume it, based on how much our bodies need. You are probably very familiar with animal sources of protein (such as meat and dairy) and plant sources as well (such as soya). As with fats and carbohydrates, the quality of proteins – including what they do in your body once they are consumed – differs considerably, as you'll soon see.

Protein is vital to life because it is the building block of all body tissues; it can also be converted into glucose for energy. Protein molecules are composed of individual amino acids linked together in a chain. Amino acids can be divided into three categories: essential, non-essential and conditional. Essential amino acids can't be produced in the body and must be obtained from the diet. Non-essential amino acids can be

Notes for this chapter may be found at ChrisKresser.com/ppcnotes/#ch7

synthesised from essential amino acids or in the breakdown of proteins during digestion. Conditional amino acids are usually non-essential, but can also be essential in certain situations (for example, in times of chronic illness or stress).

There are two considerations with protein: how much you should eat and what type. As with fats and carbohydrates, I'll cover how much protein each person should eat in Chapter 18 when we discuss further refining the diet for your particular circumstances. In this chapter we're going to focus more on what types of protein are optimal for human nutrition. The factors that determine protein quality include:

- **Amino acid profile** 'Complete' proteins contain all essential amino acids, whereas 'incomplete' proteins are lacking in one or more essential amino acids.

- **Bioavailability** No matter how much protein a food has, if we can't digest and absorb it, it won't benefit us.

- **Toxicity** Some proteins are more likely to cause an immune response or allergic reaction.

With this in mind, the best proteins are those that contain all essential amino acids in a bioavailable form and have a low potential for toxicity.

WHICH PROTEINS ARE OF THE HIGHEST QUALITY?

Over the years, several different methods have been used to measure protein quality. Although these methods provide useful information, each of them has significant shortcomings:

Protein efficiency ratio (PER) Protein efficiency ratio determines the effectiveness of a protein by measuring how much weight an animal (usually a rat) gains after being fed a test protein. The problem with PER is that the effects of a given protein on growth in rats don't necessarily correlate to the growth needs of humans.

Biological value (BV) Biological value measures how efficiently the body utilises a protein consumed in the diet. A food with a high BV indicates a strong profile of essential amino acids. BV is limited in its usefulness, however, because it does not consider several key factors that influence how protein is digested and absorbed.

Net protein utilisation (NPU) Net protein utilisation is similar to BV, but it more directly measures the retention of absorbed nitrogen (nitrogen is a by-product of protein metabolism). NPU has the same shortcomings as BV.

To address these shortcomings, the Food and Agriculture Organization and the World Health Organization created a new measure of protein quality called the 'protein digestibility corrected amino acid score' (PDCAAS). This method combines the amino acid profile of the protein (whether it's complete or incomplete) with the 'faecal true digestibility' of the protein (how much of the protein is absorbed, rather than excreted as waste). PDCAAS values are expressed on a scale of 0 to 1, with 1 being the highest. This scoring method has been the preferred method for measuring protein value in scientific studies since it was introduced in 1989.

The table opposite lists the PDCAAS of some common animal and plant proteins.

Protein digestibility corrected amino acid score of proteins

Protein type	PDCAAS
Casein	1.00
Egg	1.00
Milk (casein and whey)	1.00
Whey protein	1.00
Chicken (light meat)	1.00
Turkey (minced)	0.97
Fish	0.96
Beef	0.92
Soya beans	0.91
Chickpeas	0.78
Black beans	0.75
Vegetables	0.73
Pulses (average)	0.70
Kidney beans	0.68
Fruit	0.64
Rolled oats	0.57
Lentils	0.52
Peanuts	0.52
Tree nuts	0.42
Whole wheat	0.40
Wheat gluten	0.25

As you can see, without exception, animal proteins are of higher quality than plant proteins such as pulses, grains, fruit and vegetables. It would appear that soya beans are nearly as high quality a protein as beef.

Although the PDCAAS is the most accepted method of measuring protein quality, one of its shortcomings is that it does not take anti-nutrients into account. Soya contains substances that have been shown to decrease protein absorption in the small intestine. These anti-nutrients are also present in other pulses (such as lentils and kidney beans) and cereal grains (such as wheat, corn, oats, and so on) and they've been shown to decrease assimilation of amino acids in these foods by as much as 50 per cent. If the PDCAAS took this data into account, the scores for soya protein, other pulses and cereal grains would be significantly lower than those listed in the table.

It's clear that animal protein is superior to plant protein in terms of amino acid composition and bioavailability, but within the animal protein category, some foods have more proteins than others. For those wishing to boost their protein intake (I'll discuss who might fall into this category in later chapters), it's helpful to know which animal products are the most concentrated protein sources. The table below lists the protein content of various animal foods, based on a typical serving size.

Protein content of selected foods

Food	Measure	Protein, g
Duck	½ duck	52
Sockeye salmon	½ fillet	43
Halibut	½ fillet	36
Rock salmon	1 fillet	33
Beef, silverside	85g	30
Chicken, light meat	85g	28
Lamb loin	85g	26
Beef, sirloin	85g	25

Food	Measure	Protein, g
Ham	85g	25
Swordfish	85g	25
Yellowfin tuna	85g	25
Pork spare ribs	85g	25
Chicken, dark meat	85g	24
Turkey, light meat	85g	23
Cottage cheese	110g	14
Yoghurt (whole milk)	250g	8
Milk, whole	250ml	8
Gruyère cheese	25g	8
Egg, whole	1 large	7

As you can see, seafood, poultry and red meat are the most concentrated sources of protein. Although dairy and egg proteins score highest on the PDCAAS, they are generally much lower in protein per serving than fish and meat.

'I ate all the time, but I was still starving'

Emily, aged 32, came to see me complaining of severe fatigue. She could hardly get up in the morning and she crashed in the afternoons. Up until about six months before our visit she had been a competitive cyclist, but she had stopped competing because her performance and ability to recover after races and workouts had declined so rapidly. She began to notice extra fat around her waist and in her thighs for the first time in her life. She also had dark circles under her eyes and her hair was falling out.

'I feel like I've aged about 25 years in the past two years,' she told me. 'I'm scared that I won't be able to ride again and that this will just get worse.' She had become a vegan about two years ago. (She had been eating a standard Western diet prior to going vegan.) At first she felt fantastic, and her performance and energy levels actually improved, but after about nine months she noticed some fatigue and a decline in her performance. She was also hungry all the time and, despite eating every two to three hours, she never felt fully satisfied. As time progressed, her symptoms worsened and she decided to get help.

I explained to Emily that vegan diets were low in bioavailable, complete proteins. Although it's possible to get enough protein 'on paper' by eating pulses, grains and soya products, those proteins are not well absorbed or are lacking in essential amino acids. As a competitive athlete, her needs for highly digestible, complete protein were even higher than the average person, which is why she was feeling so poorly.

After a lot of consideration, Emily decided to begin eating eggs, fish and chicken again. Almost immediately she noticed an improvement in her energy and well-being. Within a month she was back on her bike and training, and within three months she was ready to begin competing again. Her extra body fat melted away, her hair stopped falling out and the dark circles under her eyes disappeared.

Summary: proteins

• Eat the amount of protein you crave. Most people naturally eat the right amount because the brain strongly influences our craving for it depending on how much we need. In Chapter 18 we will discuss optimising protein intake based on your individual circumstances.

- Meat, poultry, seafood and eggs should form the bulk of your protein intake during the Step 1 Reset.
- Dairy products are also a source of high-quality protein and may be reintroduced during Step 2 to determine whether you tolerate them.
- Fruits, vegetables, nuts and seeds are good sources of micronutrients, but low in absorbable protein.
- Grains and pulses are poor sources of protein compared to animal products. They also contain anti-nutrients that reduce the absorption of amino acids and proteins that may provoke an immune response. That said, moderate amounts of certain grains and pulses may be tolerated when special steps are taken to reduce their toxicity, and some people may wish to reintroduce these during Step 2.

CHAPTER 8

Whole, Organic and Wild: Eat Real Food

We've looked closely at food on a biochemical or molecular level (micronutrients, macronutrients, fatty acids and toxins), and you've learned why certain foods should be a part of Your Personal Paleo Diet and why others don't make the grade. Now that you have a good grasp of what should be on your plate, it's time to take a step back and consider food quality. Before you set off to the market or shops to collect ingredients for your next meal, I want to help you understand the importance of eating what I call 'real food'. Real food is:

- Whole, unprocessed and unrefined.

- Local, seasonal and organic.

- Pasture-raised (animal products) and wild (fish).

Let's look at each of these in turn.

Notes for this chapter may be found at ChrisKresser.com/ppcnotes/#ch8

WHOLE, UNPROCESSED
AND UNREFINED

(Or, if it comes in a bag or a box, don't eat it!)

Industrial food processing has had more detrimental effects on our health and well-being than any other factor in the last few hundred years – and possibly in the entire history of humankind. Food refining has brought us food toxins destroying our health: wheat flour, industrial seed oils, artificial trans-fats, and table sugar and high-fructose corn syrup. It has also brought us chemical additives and preservatives, some with known negative effects and others with effects still unknown.

New research is revealing the harm these newfangled processed foods have on us almost every day. A study in 2011 found that emulsifiers used in packaged foods, ranging from mayonnaise to bread to ice cream, increase intestinal permeability ('leaky gut' – which you'll learn more about in Chapter 10) and cause a chain reaction of inflammation and auto-immune disease. Another study showed that diet fizzy-drink consumption increases your risk of stroke and causes kidney damage, possibly because of the phosphoric acid used as an acidifying agent to give colas their tangy flavour. High intakes of phosphoric acid are associated with premature ageing, kidney and vascular disease as well as cardiovascular complications in patients with chronic kidney disease.

To avoid the harm caused by processed and refined foods, a good general rule is: 'If it comes in a bag or a box, don't eat it.' Of course not all foods that come in bags and boxes are harmful, so this isn't meant to be taken too literally. It's just a helpful guideline. Butter is packaged, and some fruits, vegetables and salad greens are sold in plastic bags. High-quality frozen organic produce is bagged. That doesn't mean you shouldn't eat butter, fruit and vegetables. But in general, if you follow this guideline, you'll avoid most common food toxins. And that's more than half the battle.

ORGANIC, LOCAL AND SEASONAL

More nutrients

Organic plant foods contain, on average, 25 per cent higher concentrations of micronutrients than their conventional counterparts. In particular, they tend to be higher in important polyphenols and antioxidants, such as vitamins C and E, and quercetin.

Even more relevant in determining nutrient content is where your produce comes from and, in particular, how long it's been out of the ground before you eat it. Most of the produce sold at large supermarket chains is grown hundreds – if not thousands – of miles away, often in areas with longer growing seasons (warmer countries such as those in the Mediterranean or the Middle East or those with year-round tropical climates). This is especially true when you're eating foods that are out of season in your local area. Possibly weeks have passed since it was picked (hard and unripe, so that it could be shipped without bruising), packaged and transported thousands of miles through a maze of artificially refrigerated distribution centres, before it finally arrives at the supermarket, where it can sit on the shelf for even longer.

The problem with this scenario (besides the inferior taste and quality) is that food starts to change as soon as it's harvested and its nutrient content begins to deteriorate; for example, total vitamin C content of red peppers, tomatoes, apricots, peaches and papayas has been shown to be higher when these crops are picked ripe from the plant. The vitamin C content of supermarket broccoli in season has been shown to be twice as high as supermarket broccoli out of season that has been shipped from another country.

Without exposure to light (photosynthesis), many vegetables lose their nutrient value. If you buy vegetables from the supermarket that were picked a week ago, transported to the store in a dark truck and then stored in the middle of a pile in the produce section, and then you put them in your dark fridge for several more days before eating them, the chances are they will have lost much of their nutrient value; for example, a study at Penn State University found that spinach lost 47 per cent of its folate after eight days.

This is why buying your produce at markets, greengrocers who buy local produce, local farmers' markets, through a green box scheme or, even better, picking it from your own garden are better options than buying conventional produce shipped from hundreds or thousands of miles away. Fruit and vegetables from local farms are usually sold within one or two days of picking, which means their nutrient content will be higher. And, as anyone who's eaten a fresh tomato right off the vine will tell you, local produce tastes so much better than produce shipped from afar that it might as well be considered a completely different food.

Fewer chemicals

A main benefit of organic produce is that it's grown without pesticides, herbicides and other harmful chemicals that have been shown to cause health problems – especially in vulnerable populations such as children. A study published in the journal *Pediatrics* concluded that children exposed to organophosphate pesticides at levels typically found in conventional produce are more likely to develop attention deficit hyperactivity disorder (ADHD).

In 2010, scientists who studied possible links between environmental toxins and cancer concluded that Americans should aim to eat organic produce grown without pesticides, fertilisers or other chemicals. Their report states that the US government has grossly underestimated the number of cancers caused by environmental toxins. They also highlight the risk of toxins in conventionally grown foods to unborn children. Exposure to harmful chemicals during this critical period (through a pregnant woman's consumption of produce grown with toxins) can set a child up for lifelong endocrine disruption, hormone imbalances and other problems.

The 'Dirty Dozen Plus' and 'Clean Fifteen'

Each year the Environmental Working Group publishes a list of the 12 fruits and vegetables highest in pesticide residues (Dirty Dozen) and the 15 fruits and vegetables lowest in pesticide residues (Clean Fifteen). Starting in 2012 they added two crops to the Dirty Dozen (making it the Dirty Dozen Plus) that didn't meet their typical criteria but were commonly contaminated with pesticides that are especially toxic to the nervous system.

  If you're on a tight budget and can't afford to buy organic produce exclusively, you'll get the benefits of a diet rich in fruit and vegetables while minimising the risk of pesticide exposure if you buy organic foods that appear on the Dirty Dozen list. As of 2013, the Dirty Dozen Plus includes:

Apples	Kale/spring greens
Celery	Nectarines
Cherry tomatoes	Peaches
Chillies	Peppers
Courgettes and other summer squash	Potatoes
Cucumbers	Spinach
Grapes	Strawberries

The Clean Fifteen includes:

Asparagus	Mangos
Avocados	Mushrooms
Cabbage	Onions
Cantaloupe melon	Papayas
Corn	Pineapples
Aubergine	Peas (frozen)
Grapefruit	Sweet potatoes
Kiwi fruit	

Many supermarkets and independent shops stock organic produce. Note that this list is also available as a free, downloadable app from EWG's website (www.ewg.org/foodnews). Now you can have this list at your fingertips while you shop.

Supporting local economies and preserving resources

Apart from having more nutrients and fewer chemicals, there are other non-nutritional reasons to eat local produce. These were summarised well in Cornell University's Northeast Regional Food Guide:

Community food systems promote more food-related enterprises in proximity to food production, marketing, and consumption. Such systems enhance agricultural diversity, strengthen local economies (including farm-based businesses), protect farmland, and increase the viability of farming as a livelihood. Local food systems mean less long-distance shipment of the produce we enjoy, which means decreased use of non-renewable fossil fuels for food distribution, lower emission of resulting pollutants, and less wear on transcontinental highways.

How can you argue with that? I've also found that forming relationships with the people that grow my food leads to a greater sense of community and connection. In an increasingly techno-obsessed, hyperactive world, that is especially welcome.

PASTURE-RAISED AND WILD-CAUGHT: AS NATURE INTENDED

Although the reasons to eat pasture-raised animal products and wild-caught fish span social, political, economic and health considerations, I'm going to focus on health factors. Several studies have been done comparing the nutrient content of pasture-raised to that of intensively reared grain-fed animal products (specifically regarding confinement animal feeding operations, or CAFOs, in the US). Pasture-raised is superior to intensively reared in two primary respects: 1) a better fatty acid profile; and 2) higher levels of vitamins and other micronutrients.

Omega-6 and omega-3 content

Studies have shown that grain-feeding animals deplete their omega-3 levels, thus raising the ratio of omega-6 to omega-3. As you'll recall from reading about these fats in Chapter 5, too much omega-6 and not enough omega-3 can be problematic. The more grain in a cow's diet, the lower the omega-3 levels in the beef. A 2010 paper published in the *Nutrition Journal* reviewed seven individual studies comparing omega-6 and omega-3 levels in grass- and grain-fed beef. Every study found significantly higher levels of omega-3 in grass-fed beef and in some cases the difference was almost tenfold. On average, grass-fed beef had an omega-6 to omega-3 ratio of 1.5:1, compared to 7.7:1 for grain-fed.

Another study compared the omega-6 to omega-3 ratios of several different types of meat, ranging from pasture-raised bison and beef to wild elk and conventional chicken. They found the following ratios (expressed as omega-6 to omega-3):

Pasture-raised bison: 2.1:1

CAFO bison: 7.2:1

Pasture-raised beef: 2.1:1

CAFO beef: 6.3:1

Wild elk: 3.1:1

CAFO chicken breast: 18.5:1

What is apparent from both studies is that pasture-raised beef is much closer to the historical omega-6 to omega-3 ratio of between 2:1 and 1:1 (what our Paleo ancestors consumed) than beef raised in confinement animal feeding operations. In fact, the ratio for pasture-raised beef is even better than wild elk's. This means that pasture-raised beef falls within evolutionary norms for the fatty acid content of animals that humans have eaten throughout most of our history. CAFO/ intensively reared beef does not.

You may also have noticed that the ratio of omega-6 in chicken is about nine times more than that of pasture-raised beef. I don't see this as a reason to avoid chicken, but it does suggest that the fatty acid profiles of beef and lamb are superior and they should be favoured in the diet. Studies have shown that meat from pasture-raised animals can actually raise levels of EPA and DHA in the blood, making it the only other dietary source of these important long-chain omega-3 fats apart from cold-water, oily fish.

Pastured eggs

We see a similar difference between eggs from hens raised on pasture and those raised in confinement. Eggs from pasture-raised hens contain as much as ten times more omega-3 than eggs from factory hens. Pastured eggs are higher in B_{12} and folate. They also have higher levels of fat-soluble antioxidants such as vitamin E and a denser concentration of vitamin A. (See also 'Eggs and dairy' on page 83.)

Wild-caught fish

Farmed fish contains excess omega-6 compared to wild-caught fish. Tests conducted in 2005 show that wild-caught salmon contained ten times more omega-3 than omega-6, whereas the ratio for farmed salmon was less than 4:1 (despite having more omega-3 fat overall). Another study found that consuming standard farmed salmon, raised on diets high in omega-6, raises blood levels of inflammatory chemicals linked to an increased risk of cardiovascular disease, diabetes, Alzheimer's and cancer. Wild salmon also contains four times as much vitamin D than farmed salmon, which is especially important since up to 50 per cent of people following a standard Western diet are deficient in this important vitamin.

Conjugated linoleic acid (CLA) content

Meat, fat and dairy from pasture-raised animals are the richest sources of another type of good fat, called conjugated linoleic acid (CLA). CLA may have anti-cancer properties, even in very small amounts. In animal studies, CLA at less than one-tenth of 1 per cent (0.1 per cent) of total calories prevents tumour growth. In a Finnish study on women, those who had the highest levels of CLA in their diet had a 60 per cent lower risk of breast cancer than those with the lowest levels. In another study, people with the highest levels of CLA in their tissues had a 50 per cent lower risk of heart attack than those with the lowest levels.

Pasture-raised animal products are the richest known sources of CLA in the diet and are significantly higher in CLA than grain-fed animal products. When ruminant animals like cows and sheep are raised on fresh pasture alone, their products contain three to five times more CLA than products from animals that are fed grain.

Mineral, vitamin and micronutrient content

Grass-fed beef is also much higher in key micronutrients than grain-fed beef, including:

- Seven times more beta-carotene
- Three times more vitamin E
- Higher levels of glutathione
- Twice as much riboflavin (vitamin B_2)
- Three times as much thiamin (vitamin B_1)
- Thirty per cent more calcium
- Five per cent more magnesium

Grass-fed meat also has more selenium than grain-fed products. Selenium plays an important role in thyroid function, has antioxidant effects and protects the body against mercury toxicity. Grass-fed bison has four times more selenium than grain-fed bison. (Grass-fed bison is now available in the UK.)

Super-bugs in conventionally raised meat

Here's a good reason to put some thought into how you shop for meat. A 2013 analysis of data by the US Environmental Working Group (EWG) found significant levels of antibiotic-resistant bacteria in conventionally raised meat being sold in supermarkets across the US. These so-called 'super-bugs' can cause serious food-borne illnesses and infections that are becoming increasingly difficult to treat. The EWG reports that antibiotic-resistant bacteria was found in:

- 81 per cent of minced turkey

- 69 per cent of pork chops

- 55 per cent of minced beef

- 39 per cent of chicken breasts, wings and thighs

Note These are figures for the US.

Researchers also found that 87 per cent of raw meat samples were contaminated with both normal and antibiotic-resistant enterococcus bacteria, which indicates that most of this meat came into contact with faecal matter. (In the US, cattle reared in CAFOs will usually be standing in excrement, which is then carried with the carcass after slaughter and gets onto the meat. In the UK, intensively reared cattle are not kept in such large numbers and faecal contamination to that degree may be less of a problem.)

Industrial livestock producers routinely give their animals antibiotics to encourage more rapid growth or prevent infection in overcrowded, stressful and unsanitary living conditions. Today, 80 per cent of the antibiotics manufactured each year in the US are given to food-producing animals.

Super-bugs that have evolved because of misuse of antibiotics (in both humans and livestock) have increased the risk that people will succumb to severe infection. An increase in antibiotic-resistant bacteria means that problems as common as strep throat or a scraped knee could be fatal.

The EWG report recommends the following steps to reduce your exposure to super-bugs in meat:

- Choose organic, pasture-raised meat raised without antibiotics. If you're budget-conscious, buy cheaper cuts such as beef skirt, beef shin, brisket, chuck steak, mince, bone-in chicken thighs and breasts.

- Put raw meat into a bag before it goes in your grocery trolley and be especially careful with minced meats.

- Store meat on the lowest rack in the fridge, away from fresh produce. Thaw it in the fridge, not on the kitchen worktop.

- Use separate cutting boards for meat and other produce. Don't wash meat – splashes spread bacteria.

- Use a food thermometer to ensure that roasted meat is adequately cooked, which will destroy any bacteria. See http://foodsafety.gov for more about how to cook meat safely.

Summary: eat real food

- As a general rule, avoid food that comes in a bag or a box. Focus on fresh ingredients.
- Buy organic, locally grown produce as much as possible. Shop at farmers' markets or local shops, or join a green box scheme to have vegetables delivered. Consider buying organic varieties of the foods in the Dirty Dozen Plus list; save money by buying conventional varieties of foods listed in the Clean Fifteen.
- Buy pasture-raised meat, dairy and eggs whenever possible. They will have more nutrients and fewer toxins – especially antibiotic-resistant 'super-bugs'. Choose tougher, cheaper cuts (which are among the most flavourful and can be made more tender by slow cooking methods) and buy in bulk or directly from a local farmer, if possible, to save

money. If pastured meat isn't available locally, buy it from online vendors.

- Buy wild, sustainably caught fish. If fresh, wild fish is not available locally, you can buy it canned from online vendors.

CHAPTER 9

Cheaper, More Nutritious and Better Tasting: Cooking and Eating From Nose to Tail

One of the most remarkable things about traditional diets is that they often provided all of the nutrients required for optimal health – without the benefits of modern science or even the concept of micronutrients. Our ancestors learned which nutrients we need, in what amounts and in what combinations with other nutrients, the old-fashioned way: through experimentation over thousands of generations.

Weston Price, the Ohio dentist-turned-documentarian of traditional peoples and their diets (see Chapter 1), recounts the experience of a prospector who went blind while crossing a high plateau in the Rocky Mountains, in his book *Nutrition and Physical Degeneration*. The prospector was discovered by a Native American, who fed him 'the flesh and the head and the tissues of the back of the eyes, including the eyes' of a

Notes for this chapter may be found at ChrisKresser.com/ppcnotes/#ch9

trout. Within a few hours the prospector's sight began to return, and within a few hours his sight was normal. Today, we know that this type of temporary blindness can be caused by a deficiency of vitamin A. We also know that the eyes and the heads of fish are rich in retinol: pre-formed vitamin A.

Another example is the use of special pre-conception diets of mothers-to-be (and sometimes fathers-to-be) in traditional cultures like the Masai (see Chapter 5), who allowed marriage and pregnancy only after couples spent months drinking nutrient-rich milk from cows who grazed during the lush wet season. Other cultures used special foods such as fish eggs, animal glands, spider crabs, or even the ashes of certain plants, to supply additional amounts of nutrients that are important for foetal development, such as choline, iodine, vitamins A, D and K_2 and EPA and DHA. And almost all traditional diets contained liver and other organ meats, bones and skin, fats, seafood and wild plants, which are also high in nutrients crucial for pregnancy and lactation.

Today, unfortunately, much of this ancient and time-tested wisdom has fallen by the wayside. Organ meats, bone broths, skin and cartilage, fish eggs, egg yolks and many other nutrient-dense parts of animals have all but disappeared from the modern diet. Your grandparents may have eaten these foods, but the chances are you don't. This has happened in large part because of the misguided campaigns against saturated fat, cholesterol and red meat. But it's also a consequence of our love for all things modern and our tendency to discount the knowledge of the past.

The problem is that these now-unpopular foods provide nutrients that work synergistically with those found in more commonly eaten foods and are difficult to obtain elsewhere in the diet. In other words, we may be well fed, but we're undernourished. The solution is to return to the practice of our ancestors and to 'eat from nose to tail'. This means eating not only the lean muscle meat (such as steak or chicken breast) of

Libraries NI
Antrim Library
10 Railway Street
Antrim
BT41 4AE
Tel: 028 9446 1942

Borrowed Items 23/03/2017 13:05
XXXXXX8527

Item Title	Due Date
Your personal paleo diet : feel and look great by eating the foods that are ideal for your body	13/04/2017

Email Antrim@librariesni.org.uk
www.librariesni.org.uk
Your library doesn't end here
Get free eBooks and Audiobooks
www.librariesni.org.uk/pages/Iniebooks
andmagazines.aspx
Or ask staff for details.

the animals we consume, but also the organs, skin, cartilage, bones and fattier cuts.

These parts of the animal contain nutrients that are difficult to obtain elsewhere in the diet, as well as nutrients that act synergistically with the nutrients found in muscle meats and other lean proteins; for example:

- The amino acid methionine, which is abundant in lean proteins, can't fulfil its important functions without adequate amounts of B vitamins (especially B_6, B_{12} and folate), choline and glycine.

- Vitamin A is crucial for a variety of biochemical processes in the body, yet it is only found in significant amounts in the livers of land mammals and the liver oils of fish. Beta-carotene, which is found in vegetables such as carrots and red peppers, is often mistakenly referred to as vitamin A. However, although some beta-carotene can be converted into vitamin A in humans, that amount is very small: about 3 per cent in the case of raw carrots.

- Too much vitamin A without enough vitamin D promotes bone loss, whereas too much vitamin D without enough vitamin A leads to kidney and bladder stones and calcification of the arteries. Vitamin K_2 works in concert with both vitamins A and D to regulate calcium metabolism.

With this in mind, I suggest balancing your intake of lean meats and fish with liberal amounts of choline, glycine, B vitamins, vitamin A, vitamin D and vitamin K_2. You can do that by following these guidelines:

- **Consume 125–250ml of home-made bone broth daily,** in soups, sauces, stews or as a beverage (recipe on page 447); **eat tougher cuts of meat,** such as brisket, chuck steak, oxtail and shin; and **don't shy away from skin and cartilage.** These are all excellent sources of glycine.

- **Eat one to two 85g servings of chicken and/or beef liver per week.** See page 175 in this chapter for tips on how to prepare it. Liver is rich in B vitamins, vitamin A and several other nutrients.

- **Eat at least four to five egg yolks per week,** preferably from pasture-raised chickens. You're free to eat more if you'd like, since dietary cholesterol does not have a significant impact on blood cholesterol levels or heart disease risk. Egg yolks are the highest source of choline in the diet. You can eat the eggs with or without the whites.

- **Take ½ teaspoon of high-vitamin cod liver oil per day.** Cod liver oil is the richest source of vitamin A, but it also contains vitamin D, EPA and DHA and – in the case of fermented cod liver oil (see the bonus chapter on supplementation on the website for more info) – vitamin K_2.

- **Eat two servings per day of fermented foods** (for example, sauerkraut, kefir, natto), **cheese and butter** (from pasture-raised cows) and/or **eggs** (from pasture-raised chickens) to obtain adequate amounts of vitamin K_2.

How a simple dietary change cured Aaron's depression

Aaron, aged 34, came to see me complaining of depression. He had suffered from it on and off for years, but it had become worse during the year leading up to his visit. He had tried over-the-counter remedies such as St John's wort and SAMe, but they didn't help. Aaron wanted to avoid drugs, if possible, so he asked me if there was anything else he could do.

I noticed that he had started a strict Paleo diet right around the time his symptoms started to worsen. Aaron was passionate about CrossFit – an intensive strength and conditioning pro-gramme – so he was eating large amounts of protein to support his workouts. He had been told by the personal trainer who introduced him to Paleo to focus on lean meats and avoid saturated fat. He also consumed whey protein shakes and avoided egg yolks, because he had a family history of heart disease and was worried about his cholesterol.

I explained to Aaron that his diet was rich in methionine and low in glycine, and that such an imbalance could be con-tributing to his depression. His body wasn't able to produce adequate serotonin on such a diet. I asked him to start eating fattier cuts of meat and egg yolks and to reduce his con-sumption of whey protein. I also prescribed a grass-fed gelatin supplement to provide extra glycine, as well as high-vitamin cod liver oil to provide fat-soluble vitamins. Aaron was scep-tical that such simple dietary changes could have any effect, after everything he had already tried. Yet after six weeks of this new regimen, his mood had improved significantly. After three months, his depression was completely gone. His sleep had also improved and he felt calmer and more at ease through-out the day.

ECONOMY, FLAVOUR AND CONVENIENCE

There are two other reasons to 'eat from nose to tail'. The first is economy. Organ meats, more gelatinous cuts such as brisket, chuck steak, oxtail, chicken breast or legs with the bones and skin, and fish heads to make into stock, are typically less expensive than muscle meats, boneless (and skinless) chicken breasts or fish fillets. Some butchers will even give beef bones away, if you ask. Grass-fed (pastured) animal products are often more expensive than conventional, grain-fed alternatives.

But choosing the more gelatinous cuts and organ meats of grass-fed animals is one way to make them more affordable. Including these cuts in your diet is less wasteful, as they often go unconsumed, an important consideration in a world with a growing population and dwindling natural resources.

The second reason is flavour. In many cases, to save money you have to sacrifice quality or flavour. Not so with these cuts: they are some of the most flavourful, tender and delicious cuts on the animal if they're prepared properly. This was no secret to our grandparents and their ancestors, who regularly included them in their diet. But today, many people have forgotten how to cook them. Fortunately, there's a 'nose to tail' revival happening in culinary circles, and numerous books are available that provide instruction. For some excellent inspiration and recipes, look for two of my favourite books: *The Whole Beast: From Nose to Tail Eating* (Ecco, 2004), by Fergus Henderson, and *Odd Bits: How to Cook the Rest of the Animal* (10 Speed Press, 2011), by Jennifer McLagan and Leigh Beisch.

The third reason is convenience. Let's face it: most of us are busy and don't have time to cook from scratch at every meal. One of the advantages to the fattier cuts of meat is that they tend to be larger and will feed you or your family for more than a single meal. This can save you both time and money.

If you're new to preparing these cuts, here are a few ideas to get you started. Look at my website for recipes.

- **Make a stew** Chuck steak, silverside, shin, and a boneless beef joint, such as rump, are good cuts for stew.

- **Make a pot roast** Pot roast cuts come from the fore- and hindquarters of the cow. You can also use the cuts listed above for pot roast.

- **Make chicken broth** Roast a chicken and eat the meat for dinner. Then put the carcass in a large pan with water and flavourings and make some home-made stock. It's one of the most healing foods you can eat and it's rich in glycine and minerals. Use it for soups, sauces or just drink it warm like tea.

- **Make fish-head soup** Another time-tested remedy, fish-head soup is rich in glycine, iodine, selenium and other minerals. It can also be used for soup and as a base for sauces, especially in Thai food. (Oily fish are not usually recommended for making into stock, however.)

- **Make oxtail soup** Oxtails have lots of flavour. They're incredibly gelatinous and thus high in glycine, as well as all the other vitamins and minerals beef contains. The segments are vertebrae, so they're also rich in nutrient-dense bone marrow.

A slow cooker is a good way to prepare stocks, soups and slow-cooked meats of all kinds.

Organ meats can be prepared in numerous ways. It's worth pointing out that whereas some people love the stronger flavour of organ meats, others don't. In that case, here are four ideas for how to include liver (which is one of the most nutrient-dense foods by weight you can eat) in your diet:

1 Choose recipes that mask or mellow the strong flavour.

2 Mix liver into other meat dishes. See page 48 for instructions.

3 Dice fresh liver into 'pill-size' pieces. Arrange them flat on a small baking sheet that will fit in your freezer. Freeze them for at least two weeks to kill any potential pathogens in the raw meat. Then simply swallow several frozen 'liver pills' each day. Aim for about 85–175g a week in total.

4 Eat liver pâté, either home-made or bought if made in the traditional manner without preservatives.

One frequent objection to eating liver that I hear is that it is 'toxic', because it is the primary organ of detoxification. Although it's true that the liver is in charge of detoxification, most of the toxins in the body are stored in the fat tissue – not the liver. (For this reason, it's best to buy pasture-raised and organic when you're choosing high-fat animal products, such as fattier cuts of meat, as well as butter, whole milk, or yoghurt.)

When organ meats shouldn't be on the menu

Haemochromatosis is a hereditary condition that causes excess storage of iron in the body. It's the most common genetic disease in North America and the UK, affecting as many as one in 200 people – a prevalence ten times that of cystic fibrosis. It's associated with a wide variety of diseases, such as diabetes, cardiovascular disease and Alzheimer's and, if untreated, can literally rust the organs (especially the liver, pancreas, heart and brain) and cause early death. Unfortunately, haemochromatosis is often misdiagnosed or simply just missed. A 1996 Centers for Disease Control and Prevention study found that the average haemochromatosis patient had seen three doctors over a period of nine years before being properly diagnosed. What's more, even mild iron overload that isn't associated with haemochromatosis can cause serious problems, including metabolic disease, male infertility and severe fatigue.

Iron overload is more common in men and post-menopausal women than in pre-menopausal women. Why? The only way to get rid of excess iron once it's stored in the body is through bleeding or chelation therapy. Pre-menopausal women lose a little bit of iron (in the blood) through menstruation each month, whereas men and post-menopausal women simply accumulate iron without losing it.

Ask your doctor to test your iron levels. If they're high, I'd recommend the following steps:

- Avoid consuming organ meats, clams and oysters, which are very high in iron.
- Moderate your intake of red meat – beef, lamb and wild game such as venison – which are also relatively high in iron.
- Donate blood three to four times a year. Men and post-menopausal women can do this as a preventive measure. Studies have shown that frequent blood donors have better blood sugar control and lower levels of hypertension.
- Ask your doctor about phlebotomy (the therapeutic removal of blood), the treatment of choice for iron overload.
- Avoid high doses (over 300mg per day) of vitamin C or betaine HCL, both of which increase iron absorption.
- Don't consume alcohol with meals containing iron; alcohol also increases iron absorption.

WHAT ABOUT DAIRY?

Dairy often gets a bad rap in the health and nutrition world. It's either maligned for its high saturated fat content or criticised as being 'unfit for human consumption'. Let's take a closer look at each of these arguments.

Does full-fat dairy contribute to disease?

In the conventional nutrition world, dairy is recognised as an important part of a 'healthy, well-balanced diet', because it's a good source of protein, calcium and added nutrients such as vitamins A and D; however, dairy fat is typically portrayed as being harmful, mostly due to its saturated fat and choles-terol content. Mainstream organisations like the American Heart Association and American Diabetes Association rec-ommend using non-fat, low-fat and reduced-fat dairy products, steering consumers away from full-fat or whole dairy for the most part. But does the evidence support this recommendation?

A 2012 paper published in the *European Journal of Clinical Nutrition* reviewed 16 studies examining the relationship between high-fat dairy, obesity and cardiovascular and meta-bolic disease. In the majority of studies reviewed, high-fat dairy was either inversely associated with obesity and cardiometabolic disease (that is, those who ate the most high-fat dairy had the lowest risk of these conditions), or not associated at all.

Some compounds in high-fat dairy products – such as butyrate, phytanic acid, trans-palmitoleic acid and conjugated linoleic acid – have been shown to have beneficial effects. Butyrate provides energy to the cells lining the colon, inhibits inflammation in the gastrointestinal tract and may prevent colonic bacteria from entering the bloodstream. In fact, butyrate's anti-inflammatory effect is so strong that a dose of 4g per day for eight weeks induced complete remission in a group of Crohn's disease patients. Phytanic acid, one of the fatty acids in dairy fat, has been shown to reduce triglycerides, improve insulin sensitivity and improve blood sugar regulation in animal models. Another fatty acid in dairy fat, trans-palmitoleic acid, was associated with lower triglycerides, fasting insulin, blood pressure and risk of diabetes in a study of 2,600 US adults. Finally, conjugated linoleic acid (CLA), a natural trans-fat found in dairy products, may reduce the risk of heart disease, cancer and diabetes.

Dairy is also a good source of fat-soluble vitamins such as retinol (active vitamin A) and vitamin K_2, which are difficult to obtain elsewhere in the diet.

Is dairy 'unfit for human consumption'?

One of the main arguments against dairy, advanced by vegans, raw foodists and even advocates of the Paleo diet, is that dairy isn't an appropriate food for humans. They support this argument by pointing out that most humans don't produce lactase after childhood and that no other mammal aside from humans consumes the milk of another animal.

These may seem like compelling arguments on the surface, but they don't hold up under scrutiny. As I mentioned in Chapter 1, human evolution didn't stop in the Palaeolithic era. Although it's true that most of our genes are the same as they were hundreds of thousands of years ago, some of them have adapted in a relatively short period of time. Lactase persistence is perhaps the best example of this. Our hunter-gatherer ancestors breast-fed until around age four. Mother's milk was virtually the only food they consumed which contained lactose, or milk sugar, and there was no need for the body to continue producing lactase (the enzyme that digests lactose) after early childhood. But when humans began consuming cow's milk, natural selection went to work and a genetic mutation that continued the production of lactase into adulthood began spreading through the population about 8,000 years ago. Now, a third of the world's population produces lactase into adulthood (and that figure approaches 100 per cent in some parts of Northern Europe).

Humans have also developed technology that addresses some of the potential disadvantages of dairy consumption; for example, fermentation of milk into yoghurt and kefir can reduce the lactose content to less than 1 per cent – an amount that even someone who doesn't produce lactase should be able to tolerate. Some studies have even shown that consuming fermented dairy products like yoghurt may reverse lactose tolerance by increasing levels of lactose-digesting bacteria in the gut.

What about the idea that humans shouldn't drink milk because no other animal drinks the milk of another animal? By this logic, we humans should also avoid cooking our food, drinking coffee or consuming alcohol. I don't know of any other animals doing these things, but that alone is not a sufficient reason for us not to do them. We've developed both technological (that is, fermentation) and genetic (that is, lactase persistence) adaptations that enable us to enjoy and benefit from dairy products that other animals don't have, so comparing ourselves to them in this case doesn't make sense.

All of this said, there's no doubt that dairy doesn't work for everyone. Some people are allergic or intolerant to casein, the protein in dairy, or highly sensitive to lactose. In these cases dairy must be strictly avoided, or additional steps must be taken to make it tolerable. Since there's still no gold-standard test for dairy intolerance, I recommend removing it from your diet during the Step 1 30-Day Reset and reintroducing it in Step 2. See Chapter 11 for guidelines on how to properly reintroduce dairy products to determine whether you tolerate them.

Is dairy right for you?

Although milk proteins are very well absorbed by most people, they can cause serious issues in a minority of the population. Studies suggest that between 1 in 1,000 and 1 in 200 adults are allergic to milk proteins (which include casein, whey, alpha-lactalbumin, beta-lactoglobulin and bovine serum albumin, among others). It's also likely that a larger, but undefined, number of people suffer from intolerance to milk proteins. An intolerance is different from a true allergy in that the body does not produce antibodies to the antigen (milk protein, in this case) — but it can still cause serious symptoms.

Unfortunately, there's no accurate and reliable way of testing for milk-protein intolerance, which is why I suggest that every-one removes dairy entirely for at least 30 days during the Step 1 Reset. In Chapter 11, I provide instructions for how to add dairy back into your diet, if you wish, and how to determine if the proteins or the sugar (lactose) is to blame if you have a bad reaction. This is important to know, because if you're reacting to the proteins you won't be able to tolerate most dairy products (with the possible exception of ghee and butter, which are low in protein); however, if you're reacting to lactose you will likely still be able to enjoy dairy products low in lactose, such as ghee, butter, yoghurt, kefir, hard cheeses and, possibly, cream.

Parents should also be aware that milk protein is one of the most common allergens for babies and young children, with a prevalence ranging from 2–3 per cent depending on the study. Although most children outgrow this (as reflected in the much lower rates of milk protein allergy in adults), if your baby or child is having symptoms that resemble an allergic response to food (diarrhoea, constipation, skin breakouts, abdominal pain, insomnia, irritability, and so on), ask your paediatrician about removing dairy entirely for 30 days to see if that helps.

Summary: cooking and eating from nose to tail

- Eat at least 85g of organ meats per week. Liver is the most nutritious, but heart, kidney, tongue and even brain are all fair game! Those with iron overload should not consume organ meats.
- Eat 125–250ml of home-made bone broth (from chicken, turkey, beef, pork trotter, fish or shellfish) in soups, stews and sauces.
- Enjoy tougher, more gelatinous cuts of red meat in addition to lean cuts. Brisket, shin, chuck steak, rib steak and minced

meat with 25 per cent fat are good choices. Dark-meat poultry with skin should be consumed in moderation, because of its high omega-6 linoleic acid content.

- Eat at least 4–6 egg yolks (alone or in whole eggs) per week. They are excellent sources of several nutrients, especially choline, which is hard to find elsewhere in the diet. Choose pastured eggs, or organic and truly free-range eggs, whenever possible.
- If you eat canned salmon, find a brand that includes the bones. They're soft and safe to eat, and they're a great source of calcium.

CHAPTER 10

Good Gut Feeling: Restore Your Gut Flora and Gut Barrier

Digestive problems have reached epidemic levels in the US – and the UK and Australia will have similar statistics; for example, irritable bowel syndrome (IBS) affects between 10 and 15 per cent of the US population and accounts for 12 per cent of total visits to primary care doctors. IBS is the second leading cause of missed working days, second only to the common cold.

Sixty per cent of the US population will experience GERD (gastroesophageal reflux disease) within a 12-month period and 20–30 per cent will have weekly symptoms. Nexium, an acid-suppressing drug prescribed for GERD, generated $6.3 billion in sales in 2010, second only to Lipitor (a statin).

Perhaps by now you've been on the Step 1 Reset Diet long enough to note that your gut is feeling better than ever, or perhaps you're still tweaking the diet a bit (with further tweaks to come later) and you're gradually getting there. The

Notes for this chapter may be found at ChrisKresser.com/ppcnotes/#ch10

point is that our Paleo ancestors – with their nourishing traditional diets of real foods – probably didn't walk around
with heartburn. In our modern world, however, it's a different story. Achieving good gut health is a major part of
improving your overall health through Your Personal Paleo
Diet, because gut problems don't just affect the gut.

We now know that the health of the digestive tract is critical to overall health and that an unhealthy gut contributes to
a wide range of diseases, including diabetes, obesity, rheumatoid arthritis, autism spectrum disorder, depression and
chronic fatigue syndrome. The gut is a distinct nervous system
in its own right; some researchers even refer to the gut as the
'second brain', because of its size, complexity and similarity –
in terms of neurotransmitters and signalling molecules – to the
brain. And recent studies suggest that approximately 70–80
per cent of the body's immune cells are in the gut.

Because of this, many researchers and clinicians (myself
included) believe that supporting intestinal health will be one
of the most important goals of medicine in the 21st century.
There are two closely related variables that determine our gut
health: the intestinal microbiota, or 'gut flora', and the gut
barrier. Let's discuss each of them in turn.

THE GUT MICROBIOTA (AKA 'GUT FLORA')

The gut contains over 100,000,000,000,000 (100 trillion!)
microorganisms, from 1,000 different species, with ten times
more microbes than there are human cells and 100 times
more genes than exist in the human genome. It's not inac-
curate, then, to say that at a cellular level we're more
microbial than we are human. Indeed, according to Stanford
microbiologist Justin Sonneberg, 'Humans can be regarded
as elaborate vessels evolved to permit the survival and prop-
agation of microorganisms.'

A hundred trillion microorganisms hitching a ride in our gut may sound like something from a creepy science-fiction film, but it turns out that these passengers are crucial to our health. Among other things, the gut microbiota promotes normal gastrointestinal function, provides protection from infection, regulates metabolism and is home to the majority of our immune cells. On the other hand, when the gut microbiota is out of balance, we get ill. Changes to the gut microbiota have been linked to diseases ranging from autism and depression to autoimmune conditions such as Hashimoto's, inflammatory bowel disease and type-1 diabetes.

The composition of the gut microbiota

The colonisation of the gut by bacteria begins immediately after birth and occurs within a few days. Although the gut of a newborn baby is exposed to some microbes in the womb (via ingestion of amniotic fluid), the vast majority of an infant's gut microbiota is acquired when it passes through the birth canal swallowing the mother's native bacteria. This explains why the method of delivery – vaginal birth or Caesarean section – has been shown to influence how the gut microbiota initially develops. In vaginal births, the baby's first exposure to bacteria is the birth canal, whereas in a Caesarean, the first exposure is to bacteria in the hospital environment. Some research suggests that this initial exposure to bacteria affects the future composition of the gut microbiota for months or even years. Other studies indicate that children born via Caesarean are at a greater risk of asthma, obesity and type-1 diabetes later in life.

After birth, the baby's diet (and perhaps to a lesser degree the mother's diet) has a strong influence on the composition of the gut flora. Babies that are exclusively formula-fed have significant differences in gut microbiota compared to babies that are exclusively, or partially, breast-fed. This is important because 'pioneer bacteria' (the first bacteria to colonise the gut in a baby) can alter gene expression to create a more favourable environment for themselves and a less favourable environment for later (and perhaps more beneficial) bacteria.

Diet also has a major influence on the composition of the gut microbiota later in childhood and into adulthood. The amount, type and balance of proteins, fats and carbohydrates, as well as the amount and type of fibre, have a large impact on the gut microbiota; for example, foods that are rich in soluble fibre, such as certain fruits, vegetables and starchy tubers (such as sweet potatoes and potatoes) increase levels of *Lactobacillus*, a class of bacteria often used as a probiotic because of its beneficial effects on the gut. (Probiotics are 'good' bacteria that help regulate the balance of the gut microbiota.)

Other factors that can negatively influence the gut microbiota at all ages include:

- Antibiotics and other medications like NSAIDs (non-steroidal anti-inflammatory drugs; for example, ibuprofen)

- Chronic stress

- Chronic infections – especially gut infections

Functions of the gut microbiota

The main functions of the gut microbiota can be broken down into three categories: metabolic, structural and protective.

1 Metabolic

The metabolic activity of the gut microbiota is so diverse and important that some researchers have proposed that this microbiota be referred to as an 'organ within an organ'.

Bacteria in the gut break down dietary compounds that could otherwise cause cancer; synthesise vitamins such as biotin, folate and vitamin K; convert non-digestible carbohydrates to short-chain fatty acids, which provide energy and benefit the cells lining the gut; and help with the absorption of minerals like calcium, magnesium and iron.

Recent research has also revealed a relationship between gut microbes and how we process and store the food we eat. Microbes help us to break down long-chain carbohydrates such as fibre and starch that we can't absorb on our own. During this process, the microbes produce short-chain fatty acids, including acetate, propionate and butyrate. Butyrate has anti-inflammatory effects; increases insulin sensitivity; may delay the development of neurodegenerative diseases; and may also be helpful in the treatment of diseases of the colon such as Crohn's, IBS or ulcerative colitis.

2 Structural

The short-chain fatty acids produced by fermentation (the breaking down of a substance by bacteria or other micro-organisms – in this case, the gut microbiota) of carbohydrates have other important effects. They stimulate the growth and differentiation of the epithelial cells – the cells that form the inner lining of the colon. Butyrate also inhibits cell proliferation in the colon, which can lead to colon cancer.

3 Protective

The gut is first and foremost a barrier designed to keep certain things (pathogens and toxins) out and let other things (beneficial nutrients) in. The mucosal lining of the intestine is the primary interface between the external environment and our immune system. Some might assume that the skin plays a more important role in this respect, given its continual exposure to the environment. But the surface area of the gut is approximately 100 times larger than that of the skin and the gut contains approximately 70–80 per cent of the immune cells in the body. These immune cells form a layer of tissue called the 'gut-associated lymphoid tissue', or GALT.

Studies have shown that the microbial composition of the gut affects the composition and function of the GALT. It's also true that bacteria in the gut form a crucial line of resistance to invasion by pathogenic microbes. Germ-free mice that have been bred to have sterile guts (with no microbes at all) are highly susceptible to infection, and antibiotics can disrupt the delicate balance of gut microbes and allow overgrowth of pathogenic species like *Clostridium difficile*.

THE GUT BARRIER

Think of the gut as a hollow tube that passes from the mouth to the anus. Anything that goes into the mouth and is not absorbed into the bloodstream will be eliminated as waste and will never enter the body. The gut barrier thus serves as a 'gatekeeper', which decides what gets into our body and what stays out.

Normally this process works very well; however, when the intestinal barrier becomes permeable (that is, 'leaky'), substances that should not escape the gut – such as large, undigested protein molecules and bacterial toxins – pass into the bloodstream. This triggers an immune reaction, since these particles are viewed as 'foreign invaders' by the body. And we now know that this immune reaction, resulting from intestinal permeability, contributes to everything from autoimmune disease, to depression, to obesity, to skin disease. In fact, some researchers such as Dr Alessio Fasano (a pioneer in the fields of coeliac disease and gluten intolerance) now believe that intestinal permeability is a precondition to developing auto-immunity. In other words, it may not even be possible to develop an autoimmune disease unless you have a leaky gut first.

The phrase 'leaky gut' used to be confined to the outer fringes of medicine, and conventional researchers and doctors originally scoffed at the concept. Yet today it's one of the hottest topics in the scientific literature. Researchers have identified a protein called zonulin that increases intestinal permeability in humans and other animals. Many, if not most, autoimmune diseases – including coeliac disease, type-1 diabetes, multiple sclerosis, rheumatoid arthritis and inflammatory bowel disease – are characterised by abnormally high levels of zonulin and a permeable gut barrier. In fact, researchers have found that they can induce type-1 diabetes almost immediately in animals by exposing them to zonulin. They develop a leaky gut and begin producing antibodies to islet cells, which are responsible for making insulin.

As you can see, the effects of a 'leaky gut' cause an immune reaction that affects not only the gut itself, but also other organs and tissues including the skeletal system, the pancreas, the kidney, the liver and the brain. This explains why people who have a leaky gut don't always have gut symptoms and why the range of symptoms they experience is so diverse, including (but not limited to):

Abdominal pain	Fatigue
Acne	Gas and bloating
Allergies	Joint pain
Anxiety and depression	Poor immune function
Asthma	Poor memory
Brain fog	Skin rashes such as eczema or psoriasis
Constipation or diarrhoea	

WHAT CAUSES LEAKY GUT?

Several factors can damage gut-barrier integrity, making it permeable.

Diet

Gliadin is a protein found in wheat responsible for the intestinal damage observed in coeliac disease. In people with coeliac disease (and perhaps in those without it), gliadin activates zonulin signalling, which in turn reduces intestinal barrier integrity and permits the passage of gliadin through the gut barrier. In these cases, wheat and other gluten-containing foods directly contribute to intestinal permeability. This is one reason I recommend that most people do not regularly consume wheat, even if they don't have gluten intolerance or coeliac disease.

Diet can also have an indirect effect on gut-barrier integrity via its impact on the gut microbiota. The standard Western diet – which is high in refined flours and sugars, and industrial seed oils, and low in whole fruits, vegetables and soluble fibre – has been shown to cause undesirable changes in the gut microbiota. These changes to the microbiota in turn make the gut barrier permeable and may increase the risk of auto-immune disease and other problems associated with a leaky gut. On the other hand, traditional diets rich in fruits, vegetables and soluble fibres with very little processed, modern food cause beneficial changes in the gut microbiota, which preserve barrier integrity and improve overall health.

Small intestinal bacterial overgrowth

SIBO, or small intestinal bacterial overgrowth, is a condition involving inappropriate growth of bacteria in the small intestine. The large majority of the bacteria in our gut should inhabit the colon; however, chronic stress, poor diet, infection, antibiotic use and other factors can cause bacteria to migrate from the colon into the small intestine. This causes malabsorption of proteins, fats, B vitamins and other micronutrients. It also causes intestinal permeability.

Chronic stress

Chronic stress has been shown to reduce gut-barrier integrity in both human and animal studies.

Infections

Infection with bacteria (such as *Helicobacter pylori*, the bacterium that causes stomach ulcers), viruses (such as HIV) and parasites (such as *Giardia lamblia*) have all been shown to disrupt intestinal barrier integrity.

Excess alcohol

Alcohol in excess can promote the growth of certain types of bacteria in the gut that, in turn, increase intestinal permeability.

Medications

NSAIDs, aspirin, proton pump inhibitors (PPIs, prescribed for acid reflux and GERD) and several other medications increase gut-barrier permeability. Antibiotics may indirectly disrupt gut-barrier function via their adverse effects on the gut microbiota.

Environmental toxins

Preliminary research suggests that some environmental toxins, such as bisphenol-A (BPA), may cause intestinal permeability.

THE GUT–DISEASE CONNECTION

The Greek physician Hippocrates once said that 'All disease begins in the gut.' By now, I'm sure you realise how true those words are. Let's look more closely at the gut–disease connection.

The gut–brain connection

The connection between the gut and the brain is deeply rooted in our language, with sayings like 'I have a gut feeling' and 'I have butterflies in my stomach.' Long before scientists understood how the gut and brain influence each other, people had experienced it first hand: a 'nervous' stomach before an important speech, or perhaps heartburn during a stressful financial situation.

Although most people are aware that stress and emotional states like anxiety affect the gut, fewer people realise that problems in the gut can affect the brain; for example, SIBO (see page 190) is strongly associated with depression and anxiety in observational studies. Other research indicates that inflammation in the gut can alter mood and cause depression. Inflammatory molecules produced in the gut travel through the bloodstream, cross the blood–brain barrier and activate specific cells in the brain, known as microglia cells. The microglia cells play an important role in repairing brain cells, but when they are chronically activated, communication between neurons (the functional brain cells) is impaired and depression results. Finally, increased intestinal permeability is much more common in autistic children and may contribute to the development of autism spectrum disorder.

I've found in my work with patients that SIBO, gut dysbiosis (an imbalance between the good and bad bacteria that colonise the gut) and gut inflammation are the most common causes of anxiety, depression and other psychological and behavioural problems. This is especially true in children.

The gut–metabolism connection

One of the hottest topics in the scientific community over the past few years has been the connection between the gut microbiota and metabolic health. There are several reasons for this link. The gut microbiota is a source of bacterial toxins that provoke inflammation and insulin resistance, both of which contribute to obesity. Changes in the gut microbiota have been shown to increase appetite, increase the rate at which we absorb fats and carbohydrates and increase the storage of calories as fat. Bad bacteria in the gut can also cause insulin resistance and inflammation of the hypothalamus in the brain, both of which are associated with obesity.

Other gut problems have also been shown to cause obesity and metabolic disease, including bacterial overgrowth in the small intestine, increased intestinal permeability, gallstones and changes in the enteric (gut) nervous system.

The gut–immune connection

Gut dysfunction is an emerging focus in the study of auto-immune disease. In fact, as I mentioned above, some researchers believe that intestinal permeability is a precondition for developing autoimmune disease in the first place. In this theory, an environmental antigen (such as a protein from a food) 'leaks' through the permeable gut barrier, where it initiates an immune response. Although this immune response is designed to protect us from foreign invaders such as bacteria and viruses, when it's continually triggered by food proteins and other environmental antigens penetrating the gut barrier, it can become overzealous and begin attacking human tissue. That's what autoimmune disease is: the body attacking itself.

In addition to contributing to autoimmune disease, disruptions in the gut barrier have been shown to increase susceptibility to infection and weaken our immune defences.

The gut–skin axis

There are clear associations between gut disorders and skin conditions in the scientific literature. Fourteen per cent of patients with ulcerative colitis and 24 per cent of patients with Crohn's disease have skin rashes, and 25 per cent of patients with coeliac disease have a skin condition called dermatitis herpetiformis. People with coeliac disease also have a higher frequency of oral mucosal lesions, alopecia and vitiligo (both autoimmune skin diseases).

One fascinating study found that SIBO is ten times more prevalent in those with acne rosacea and that correction of SIBO leads to either a complete clearing or a significant improvement of lesions in 92 per cent of these patients. Altered gut microbiota also promotes the release of substance P, a potent neuropeptide that is produced in both the gut and skin, and plays a major role in skin disorders. Finally, probiotics have been shown to improve intestinal barrier function, reduce inflammation and improve skin conditions. One Italian study involving 40 patients with acne found that probiotics plus standard care were more effective than standard care alone.

NOURISHING YOUR GUT

Now that you know how important the gut is to overall health, let's discuss some basic strategies for maintaining your digestive health.

Avoid foods that are harmful to the gut

The basic Paleo approach is an excellent starting place for maintaining gut health. Refined flour, sugar and industrial seed oils – the staples of the industrialised diet – are harmful because they cause undesirable changes in the gut microbiota and may disrupt the integrity of the intestinal barrier, among other effects.

Excess alcohol has been shown to cause intestinal permeability, so I recommend limiting alcohol consumption to four to six drinks per week (or eliminating it altogether if you have significant gut issues). Certain classes of foods (such as the nightshade family – potatoes, tomatoes, aubergines and peppers, for example) and nutrients that are well tolerated by most people can be harmful for people with digestive problems. I discuss these in more detail in the bonus chapter on digestive disorders, available on my website.

Reduce foods that may irritate an already inflamed gut

Vegetables are one of the few foods that every diet philosophy agrees are healthy. That said, vegetables (particularly non-starchy vegetables) tend to be high in *insoluble fibre*, which can irritate an inflamed gut. If you have irritable bowel syndrome (IBS), inflammatory bowel disease (IBD), or other digestive disorders, you may benefit from reducing your intake of non-starchy vegetables. These include:

Aubergine

Broccoli

Cabbage, pak choi, Brussels sprouts

Cauliflower

Celery

Green beans

Greens (spinach, lettuce, kale, spring greens, rocket, watercress, and so on)

Onions, shallots, leeks, spring onions, garlic

Peas, mangetouts, sugar snap peas

Peppers

Sweetcorn

Although, remember that these should be eaten as normal if you do not suffer from the above conditions.

On the other hand, vegetables that are high in *soluble fibre* and lower in insoluble fibre tend to have a soothing effect on the gut. These include:

Beetroot	Pumpkin and squashes
Carrots	Starchy tubers (yams, sweet potatoes, potatoes)
Celeriac	Swedes
Courgettes and other summer squash (especially peeled)	Taro
Parsnips	Turnips
Plantains	Yuca (cassava/manioc)

In addition to reducing your overall intake of vegetables high in insoluble fibre, you should reduce the variety of vegetables you eat at any given meal. Instead of stir-fries with six different vegetables, for example, have a single steamed or roasted vegetable as a side dish.

Note that I'm not suggesting you completely avoid vegetables that are high in insoluble fibre; I'm just suggesting that you limit them. Moreover, there are steps you can take to make these foods more digestible and less likely to irritate your gut. They include:

1 Never eat insoluble fibre foods on an empty stomach. Always eat them with other foods that contain soluble fibre.

2 Remove the stems and peels from veggies (that is, broccoli, cauliflower and cabbage) – and fruits – high in insoluble fibre.

3 Dice, mash, chop, grate or blend high-insoluble fibre foods to make them easier to break down.

4 Insoluble fibre foods are best eaten well cooked: steamed thoroughly, boiled in soup, braised, and so on. Avoid consuming them in stir-fries, and if you do eat them raw, prepare them as described above.

Finally, fermenting vegetables that are high in insoluble fibre is another option for making them more digestible – since fermentation is essentially a process of 'pre-digestion'. Many of my patients who can't tolerate unfermented cabbage (raw or cooked) are able to eat fermented cabbage (sauerkraut) without a problem. See the Fermented Foods Guide on my website for more information about how to make fermented foods. If you choose to buy fermented foods from a shop, make sure that it says 'raw' on the jar and that they're in the chiller section. The sauerkraut you can buy in the condiments section has been pasteurised and won't have the same beneficial effect as raw or unpasteurised sauerkraut. (For more on fermented foods, see page 199.)

Eat foods that nourish the gut

In addition to avoiding foods that harm the gut, it's important to focus on foods that nourish the gut. These can be broken down into three categories: bone broth, fermentable fibres and fermented foods.

Bone broth

Bone broth is made from water and the meat and bones of animals (and may also contain vegetables and seasonings). It's considered a healing food in many traditional cultures and it's rich in glycine and gelatin, both of which support digestive health. The nutrients in bone broth are particularly helpful for restoring the integrity of the gut barrier when it's damaged. I recommend consuming 125–250ml of bone broth per day in the form of soups, stock, stews or sauces (bone broth makes an excellent base for sauces and stews – see page 447 for the recipe).

Fermentable fibres

Soluble fibres naturally found in fruits, vegetables, starches (for example, potato, sweet potato, plantain, and so on) and nuts and seeds provide a food source for the beneficial bacteria in the gut. These bacteria ferment the fibre and produce short-chain fatty acids such as butyrate, which has anti-inflammatory properties, promotes the development of healthy cells in the colon and may protect against colon cancer. Starches like potatoes, sweet potatoes, plantains, taro root, yuca (cassava/manioc), celeriac and parsnip are particularly good sources of soluble fibres.

Another option for fermentable fibre is resistant starch. The suggested amount is between 20g and 40g. Unfortunately, it's not easy to come by in whole foods, because cooking tends to destroy it, and foods that contain it in large amounts can't be eaten raw. With this in mind, here are a few ways to add resistant starch to your diet:

- Mix 4 tablespoons of raw, unmodified potato starch (Bob's Red Mill is a good brand) with water or other food or a beverage at room temperature – 4 tablespoons of potato starch provides about 32g of resistant starch.

- Make plantain chips by cutting a large, green (unripe) plantain into thin slices and putting them into a food dehydrator or use the dehydrating function on the oven, if you have this. Eat these as a snack. A single, large, unripe plantain contains about 40g of resistant starch.

- Eat a green (unripe) banana, which contains about 15g of resistant starch, depending on ripeness.

Note Some people with gut issues may benefit from reducing their intake of fibre for a period of time.

Fermented foods

These include fermented vegetables such as raw (unpas-teurised) sauerkraut, kimchi and pickles, fermented dairy, such as yoghurt and kefir, and fermented beverages such as beetroot kvaas, kombucha and water kefir. Fermented foods contain beneficial microorganisms, which in turn have positive effects on several different aspects of gut health. I suggest consuming 1–2 tablespoons of sauerkraut or other fermented vegetables with each meal and additional fermented foods such as yoghurt, dairy kefir, water kefir or beetroot kvaas throughout the day. (**Note** Although cheese, soured cream and alcohol are fermented, they do not have a therapeutic effect like the fermented foods I've listed above.)

Avoid antibiotics as much as possible

We've known for some time that antibiotics kill beneficial bacteria in the gut; however, more sensitive DNA sequencing technology that has been developed in the past few years has increased our understanding of just how far-reaching the effects of antibiotic use on the gut microbiota can be; for example, two separate studies published in the last five years have shown that a single course of antibiotics may cause irreversible, permanent changes to the gut microbiota. The clinical significance of these changes is not yet well understood, but given what we know about the importance of the gut microbiota to health, it's likely they aren't harmless.

Antibiotics are potentially life-saving and certainly necessary in some cases, and I'm not suggesting that you avoid them. But they are often prescribed (or requested by patients) when there's no evidence that they help, such as for colds and flu and other infections that are viral in origin. Even in the case of bacterial infections like strep throat, studies have shown that antibiotics don't shorten the duration of the infection, although they may improve symptoms and reduce the time the patient is contagious.

Treat gut infections

Gut infections are far more common than most people believe and you don't have to travel to a foreign country to get one (although that can help!). *Helicobacter pylori*, the bacterium that causes gastritis and ulcers, is thought to infect up to half the global population, with significantly higher rates in developing countries. Parasite infections are more difficult to track, because conventional testing does a poor job of identifying them. But using more sensitive lab methods in my practice, I've found them to be quite common.

Manage stress

Chronic stress can cause bacterial overgrowth in the small intestine, inflammation and intestinal permeability. It also increases disease activity in IBS and IBD. On the other hand, mindfulness-based stress reduction, hypnotherapy, biofeedback and other stress-reduction techniques have been shown to improve gut function and reduce gut symptoms. Please see Chapter 14 for specific recommendations for stress management.

Summary: gut health

- Understand the causes of gut dysfunction, including 'leaky gut' and intestinal dysbiosis.
- Avoid foods that harm the gut, including refined flour, industrial seed oils and sugar.
- Eat foods that nourish the gut, including bone broths, fermentable fibre and fermented foods.
- Avoid antibiotics whenever possible.
- Treat gut infections if they are present.
- Practise stress management on a daily basis.

STEP 2

Rebuild Your Life

CHAPTER 11

Reintroduce
'Grey Area' Foods

Now that you've finished the 30-day Reset and know how your body feels on a strict Paleo diet, it's time to add back into your diet some of the 'grey area' foods you removed in Step 1. These are foods that were not a part of the original human dietary template, but are nevertheless nourishing and health-promoting *when they're well tolerated*. The important thing to understand about these grey area foods is that different people respond to them in different ways; for example, some people (I happen to be one of them) thrive on dairy products like butter and yoghurt; however, those same foods can give another person stomach cramps or make them break out in hives. We don't know why people can react so differently to the same food, but genetics, gut microbiota ('gut flora'), immune health, stress and emotional and psychological factors all play a role.

Before we get into details about how to reintroduce these

Notes for this chapter may be found at ChrisKresser.com/ppcnotes/#ch11

foods safely, we should answer the question: *why reintroduce them at all?* If you're like most of my patients and readers, you're probably feeling better than you have in many years after the Reset phase – or perhaps better than you've ever felt in your life. If that's the case, why rock the boat? That's certainly a valid question. If you are feeling better than ever and you don't miss any of the grey area foods, then by all means continue with the 30-Day Reset Diet. There's no risk in doing so. That's how our ancestors ate for hundreds of thousands of years. The foods permitted in Step 1 are loaded with all the nutrients you need to be healthy, vital and avoid disease. You could keep eating that way for the rest of your life (which is likely to be a lot longer than if you stayed on the standard Western diet) – and many who embrace the Paleo diet do just that.

If you're like most of my patients, however, you might be missing some of your favourite foods that were prohibited during Step 1. I'm sorry to tell you this, but if crisps and cheese puffs are two of your favourite foods, you won't be reintroducing them in Step 2. The good news is that if you've been missing butter on your sweet potato, or that morning bowl of yoghurt with berries you love so much, or that occasional Thai meal with white rice, you're in luck. Those are some of the foods you will be reintroducing during Step 2. They're perfectly healthy foods – provided you tolerate them well.

But how do you know if you tolerate them? I've developed a very specific programme – tested and refined with thousands of patients and readers of my blog – that will help you answer that question. And in my opinion, doing a controlled food reintroduction like the one I'm about to teach you is the only way you can accurately determine how a particular food affects you. There are many food-sensitivity tests on the market, but all of them have serious limitations or problems that limit their usefulness. It would be nice if we could take a test that told us exactly which foods we tolerate and which ones we don't, but so far that test doesn't exist.

Although the food reintroduction does require some time and effort, by the end you'll know exactly what does and what doesn't work for *you* – which is much better than relying on the experience or advice of others. Just because something works for me, your best friend, or a total stranger on an internet forum, that doesn't mean it will work for you.

In the sections that follow, I'll explain some general guidelines about how to successfully reintroduce foods. I'll also tell you which foods I think are safe to reintroduce and provide specific advice about the order in which to reintroduce certain foods.

GENERAL GUIDELINES FOR FOOD REINTRODUCTION

Food reintroduction requires a methodical approach and there's both a right and wrong way to do it. The method I'm going to share below has been tested with hundreds of patients and thousands of readers and listeners around the world and is very effective provided you stick with it.

It's important to understand that negative reactions to food can happen in three different ways:

1 **Immediate** You eat a food and almost immediately you notice a reaction. This isn't very common, but it can happen in the case of dairy products when someone is lactose or casein (the protein in dairy) intolerant, or when they have a true allergy to a food (I'll explain the difference between allergy and intolerance below).

2 **Delayed (two to eight hours)** You eat something for breakfast and by lunchtime you notice you're not feeling so hot. This is probably the most common food intolerance reaction.

3 **Extended (eight to 24 hours)** You eat something for lunch, feel fine at dinner, but begin to feel bad the next morning. This tends to be more common in people with slow digestion and constipation, although it can happen in anyone.

The delayed and extended reactions to foods are what make it so challenging to determine how a particular food affects you; for example, let's say you've just finished the Reset phase and are ready to move on to Step 2. You decide you're going to introduce butter, since it's the food you've missed the most, so you get up in the morning and cook your eggs in butter instead of coconut oil. You feel fine at lunchtime, so you boldly decide to reintroduce white rice at dinner, which you've also missed. The next morning you wake up with terrible diarrhoea. Logic might dictate it was the white rice, since you ate it at dinner and didn't have problems until the morning after. You might even forget you had eaten butter at breakfast the morning before. It's entirely possible, though, that the butter is what caused the problem and not the rice – but it simply took a while for the reaction to manifest. This illustrates the importance of the first guideline of food reintroduction.

Guideline 1: reintroduce only one food every three days

It's essential that you introduce only one food in each three-day period. This gives time for the immediate, delayed and extended food reactions to happen. If you don't wait this long before introducing the next food and you have a reaction, you'll never know which food caused it. When I say one food, I'm not referring to an entire category of foods (like dairy products), but a single food; for example, you could introduce butter, wait three days, then try cream, wait another three days, then yoghurt, and so on. This may seem overly cautious, but it's necessary. I suggest eating one normal-sized serving per day of the food you're reintroducing. Make a note in your food diary (see below) of exactly when you eat it, so it's easier for you to track any potential reaction.

Guideline 2: keep a food diary

As you've gathered by now, it can be tricky to determine how foods are affecting you as you add them back in. This is where the food diary really shines. Sometimes it's only clear how a food affected you in retrospect, by looking back at your diary to determine a pattern. I've provided a blank diary template as part of the Personal Paleo Diet resources you'll find on my website to make this as easy as possible. You'll be recording what you ate, at what time, as well as how you felt before you ate and at various times throughout the day. If you're a little unclear as to how you're doing with a new food you've re-introduced, you can just take out your diary and study the last two to three days. Has there been any change in your energy level, mood, digestion or other symptoms compared to the days prior to when you introduced the food? If so, that's probably a sign you're not tolerating the new food very well.

Guideline 3: 'low and slow' wins the game

If you introduce a food and have a reaction to it, it's best to remove that food and wait until your body settles back to where it was before you introduced it. This usually takes somewhere between one to three days, but if the reaction was severe, it may take longer. If you introduce a food and you're not sure how you're reacting to it, remove it, wait three days and reintroduce it again. Most of my patients need only to do this twice or, at most, three times to determine whether the food is safe for them to eat.

The key is not to rush it. I know it can be frustrating, and you're excited to start eating some of those foods you missed during the Reset phase, but if you move too fast you risk having to start all over again. You've already invested 30 days or more during Step 1, so don't sabotage all that hard work. A little patience here will go a long way.

Guideline 4: context matters

You might find that you're able to tolerate certain foods well at some times but not others; for example, perhaps when you're feeling well rested and healthy overall, you can eat some yoghurt and feel fine afterwards; however, if you haven't slept well for a few nights, or you have a cold or flu, or your typical symptoms are flaring up, even a small amount of yoghurt might make you break out or hurt your gut.

This is why context matters. If you're systemically inflamed due to sleep deprivation, an infection or an autoimmune flare-up, your body won't respond in the same way to food as it does when you're feeling relatively healthy. Avoid reintroducing any new foods if you're sick, stressed or otherwise unwell, and consider returning to a more basic 30-Day Reset Diet during these times in the future, even after you've worked out your own Personal Paleo Diet.

COMMON FOOD REACTIONS

Here's a list of typical symptoms people experience when they are sensitive to a particular food:

Acid reflux	Depression
Acne	Fatigue
Anxiety	Gas
Bloating	Insomnia or excessive sleep

Brain fog   Itchy skin

Changes in stool consistency   Malaise
(dry, hard stool or loose stool)

Changes in stool frequency   Muscle or joint aches
(diarrhoea or constipation)

Skin rashes

This is just a partial list. You also want to look out for an increase of any symptoms that lessened during the Reset phase but were typical for you prior to starting it. If you do experience a reaction, stop eating that particular food and wait a few days for things to settle. This is important. At that point, you can try reintroducing that food again (if you're uncertain whether it was responsible for the reaction), or you can move on to the next food. But do not move on to a new food when you're still in the midst of a negative reaction to something you just introduced.

One last thing: it's important to distinguish between 'food intolerance', which is what we're talking about here, and true allergy. A food allergy involves an immune response to an antigen. An antigen is a substance (in this case a food) that provokes the production of one or more antibodies by the immune system, just as it would in the case of a pathogen like a bacteria or virus. The reactions in true food allergies can be very severe and in some cases can even cause anaphylactic shock and death. The most common food allergens are peanuts, tree nuts (for example, walnuts, pecan nuts, almonds), fish, shellfish, milk, eggs, soya products and gluten-containing products. Fortunately, true food allergies are relatively rare.

Food intolerances are much more common. They involve an adverse reaction that isn't necessarily characterised by an antibody-driven immune response. (One exception to this is gluten intolerance, which does often involve the production of antibodies against gluten.) A food intolerance occurs when something in a food irritates your digestive system or when you're unable to properly digest or break down the food. Intolerance to lactose is the most common food intolerance.

When we talk about reintroducing foods in this section, we're attempting to discover food intolerances more than food allergies. If you have an allergy to something like peanuts or shellfish, it's likely you already know that. Do not attempt to reintroduce foods that you have a known allergy to. Those foods should be avoided for life. On the other hand, it's relatively safe to reintroduce foods you suspect you might be intolerant to – in order to see if you really are – because the reactions are not life threatening. They can be very uncomfortable, but are rarely serious.

FOODS TO CONSIDER REINTRODUCING

I believe the foods below are generally healthy and nourishing when they are well tolerated by the individual. Remember, these aren't mandatory. If you feel great on the 30-Day Reset Diet and have no urge to add these foods back in, by all means continue!

Dairy products

Although it's true that dairy products have the potential to cause problems, recent genetic adaptations have enabled some people – particularly those of northern European descent – to digest them without a problem (see pages 36–37). In addition, there are several reasons you might wish to bring dairy products back into your diet:

• They're delicious. Most people love the taste of dairy products such as butter, cheese and yoghurt, and they are common ingredients in several different types of cuisine.

- They're nutritious. They contain calcium, high-quality protein, potassium, phosphorus, vitamin B_{12}, vitamin B_6, riboflavin, niacin and, most importantly, the fat-soluble vitamins A and K_2 (in the case of raw milk).

- They're health-promoting. As you learned in Chapter 9, full-fat dairy products have several beneficial impacts on health, including reducing the risk of heart disease, diabetes and cancer.

- They're a good source of probiotics (when raw or fermented). Fermented milk products such as yoghurt and kefir contain probiotic bacteria and yeast that improve digestive function and strengthen the immune system. Raw milk also contains beneficial bacteria, albeit in lesser amounts than fermented milk products. (Raw milk is not available in all areas, but organic, raw milk can be obtained direct from approved farms or by mail order in parts of the UK.)

Of course, as with all of the foods in this section, if you don't care for dairy or you already know you're intolerant there's no need to reintroduce it; however, it's worth mentioning that many of my patients who can't digest pasteurised milk are able to tolerate dairy products with little or no lactose (like ghee, butter, hard cheeses and yoghurt or kefir), or raw dairy products. See the next section in this chapter for a specific method of reintroducing dairy that will help you determine which dairy products, if any, you can tolerate.

Grains and 'pseudo-cereals'

Human beings thrived for thousands of generations without eating a substantial amount of grain. There are no important nutrients in grains that cannot be obtained by eating a diet rich in animal products, fruits and vegetables. One myth I've seen perpetuated by mainstream nutritionists is that we need to eat grains for fibre. This is not true. We can get all the fibre we need from starchy tubers, fruit, vegetables, nuts and seeds.

As I explained in Chapter 4, grains contain a number of problematic chemical compounds that can damage the human intestinal tract, provoke immune reactions and interfere with absorption of key nutrients. They are also lower on the nutrient-density scale than meat, fish, vegetables, fruit, nuts, seeds and dairy products. With this in mind, it might be easy to conclude that we should avoid eating grains entirely. I think that's a valid choice, and many people simply feel better when they eliminate grains completely.

That said, there are ways of preparing grains that reduce their toxicity, break down anti-nutrients, like phytic acid, and improve the bioavailability of the nutrients they contain. (The exceptions to this are gluten-containing grains such as wheat, rye, barley, spelt and kamut. If you have coeliac disease or are gluten-intolerant, no amount of preparation will render gluten harmless for you.) Indigenous cultures worked out very early on in the history of agriculture that certain steps taken beforehand made these foods easier to digest. They went to extreme lengths – including soaking, sprouting, fermenting, pounding, mashing and roasting – to process their grains to break down the food toxins and make them healthy to eat. Those methods are time-intensive, to say the least.

In the modern world, where most people can barely find the time to cook a quick dinner at home, few are willing to go to these extreme lengths to properly prepare grains. Fermenting grains in your home kitchen is a tremendous amount of work – involving soaking for up to 24 hours at specific temperatures, reserving the soaking water to use for the next round of soaking, repeating the process extensively, and so on. Even then, you may not be successful in neutralising phytic acid and other toxins, and the food-processing industry certainly isn't taking these steps. The result is that most people on the standard Western diet end up eating a diet high in unprepared grains, low in nutrients and high in anti-nutrients, and our health has suffered as a result.

Because each grain has a different botanical structure and food-toxin profile, each requires different types of preparation to make it safe to eat. And how safe grains are for you to eat varies significantly based on your genetic heritage, your age, your health (especially gut health) and what other foods you eat. If you're generally healthy and you soak or ferment grains prior to consuming them to reduce their toxicity and improve their nutrient density, consuming a modest amount of grain is unlikely to cause harm – provided it doesn't replace more nutrient-dense foods in your diet; however, in my experience, people with digestive problems, autoimmune disease or other chronic, inflammatory conditions often do poorly with grains, even when they are properly prepared – with the possible exception of white rice and buckwheat. (For links to resources on properly preparing grains through soaking/fermenting, see my website.)

You might be surprised to hear me recommend white rice. It's commonly believed that white rice is less nutritious than brown rice, but scientific research suggests otherwise. Studies that have compared the amount of nutrients actually absorbed from eating white and brown rice have shown that humans absorb more nutrients from white rice. Why? Because the anti-nutrients in brown rice, like phytic acid, interfere with the absorption of the nutrients it contains. Brown rice also reduces dietary protein and fat digestibility compared to white rice. White rice doesn't have those problems. Phytic acid and other food toxins are found in the husk or the bran (the outer covering) of the grain. In the case of white rice, the bran has been removed and what remains is mostly starch. As we have seen, humans produce an enzyme called amylase that allows us to digest starch efficiently.

This is why I believe white rice is an acceptable food and my experience with patients suggests that it is generally well tolerated. That doesn't mean everyone does well with it, nor does it mean it should comprise a significant portion of your diet or replace more nutrient-dense carbohydrate sources such as sweet potatoes and other starchy vegetables. The point of removing rice (along with all grains) during the 30-Day Reset and then reintroducing it is to find out how you tolerate it in moderate amounts. Those with blood sugar problems like hypoglycaemia, insulin resistance or diabetes may need to minimise or avoid white rice entirely, because of how rapidly it is broken down into glucose. In addition, you may need to avoid rice if you are gluten intolerant. Studies have shown that people with both coeliac disease and non-coeliac gluten sensitivity are more likely to react to the proteins in rice.

The other exception is buckwheat. Despite its name, buckwheat isn't even a distant relative of wheat. In fact, buckwheat isn't even a grain. It's a plant in the same family as sorrel (a herb) and rhubarb (a fruit). Although buckwheat does contain some phytic acid, it also contains significant amounts of phytase, the enzyme required to break down phytic acid. This means that it's relatively easy to eliminate the phytic acid in buckwheat without extensive preparation. (I do not recommend eating buckwheat without preparing it properly first, however.) On my website, I have a recipe for sourdough buckwheat pancakes that explains how to prepare buckwheat properly to make it safe for consumption. If you'd like to eat whole buckwheat (instead of making pancakes with it), simply soak it overnight, rinse and cook.

What about 'pseudo-cereals' such as quinoa, amaranth, millet and teff? In general, these pseudo-grains do contain many of the same plant toxins that other more common grains like wheat, rye, oats and brown rice contain; however, we don't have good information about how much preparation is required to neutralise the toxins they contain. For this reason, I generally recommend that people do not eat them regularly.

Pulses

Much of what I said above about grains also applies to pulses. All beans contain phytic acid and thus require significant amounts of preparation. Traditional cultures were aware of this, and reports by anthropologists indicate that they often went to great lengths to break down the phytic acid in beans before consuming them. In Central America, beans are made into a sour porridge called *chugo*, which is fermented for several days.

Simply soaking beans at moderate temperatures (24°C) overnight reduces phytic acid only by 8–20 per cent. Sprouting beans for several days and then cooking them will remove a larger amount; for example, fermenting lentils for three days at 42°C results in about a 70–75 per cent reduction in phytic acid. Soaking lentils for 12 hours, germinating them for three to four days and then souring them afterwards will probably remove most of their phytic acid.

If you're willing to go to these lengths of preparation, and you are healthy and don't have digestive issues or a chronic, inflammatory condition, moderate consumption of pulses is unlikely to cause problems. Otherwise I think they are best avoided.

Nightshades and eggs

If you removed nightshades or eggs due to arthritis or auto-immune problems in Step 1, you may want to reintroduce them in this phase to determine whether they cause problems for you. (Although these two food groups are unrelated, I will be discussing them together because they were removed from Step 1 for the same reasons.)

Eggs are an incredibly healthy food when well tolerated, although they can provoke an immune or inflammatory response in certain individuals. The nightshade family includes peppers, tomatoes, white potatoes, aubergines and spices such as chillies, paprika and cayenne pepper. Nightshades contain toxins called glycoalkaloids, the most prevalent of which are solanine and chaconine. Glycoalkaloids may cause headaches, diarrhoea, cramps, joint pain and body aches in susceptible individuals.

There's nothing wrong with these foods when they're well tolerated. In fact, contrary to popular belief, white potatoes provide substantial amounts of some nutrients, such as potassium, which is difficult to obtain elsewhere in the diet. But they do sometimes cause inflammation in people with arthritis or immune issues.

Alcohol

Alcohol is another substance that is highly subject to individual tolerance. I advise removing it in Step 1 not because of its potentially addictive properties, but because it can cause leaky gut and other problems in susceptible people.

That said, most research suggests that moderate intake of alcohol is healthy for most people. But not all alcohol is created equal! Beer has gluten, which is probably the biggest offender when it comes to food toxins in grain products. For this reason, I don't recommend reintroducing standard beer. There are, however, several gluten-free beers on the market made from sorghum, tapioca and brown rice. Some of them actually taste pretty good, but you'll need to experiment to see if you tolerate them.

Wine and spirits such as vodka, tequila and gin are a good choice for those who do wish to drink alcohol. Spirits made from grain (such as bourbon) are fermented, significantly decreasing any anti-nutrient properties they might otherwise have.

Concentrated sweeteners

One of the main considerations when choosing a concentrated sweetener is its ratio of fructose to glucose. Fructose and glucose are both simple sugars (single-molecule monosaccharides). Glucose is easily absorbed into the bloodstream and taken up as fuel by the cells. Our bodies are designed to run on glucose in moderate amounts. Fructose is a little more complicated. Although most people are able to process fructose in moderate amounts (as found in whole fruits, for example) without a problem, excess fructose in concentrated sweeteners, juices and fructose-sweetened beverages can cause metabolic problems and digestive distress.

Fortunately, glucose enhances the absorption and uptake of fructose, so when the two are found together in roughly equal amounts, the body can handle the fructose without much trouble; however, when the amount of fructose in a food or sweetener is significantly higher than the amount of glucose it contains, the excess fructose may be problematic – especially for those with gut issues.

With this in mind, here's a list of sweeteners to favour and avoid:

Recommended	Not Recommended
Coconut sugar	High-fructose corn syrup*
Maple syrup	Table sugar (sucrose)*
Molasses	Agave syrup*
Honey	Brown rice syrup**
Dextrose	Artificial sweeteners***
Stevia	

*Unfavourable ratio of glucose to fructose, or highly processed.
**Recent studies have found high amounts of arsenic, a toxic chemical, in most varieties of brown rice syrup.
***Includes sugar alcohols. Some studies suggest a link between artificial sweeteners and cancer, harmful metabolic effects and digestive problems.

Caffeine

Caffeine is another grey area food that is highly dependent upon individual tolerance. And individual tolerance is determined by several factors, including adrenal function, mood stability, quality and duration of sleep, and biological factors that we don't fully understand.

Caffeine is a compound present in a number of foods and beverages, including coffee, tea and chocolate. The amount of caffeine in each of them varies considerably depending on the type of product and the amount of it you consume. The table below lists the caffeine content of several common beverages:

Beverage	Serving size	Caffeine
Starbucks Grande	473ml	330mg
Brewed coffee	225ml	130mg
Red Bull	1 can	80mg
Black tea	225ml	55mg
Green tea	225ml	52mg
Yerba mate	225ml	43mg
Twig tea	225ml	5mg

Since a lot of people consume their caffeinated beverages at places like Starbucks, I think it's safe to say that they're getting far more caffeine than they think they are. This explains, at least in part, why I see so many patients in my clinic with burned-out adrenals and sleep problems. If you are generally healthy, sleeping well and have stable energy levels throughout the day, one to two cups of coffee (brewed at home – not a Starbucks Grande!) or tea each day is probably not going to harm you; however, if you're dealing with insomnia, anxiety, mood swings, or low energy, I'd recommend eliminating or dramatically reducing caffeine until you overcome these problems.

Chocolate

There's nothing wrong with chocolate itself. In fact, it has a number of health benefits. It's high in magnesium, it's a powerful antioxidant and it has been shown to have positive effects on the brain, and the cardiovascular and circulatory system.

The main issues with chocolate are that it is often sold as milk chocolate, which contains a lot of sugar, and that it can have a stimulating effect because of its theobromine content. Theobromine is a bitter compound found in cacao beans, which has similar effects to caffeine. Theobromine is generally not as stimulating as caffeine, but some people seem to be more sensitive to its effects than others.

Chocolate can be safely consumed by eating only dark chocolate (more than 70 per cent cocoa content, with more than 85 per cent preferred), limiting your intake to a small serving size (about a 4cm piece) and not eating it at night if you're sensitive to its stimulating effect.

FOOD REINTRODUCTION SCHEDULE

Now that we've discussed which foods you may want to reintroduce, I'm going to propose a schedule for when to do so, based on my experience with how well tolerated they are by the majority of people I work with and our understanding of their biochemical composition. Please see my website for a quick-reference cheat sheet that you can print out and put on your fridge.

Note that if you don't tolerate one food in a particular category, that doesn't necessarily mean you won't tolerate any other foods in that category. This is especially true for dairy and nightshades; for example, I have several patients who can't tolerate yoghurt, cheese or kefir, but do just fine with butter and cream. Likewise, some of my patients can't eat tomatoes or aubergines but have no problem with white potatoes.

Dairy products reintroduction

There's a specific order for reintroducing dairy products based on how likely you are to react to them, which is in turn determined by their sugar and protein content. People who are intolerant to dairy are reacting to either the sugar (lactose) or the proteins (casein, butyrophilin, lactoglobulins, and so on), or in some cases, both. But, as I mentioned, some dairy products have negligible amounts of both casein and lactose. These are usually well tolerated, even in cases where people are reacting to lactose or milk protein (provided the reaction is an intolerance, not an allergy).

Because most dairy products contain protein, I'm going to focus on the lactose content of dairy foods. As a general rule, anything below 2 per cent lactose can be tolerated by the majority of those who are lactose-intolerant, as long as they don't overdo it. If you find yourself reacting to a dairy food with very low amounts of lactose, it's likely you are intolerant to milk protein and will have to avoid cow's milk products (with the possible exception of ghee, which contains only trace amounts of protein, and butter, which contains very low amounts); however, goat and sheep dairy products contain a different type of protein than that found in cow dairy. Because of this, some people who can't consume cow dairy products are able to safely consume goat and sheep dairy. If you determine that you can't tolerate cow milk products (kefir, yoghurt, cheese, milk), then you might want to try goat or sheep dairy during the reintroduction phase.

Dairy products are listed below from the lowest to the highest in lactose content. Begin by introducing ghee, at the top of the list, and if you tolerate it well, proceed to the next item. If you don't want to reintroduce a particular item on this list, simply move on to the next.

1 Ghee (clarified butter) is butter with the milk solids removed. You can think of it as 'butter oil'. Butter has almost no lactose to begin with, and the lactose is in the milk solids, so ghee has virtually no detectable lactose. The level of protein is also nearly undetectable in ghee.

2 Butter is only 0.8–1 per cent of lactose. It is well tolerated by all but the most lactose-sensitive individuals.

3 Kefir is milk that has been fermented by strains of beneficial bacteria and yeast. (See the Fermented Foods Guide on my website for instructions on how to make it at home.) Since the yeast and bacteria consume (ferment) the lactose in the milk, the longer you ferment it, the less lactose it will have. I've seen varying estimates of the lactose content of home-made kefir ranging from 0–3.5 per cent. At 24–36 hours of fermentation it's likely to contain less than 1 per cent lactose. Kefir purchased from a shop is often not fermented for as long and is likely to be towards the upper end of the 1–3.5 per cent range.

4 Yoghurt is milk that has been fermented by strains of lactic acid-producing bacteria (again, see the Fermented Foods Guide on my website for instructions on how to make it at home). As with kefir, the longer you ferment yoghurt, the less lactose it will have. If you ferment it for 24-plus hours, it's likely to have negligible amounts of lactose and may be well tolerated even by lactose-sensitive individuals. Most varieties of shop-bought yoghurt, including Greek yoghurt, are typically fermented for only 3–4 hours, and its lactose content ranges from 4.1–4.7 per cent. If you react to shop-bought yoghurt, try making it at home and fermenting it for at least 24 hours.

5 Cheese Hard cheeses, such as Cheddar, Parmesan, Pecorino Romano, and so on, tend to be very low in lactose, ranging from 0.0–3.5 per cent. Soft cheeses often range between 0.0–5 per cent. Be aware that cheese does contain a significant amount of casein, so if you're casein-intolerant, you'll need to avoid it.

6 Full-fat (whipping or double) cream Cream is mostly fat and 2.8–3.0 per cent lactose. Although it is above the 2 per cent safe range, in my experience moderate amounts of cream are usually well tolerated even by those who are lactose-intolerant.

7 Soured cream ranges from 3.0–4.3 per cent lactose. If you don't tolerate shop-bought soured cream, you can try making it at home. See the Fermented Foods Guide on my website for instructions.

8 Ice cream Yes, I said it – ice cream! Home-made ice cream is a luxurious, but occasional, treat. It contains 3.1–8.4 per cent lactose, so it is usually not a good choice for the lactose-intolerant.

9 Buttermilk is a cultured milk product. It contains roughly 3.6–5.0 per cent lactose.

10 Milk (whole/full-fat, semi-skimmed and skimmed) contains 3.7–5.1 per cent lactose. Fluid milk (as opposed to many other dairy products, such as kefir, cheese, yoghurt and butter) is not well tolerated by most people, so I generally don't recommend it. (The exception would be raw milk. Raw milk is often well tolerated even by those who can't drink pasteurised milk.) Semi-skimmed and skimmed milks have higher lactose content than whole milk. I do not recommend consuming reduced-fat milk products for any reason – this goes for yoghurts, cheeses and other dairy products as well. If you must have milk, go for whole!

For at-a-glance information on lactose content, see the charts on my website.

What about 'fake milks'?

Over the past decade, milk substitutes, such as soya, rice and almond milk, have grown in popularity. There are two issues with the shop-bought versions of these milks that make them a poor choice for regular consumption:

1 They are usually quite high in sugar, especially compared to cow's milk or goat's milk.
2 They often contain carrageenan, a seaweed extract used to make the milks more viscous. Although there is still controversy about the relevance of this in humans, animal research suggests that carrageenan may cause inflammation and ulceration of the digestive tract, impaired glucose tolerance, and insulin resistance and cancer.

Beyond these two issues, soya milk has additional problems. It may have adverse effects on male fertility. A study at the Harvard Public School of Health found that consuming just one cup per day of soya milk decreases sperm count in men, especially in those who are overweight or obese. Other studies found that phytoestrogens in soya may adversely affect male reproductive hormones and sperm capacitation (an important process sperm must go through after being ejaculated into the female reproductive tract. Soya phytoestrogens also have potentially harmful effects on women. A large review of 47 studies found that soya phytoestrogens reduce levels of LH and FSH, two hormones essential to fertility and reproductive health, and increase the length of the menstrual cycle.

The research on soya is not black and white. Some studies (like those above) show harm, whereas others show no harm. I think the precautionary principle applies here: since there's nothing essential about soya milk, it's not especially nutrient dense and it may cause reproductive and endocrine problems (especially in infants fed soya formula), it's best avoided entirely or consumed only in small quantities.

What about rice milk and almond milk? If you can find varieties in the shop without carrageenan and with no added sweetener, they're fine in moderation. In addition, both rice and almond milk (and other nut and seed milks) can be made simply and quickly at home. Please see my website for instructions on how to make nut milk at home.

Grains, pseudo-cereals and pulses reintroduction

As I have indicated, extensive preparation is required to make grains and pulses more digestible and improve their nutrient bioavailability. If you really miss grains or pulses in your diet, you are healthy and have a strong digestive system and you are willing to take the necessary steps to prepare grains and pulses, then you may reintroduce them in modest amounts (that is, three to five servings per week) during Step 2.

I suggest starting with white rice and fermented buckwheat, since they are low in phytic acid and other anti-nutrients and are less likely to irritate the gut. Beyond white rice and buckwheat, I don't think it matters much in which order you reintroduce properly prepared grains and pulses. Just be sure to reintroduce them one at a time and carefully track your symptoms as you do. And remember, even soaked and fermented grains and pulses should never displace more nutrient-dense foods like meat, fish, vegetables, nuts, seeds and fruits.

Nightshades and eggs reintroduction

If you've been on the 'autoimmune/arthritis' version of the Step 1 Reset, where you removed eggs and nightshades, you may want to reintroduce these after you've tried dairy and/or buckwheat and white rice.

I suggest introducing eggs first, because they're one of the most nutrient-dense super-foods nature has made available to us. They're also tasty, versatile and easy to prepare. Be aware that some people react negatively to egg whites (one of the most common food allergens); however, it's far less common for people to react to the yolks. This is fortunate, because the yolks contain the majority of the nutrients and are by far the healthiest part of the egg. If you don't tolerate egg whites, you can continue to eat the yolks. You can make egg yolk omelettes or add raw egg yolks to soups or smoothies. (If you put them in smoothies, use only raw egg yolks from pasture-raised, organic chickens – not from supermarket eggs, which are sometimes contaminated with salmonella and should always be cooked.) Try hard-boiling eggs, then removing and eating the solid yolks if you want a quick source of nutrients without worrying about raw egg safety or egg-white contamination.

There is a lot of variation in how people react to nightshades, but I advise reintroducing them (after eggs) in the following order:

1 Ripe, raw tomatoes

2 White potatoes

3 Aubergines

4 Peppers

5 Chillies, cayenne pepper and paprika

Alcohol reintroduction

Which alcoholic drinks you reintroduce depends primarily on your preference. I haven't noticed one particular class being tolerated better than another. That said, wine does tend to have more sugar than spirits, so if you are sensitive to sugar, it may be wise to start with something like tequila or vodka (if you like them, that is). The reintroduction schedule could look like this:

1 Vodka

2 Tequila

3 Other spirits

4 Wine

5 Gluten-free beer (rare treat)

In general, I'd recommend limiting alcohol consumption to three to five drinks per week.

Concentrated sweeteners reintroduction

The particular order of reintroduction of the recommended sweeteners is not important, but this fact is: sugar is sugar. Yes, natural sweeteners do have a higher nutrient content than the processed sugars, but in general (with the exception of molasses) it's not high enough to make a significant contribution to the diet. Since you will be eating only minimal amounts of these sweeteners, the most important consideration in which ones you choose is their glucose-to-fructose ratio – especially if you have digestive problems. Refer back to the list on page 219 for recommended sweeteners; remember to avoid agave syrup, brown rice syrup and all artificial sweeteners.

Caffeine reintroduction

I suggest beginning with the lower caffeine-containing beverages, such as green tea and twig tea. If you do well with those, you can move on to black tea and coffee. (See the caffeine section on pages 220–221 for information on which beverages have the highest and lowest amounts of caffeine, and visit my website for information on caffeine content of specific coffees, teas, soft drinks and energy drinks.) Remember that coffee from Starbucks and other vendors can have significantly higher amounts of caffeine than coffee you brew at home! If you notice any worsening of sleep, fluctuations in energy or mood, irritability, anxiety or agitation when you drink coffee or black tea, remove it again for a few days and then try again, starting with the lower caffeine beverages. Decaf coffee is another possibility, although it is not completely free of caffeine. Most estimates I've seen suggest it has about 5mg of caffeine per cup.

Chocolate reintroduction

Start with a 4cm piece of dark chocolate (more than 70 per cent, or preferably more than 85 per cent, cocoa solids) earlier in the day – perhaps after lunch. The reason I suggest this is that some people are very stimulated by chocolate and it can interfere with sleep. If you don't notice that effect, or any other ill effects, you're free to eat one to two 4cm pieces of dark chocolate per day, if you wish. Another great way to enjoy chocolate is to add unsweetened, raw cacao nibs or powder to smoothies. Try combining nut milk, coconut milk and/or kefir with half a banana and some raw cacao powder for a special treat.

Summary: reintroduce grey area foods

- Reintroducing the foods in this chapter is optional. If you feel great without them and don't miss them, there's no need to add them back to your diet.
- Reintroduce one food every three days.
- Keep a food diary to make it easier to isolate adverse reactions to foods.
- Go slowly! If there's any doubt about how you're reacting to a food, remove it from your diet, wait a few days and then try again.
- Don't reintroduce new foods if you're experiencing unusual stress, sleep deprivation, a flare-up of a chronic health condition, or inflammation, as these things will affect your response to the new food.

CHAPTER 12

Move Like Your Ancestors

While there's no doubt that proper nutrition is crucial to health, it's not the only consideration. Getting adequate physical activity and sleep, managing stress, spending time outdoors, and other lifestyle factors also have a significant impact on our well-being. Unfortunately, just as there's a 'mismatch' between the modern diet and the diet we've evolved to eat, there's a 'mismatch' between our current lifestyles and what our bodies are designed for. Sitting for long periods, exposure to artificial light, reduced sleep time, persistent, chronic stress and living alone or in small, nuclear families are all outside of the evolutionary norm for humans, and our health is suffering as a result. In the following chapters, I'll teach you the essentials for an overall 'code' of living that is closer to what's natural – and healthy – for humans.

Notes for this chapter may be found at ChrisKresser.com/ppcnotes/#ch12

Questionnaire: Movement

Complete the questionnaire below and add up the total of points for those questions you answered 'yes' to, then use the answer key to determine your movement score.

	Points
I sit for less than 6 hours per day.	2
I get at least 30 minutes of moderate-to-vigorous physical activity each day.	2
I walk or bike to work.	2
I do activities to increase muscle strength, such as lifting weights or calisthenics, once a week or more.	1
I do activities to improve flexibility, such as stretching or yoga, once a week or more.	1
I use a standing desk at work, or spend several hours standing daily.	2
I typically walk at least 10,000 steps per day (about 5 miles/8km).	3
I do not have any injuries or health conditions that restrict my ability to exercise (such as asthma, chest pain, fatigue, and so on).	1
I enjoy being physically active.	1
I watch less than 2 hours of television per day.	1
TOTAL	

Answer key:

Total points	What your points mean	Your aim
6+	You are probably getting adequate and healthy levels of physical activity	Complete Your Personal Paleo Diet 3-Step programme. No additional personalisation is required
3–5	You may benefit from incorporating additional movement into your day	Complete Your Personal Paleo Diet 3-Step programme and add the recommendations in this chapter
0–2	You are likely getting an inadequate amount of physical activity	Complete both steps above and consider working with a fitness professional for additional assistance. This should be a major focus for you, and ignoring this area may stand in the way of improvement elsewhere

Our Palaeolithic ancestors didn't worry about cardio versus weight training, doing Pilates to strengthen their cores versus squats to sculpt their glutes. They didn't 'exercise' or 'work out' – they just 'lived'. For the vast majority of our evolutionary history, we humans had to exert ourselves – often quite strenuously – to survive. We naturally spent a lot of time outdoors in the sun, walking, hunting and gathering, among other activities.

Anthropological research suggests that our ancestors sprinted, jogged, climbed, carried and jumped intermittently throughout the day. They walked an average of 6 miles (9.6km) and ran an average of 0.5–1 mile (0.8–1.6km) per day. Women were as active as men; although they rarely took part in large-game hunting, they spent hours walking to and from sources of food, water and wood and carried their children (until up to four years of age!) for extended distances. At the same time, our ancestors alternated days of strenuous and demanding activity with days of rest. This instinctual response protected them from injury and fatigue, which in turn improved their chances of survival.

Contemporary hunter-gatherers are also active. Studies show that they walk an average of 10,000 steps (about 5 miles/8km) per day, with frequent bouts of more intense activity. Anthropologist Kim Hill spent 30 years living with and studying the Ache hunter-gatherers of Paraguay. His GPS data indicated that they covered more than 6 miles a day on average while they hunted, running in hot pursuit of their quarry for 0.5–1 mile (0.8–1.6km) – all while 'ducking under low branches and vines about once every 20 seconds all day long and climbing over fallen trees, moving through tangled thorns, etc.' Closer to home, contemporary Amish people who have retained their traditional ways take between 14,000 and 18,000 steps per day.

One way of measuring fitness is VO_2 max, the volume of oxygen that can be consumed while exercising at maximum capacity (VO_2 max is measured in millilitres of oxygen used in one minute, per kilogram of body weight). Today, the average sedentary person has a VO_2 max of 35ml/kg/min and the average elite endurance athlete has one around 70ml/kg/min. The estimated VO_2 max in modern hunter-gatherers is 52, which places them in the 'excellent to superior' fitness category; it's likely our ancestors were equally fit. If we want to get and stay highly physically fit, in other words, we should move more like our ancestors.

Many concepts in this chapter were inspired by the Enduring Mover framework created by Dan Pardi, a researcher on human behaviour and CEO of Dan's Plan. As

Enduring Movers, we maintain optimal health and fitness by incorporating both low- and high-intensity activity into our daily lives – just as our ancestors did. I'll have more to say about the Enduring Mover framework and Dan's Plan later in the chapter.

AN EPIDEMIC OF INACTIVITY

In most Western societies, people were highly physically active until relatively recently. In the 1800s, approximately 90 per cent of jobs required manual labour; today only 2 per cent do. Now, thanks to dramatic changes in the way we live, communicate, travel, use technology, and get and consume our food, the typical American, British or Australian adult walks only about 5,900 to 6,900 steps per day.

Simply put, we've become a nation of sitters, whether we're working at our computers, watching TV, playing video games, or commuting. The typical US adult is now sedentary for 60 per cent of his or her waking hours and sits for an average of six hours (and often much more, in the case of those who work primarily on computers). A sedentary office worker today expends only 10 calories per 450g eaten each day, down from an average of 43–55 calories per 450g in our hunting and gathering days.

Why sitting is dangerous for your health

We weren't born to sit all day. We're genetically adapted to be physically active. All this increased sitting and decreased physical activity has a profound, negative effect on almost every aspect of our health, from our cardiovascular and pulmonary systems to our immunity. In fact, a whole new field called 'sedentary physiology' has evolved to address the health risks of being too sedentary. There are a few specific ways in which being sedentary harms us.

Sitting wrecks our metabolic function

Sitting decreases the activity of an enzyme called lipoprotein lipase (LPL), which is associated with higher triglyceride levels, lower HDL levels (the 'good' cholesterol) and increased risk of cardiovascular disease. Even a single day of prolonged sitting has been shown to reduce insulin action.

Sitting weakens our bones

Up to two-thirds of professional cyclists, who spend long hours in a seated position, have lower levels of bone mass, studies have shown. Both humans and animals experience dramatic reductions in bone mass following spinal cord injuries, long-term bed rest and time in zero gravity. After just 12 weeks of bed rest, healthy men and women experienced reductions in specific bone mineral density of 1–4 per cent. What's more, studies suggest that vigorous exercise alone isn't enough to prevent the changes in bone metabolism caused by too much sedentary behaviour.

Sitting harms our blood vessels

Although the research in this area isn't as robust as it is with metabolic and bone health, initial findings suggest that sedentary behaviour has harmful effects on the vascular system. Just five days of bed rest have been shown to increase blood pressure and decrease arterial diameter. Other studies have found that two months of bed rest led to decreased blood flow and increased damage of the cells in the fragile lining of the blood vessels.

Sitting increases our risk of death

In an Australian study that followed participants over a six-and-a-half-year period, researchers found that high levels of

TV time were significantly associated with an increased risk of death from both heart disease and all causes. Each additional hour of TV daily was associated with an 11 per cent and 18 per cent increase in all-cause and cardiovascular mortality, respectively. On the other hand, compared to those who watched more than four hours of TV a day, those who watched less than two hours had an 80 per cent lower risk of death from cardiovascular disease and a 46 per cent lower risk of death from all causes. These associations were independent of exercise and traditional risk factors such as smoking, blood pressure, cholesterol levels, waist circumference and diet.

A US study based on 21 years of follow-up of 7,700 men found that those who reported spending more than ten hours a week sitting in automobiles and more than 23 hours a week of combined TV and automobile time had an 82 per cent and 64 per cent greater risk of death from cardiovascular disease, respectively.

Regular physical activity is one of the best predictors of long-term health and survival in large, observational studies. In fact, your fitness level (as measured by performance on a treadmill exercise test) has been shown to be a better predictor of how and when you'll die than age, body mass index, or even cardiovascular risk factors.

In other words, if you want to live longer, you have to be physically active on a regular basis. And if you want a better quality of life, physical activity's the answer too. Adults who exercise report a higher quality of life, and studies have shown that physical activity improves cognitive function in the elderly. These changes are evident from our earliest years; physically active children report greater body satisfaction and self-esteem than their sedentary peers. Finally, getting adequate exercise during the day promotes deeper and more restful sleep at night and reduces pre-sleep anxiety and insomnia.

Working out isn't the answer
(or, the active-couch-potato problem)

Perhaps you're thinking, 'OK, I sit a lot – but I also work out a lot, so I'm OK.' Here's the shocker: too much sitting and sedentary time is harmful, even if you're getting enough exercise. This means you could be meeting the recommended government guidelines for exercise (that is, 30 minutes of moderate to vigorous activity five days a week), but still be at higher risk of disease if you sit for long periods each day. In fact, a large study involving over 100,000 US adults found that those who sat for more than six hours a day had up to a 40 per cent greater risk of death over the next 15 years than those who sat for less than three hours a day regardless of whether the participants exercised. Canadians who reported spending the majority of their day sitting had an increased risk of death compared to those who reported less time sitting. As with the American study, this association was apparent even among those who exercised regularly.

Perhaps you're one of these 'active couch potatoes'. If you work in an office, commute by car and watch a few hours of TV each night, it's not difficult to see how you could spend the vast majority of your waking hours sitting on your butt. Imagine the following hypothetical day:

7.00am: wake up

7.15–7.45am: go for a jog (exercise)

8.00–9:00am: breakfast and drive to work (sitting)

9:00am–12.30pm: work on computer (sitting)

12.30–1.00pm: lunch (sitting)

1.00–5.00pm: work on computer (sitting)

5.00–6.30pm: drive home and eat dinner (sitting)

6.30–9.30pm: watch TV, read, check email (sitting)

10.00pm: go to bed

If you did this routine five days a week, you'd meet the typical guidelines for exercise (at least 150 minutes of moderate exercise a week), but you'd also be sitting for at least 12 hours a day.

Other problems with exercise as an 'intervention'

The evidence clearly indicates that sitting too much is harmful in its own right and that exercise alone isn't enough to reverse those harmful effects. But there are other problems with looking at exercise solely as an intervention.

In an effort to overcome inactivity when they're not exercising, some people are overtraining. Exercise is a stressor. Not all stress is harmful; in the right dose, it can cause a positive adaptation and better equip us to face that stressor in the future. This is referred to as 'hormesis'. Weightlifting is a great example of the hormetic effects of stress. When you lift weights, you stress the muscles and this causes them to get stronger.

When stress exceeds our capacity to adapt, however, it stops having a beneficial, hormetic effect and begins to cause damage. (See 'Are you overtraining?', pages 251–253.) Just as we didn't evolve to sit so much, we're not adapted to excessive amounts of exercise. A large and growing body of evidence has demonstrated that excessive exercise, such as marathons, ultra-marathons, full-distance triathlons and very long-distance bicycle rides, is associated with damage to the heart, muscles and joints. Overtraining has been associated with increased injury, oxidative damage, inflammation and cognitive decline, and decreased immune function, fat metabolism and cardiovascular health. Consider the following:

- A study of 100 middle-aged marathon runners found higher levels of coronary calcium (a marker of heart disease risk) compared with non-runners, and their risk of cardiovascular events during the follow-up period was similar to that of people with pre-existing heart disease.

- A study of elite runners found that those who participated in a large number of long-distance races had increased scarring (fibrosis) of heart tissue and the degree of scarring was directly correlated with the number of marathons or ultra-marathons completed and number of years spent training.

- Finally, a study of marathoners between 50 and 72 years of age who ran an average of 35 miles a week found that they were more than three times more likely to have heart damage than non-runners.

Too much exercise may harm us in less obvious ways as well. If you get up 30 minutes early to exercise to offset all that sitting, that's better than doing nothing, of course, but you're also cutting into valuable sleep time. You may simply trade one problem (too much sitting) for another (chronic sleep deprivation). As you'll see in the next chapter on sleep, that's not a good trade! Some research suggests that people who exercise intensely (like marathon runners) are actually more likely to be sedentary when they're not exercising. They may assume – incorrectly – that their exercise regimen protects them from the harmful effects of too much sitting outside of their exercise sessions.

THE SOLUTION: SWAP YOUR
WAY TO HEALTH

So how do we find the sweet spot that ensures we get enough – but not too much – physical activity? Once again, we can look to our ancestors for clues on how to be naturally active throughout the day: sitting less, incorporating more movement into our daily routines and engaging in moderate-to-vigorous exercise periodically.

The best way to accomplish this is by becoming what Dan Pardi of Dan's Plan calls an Enduring Mover. The Enduring Mover framework involves three elements that can be expressed in the acronym SWaP: Stand, Walk and Push. (Please see my website for a great infographic that Dan created to inspire the Enduring Mover in you and a link to Dan's Plan, where you can find additional information about this approach.)

Stand

To undo the harmful effects of sitting, stand up! Standing engages postural muscles that increase helpful LPL activity, among other beneficial changes. Standing and walking slowly increase energy expenditure 2.5 times; employees who stand while they work burn up to 75 per cent more calories per day than people in sedentary jobs. An analysis by Dan Pardi showed that, compared to sitting, simply standing and engaging in light activity throughout the day burns as many calories over the course of a week as one to three intense spinning classes!

Studies show that the more breaks you take from sitting, the lower your waist circumference, body mass index, triglycerides and the more stable your blood sugar. In fact, some research suggests that regular light physical activity throughout the day – including standing and walking – is more effective than short periods of vigorous exercise in reversing the harm caused by too much sitting.

If your day typically involves sitting for long periods, here are a few ways to reduce your sitting time:

- Follow the guidelines for 'How to make your workspace Paleo-friendly' on pages 245–246.

- Take standing breaks. Stand up for at least two minutes every 30–45 minutes. Take a brief walk or do some light stretching. Even short breaks like this can make a big difference. (They're great for relieving eyestrain too.) Try setting an alarm on your phone each time you sit down again until this break becomes second nature.

- Stand up at long meetings. If you're worried about what your colleagues might think, just tell them you have a bad back!

Goals:

- Stand for about half the day.
- Take a standing break every 30–45 minutes.

Walk

Again, let's keep it simple: walk more, sit less. Of course, light physical activity, such as gardening or performing household chores, is also beneficial. In fact, all that fidgeting your parents and teachers told you to stop – pacing around, being restless, doing a whole lot of nothing – is actually good for you. Studies show that fidgeting alone can increase energy expenditure by 50 per cent compared to sitting motionless; that translates to burning off an extra 350 calories a day – the equivalent of 2½ stone–2 stone 12lb (15.8–18kg) a year! Besides, it's easier (and cheaper) to integrate low-intensity activity into your daily life than it is an intensive, formal workout (like that pricey class at a gym you have to drive to).

You don't have to do intensive exercise to improve fitness. Even a relatively low-to-moderate level of physical activity will lower your post-meal blood sugar, insulin levels, triglycerides and waist circumference. People who are lean tend to be physically active for more than 50 per cent of their day, whereas people who are obese tend to be active for less than 40 per cent of their day.

The benefits of incorporating more activity and walking into your day don't stop with fitness. For years, I suffered from back pain and persistent muscle aches. I tried numerous treatments, from acupuncture to anti-inflammatory nutrients (like curcumin) to yoga. Nothing seemed to work. When I started writing this book, the pain got even worse; I was now spending two or three additional hours sitting at my computer – and I was only on the first chapter! I also had a 15-month-old daughter, a busy private practice and several other obligations encroaching on my exercise and physical activity time. I had to do something.

My first step was to install a standing desk in my office and begin alternating between standing and sitting as I wrote. (I'll talk more about the benefits of this routine later in this chapter.) It took me only about half a day to get used to writing while standing. My back pain improved slightly, but my muscles still ached. So I installed a treadmill under my standing desk. In the beginning, I averaged about 8,000–10,000 steps a day as I wrote. I felt a little sore at first, simply because I wasn't accustomed to walking this much, but I also noticed a decrease in muscle pain at other times of day, and my back pain was significantly reduced. Encouraged, I slowly increased the amount of time I spent working at my treadmill desk. After a couple of weeks, I settled into an average of between 15,000 and 18,000 steps per day.

The improvements were nothing short of miraculous. Back pain? Gone. Muscle pain? Gone. I noticed other benefits as well, from an increase in mental clarity and sharpness to an improvement in the quality of my sleep.

You don't need to match my steps to see a major improvement – just aim for 10,000 steps a day for optimal health. Walking that distance – about 5 miles (8km) a day – might seem impossible if you commute by car to work and spend most of the day at a computer, but here are a few tips for increasing your steps:

- Take walking meetings. If you have a meeting scheduled with someone in your office, why not suggest taking a walk while you do it?

- Use the stairs whenever possible. You might want to take the lift if you work on the 20th floor of a building (at least some of the time), but do you really need to take it if you work on the third floor?

- Walk or bicycle to work. Get creative. If you live too far away to walk or ride exclusively, consider driving part of the way and walking or cycling for the remainder.

- Do your own chores. Rather than outsourcing cleaning, laundry, gardening, washing the car, or other household chores, do them yourself.

- Get a dog. Dogs need to be exercised regularly for optimal health, just like people. You might not be motivated to take a walk yourself, but if you have a dog, you're more likely to do it.

- Choose a hobby that requires physical activity. Ballroom dancing, bowling and cooking are fun choices, but it's especially great to pick a hobby that gets you outdoors, like bird-watching, gardening, snorkelling or camping.

- Extra credit: work at a treadmill desk! See 'How to make your workspace Paleo-friendly' on pages 245–246.

Goals:

- Aim for 10,000 steps each day.
- Integrate light activity throughout your daily routine.

How to make your workspace Paleo-friendly

The most important change you can make in your work-space is to decrease the amount of time you spend sitting and to sit more actively when you do sit. Here are five of the best ways I've found to accomplish this goal. I realise, though, that unless you are self-employed you probably won't have much flexibility when it comes to purchasing different office furniture.

- **Use a standing desk** There are several types available, ranging from stationary models to adjustable desks that move from seated to standing work positions. I generally suggest alternating between sitting and standing, to avoid long periods of standing, which can also be harmful. Many standing desks are 'convertible' and can double as sitting–standing desks. Other options are taking sitting breaks. See my website for more information on standing desks (including how to make one yourself).
- **Use a treadmill desk** Treadmill desks are similar to standing desks, except that they have a treadmill underneath them. I use one daily and it allows me to walk while I'm working. You can buy a treadmill for your existing standing desk, as I did, or buy a desk that fits above your existing treadmill; however, if you're just starting out, the best option might be to buy a preconfigured treadmill desk. (See ChrisKresser.com for an article I wrote on treadmill desk options.)

- **Sit on a balance disc** Balance disks are squishy cylinders about 10cm thick. When you slip one onto your chair and sit on it, you'll find it's almost impossible to slouch. The disc forces you (in a good way) to engage your sitting muscles and to continually readjust your position. There are several different brands of balance discs on the market. I use one made by Fitter First.
- **Sit on a yoga ball** Try using a yoga ball in place of your chair for certain periods throughout the day. Like balance discs, they also require you to make small postural adjustments while sitting. I like my Natural Fitness Professional yoga ball, because it's so sturdy, but there are several other good brands.
- **Take frequent breaks** I recommend taking a 'micro-break' every 10–15 minutes, where you look away from the computer screen and shift your position, and 'macro-breaks' every 30–45 minutes where you stand up, walk, do a set of strength-training or conditioning exercises or perhaps some stress reduction. If you have trouble remembering to take breaks, you can use an app like Time Out (Mac) or Work Rave (Windows) to remind you.

The ideal approach would be to alternate between standing, walking, sitting in your chair, sitting on a balance disc in your chair and sitting on a yoga ball throughout the day. If you do that, even if you have to work for 10 hours straight, you'll be sure to get plenty of physical activity and continue to burn calories.

Push

The word 'push' here is short for 'push yourself'. The goal is to include intense physical activity in addition to standing and walking throughout the week.

Modern research has confirmed that intense, intermittent exercise results in reductions in weight and improvements in blood sugar regulation that are similar to the results of equivalent lower-intensity continuous activity. In fact, some studies suggest that high-intensity, intermittent strength training is even more effective at improving resting metabolic rate (which helps burn fat) than lower-intensity, traditional strength training.

On the other hand, our ancestors didn't overdo it. They instinctively conserved their energy, strength and stamina for the daily tasks they needed to perform to survive. As one researcher put it, 'Retirement was not an option for hunter-gatherers.' Studies of contemporary hunter-gatherers indicate that they likewise alternate difficult or strenuous days with easier 'rest days' whenever possible. Modern research suggests that the same pattern of a strenuous workout day followed by a less demanding one leads to superior fitness and a lower risk of injury.

With this in mind, I recommend following Dan Pardi's guidelines for moderate-to-vigorous activity:

- 150 minutes of moderate-intensity activity per week (for example, jogging, yoga or dancing).

Or

- 75 minutes of vigorous-intensity activity per week (for example, running, Zumba or playing sports).

Or

- 30 sets of highest-intensity exercise per week (for example, sprinting, rope jumping, or resistance training – see 'How to strength train in your home or office', pages 249–250).

Or

- A combination of the above.

Moderate-, vigorous- and highest-intensity exercise are defined follows:

- Moderate: 50–70 per cent of maximum effort
- Vigorous: 70–90 per cent of maximum effort
- Highest: more than 90 per cent of maximum effort

I use these percentages because *your* 'moderate' activity might be someone else's all-out, 'highest' effort. If you've been completely sedentary, you might consider even a leisurely jog or a yoga class to be 'high intensity', whereas a fit person would likely classify them as 'moderate intensity'. A set of squats or bench presses performed to failure – that is, until you can't do one more repetition – would always be considered highest intensity, since by definition you've exerted maximum effort.

You can do your Push activity in designated workouts or simply integrate it into your daily routine throughout the day (see box 'How to strength train in your home or office'), as part of SWAP. (I incorporate SWAP into my day through working at my treadmill desk and taking regular micro- and macro-breaks. I use micro-breaks to look away from the computer monitor and give my eyes a rest and do some light stretching; during longer macro-breaks, I do some sets of pull-ups or other exercises, or go outside and jump over a rope. By the time my work day is done, there's no need for me to go to a gym!)

Most of my patients and readers report huge improvements in energy levels and cognitive function, and reductions in muscle and joint pain, and soreness, when they sneak in moderate-to-vigorous activity throughout the day. Of course, if you can't do this at work or if you simply prefer a predictable workout schedule, that's fine too. The important thing is to Push!

Goal:

- Push it for 150 minutes of moderate-intensity activity, 75 minutes of vigorous activity or 30 minutes maximal, or near maximal, activity each week.

How to strength train in your home or office

Resistance, or strength, training is a proven way to build up and maintain muscle, which helps keep your metabolism revved, keeps you mobile and helps to prevent injuries. Stressing your body with a load makes it stronger, whether that 'load' is a dumb-bell or your own body. Lifting weights at the gym a few times a week is a great option, but for those of you with less time or without gym access, or if you wish to pursue a more natural pattern of movement, try incorporating your strength training throughout the day using relatively affordable tools you can keep in your home or office. This is the strategy advocated by Dan's Plan with its inTUNE daily movement practice. inTUNE stands for 'integrative and opportunistic training'. The concept is to integrate short bursts of physical activity through-out your day. You might, for example, do three sets of push-ups, three sets of pull-ups and three sets of lunges interspersed with periods of sitting or standing at your desk (or walking if you have a treadmill desk).

With this approach, you'll reap great health benefits in very little time, without leaving your home or office. You're far more likely to find multiple two-minute opportunities for exercise across your day than you are to find one larger chunk of time. Also, it's no cost (if you use your body, as when you do push-ups or lunges) or low cost – no need for an expensive gym membership. And the more time-efficient and convenient your exercise routine is, the more likely you are to stick with it. You will probably find it difficult to follow the fitness ideas in most work situations unless you are self-employed, but perhaps you can educate your employers on the benefits of exercising during the day.

Here are some of my favourite tools that make incorporating exercise throughout the day easier than ever:

- **Push-up handles** to amp up the intensity of push-ups.
- **Pull-up bar**, which you can attach to a doorframe to do pull-ups and chin-ups.
- **Powerblocks** – adjustable dumb-bells which adjust from a range of weights, so that you don't need a whole set of weights taking up room (they are quite expensive though).
- **Abdominal wheel** to give your abs a super-intense workout.
- **Weight bench** to add more range to your strength-training workouts.
- **Weight vest** to make pull-ups, push-ups and dips more intense.
- **Suspension training straps**, such as TRX or Jungle XT straps, are pricey but they turn a doorway into an instant gym – and they're portable. I take mine along when I travel.

TRACKING YOUR PROGRESS

If you want to make a change last, track your progress. Getting visual confirmation that you're meeting, or even exceeding, your goals is one of the best ways to stay motivated and inspired. Tracking your SWAP programme is easy if you've got the right hardware and software.

There are lots of hardware gadgets to choose from: FitBit, Nike+ FuelBand, Jawbone's Up, Striiv or a simple pedometer can all do the job. I use a FitBit every day and I get a lot of value from it. The FitBit includes a pedometer that measures the number of steps you take each day. (It can also track sleep and calories.) It then syncs up wirelessly to the FitBit dashboard, which emails you progress reports.

There are a zillion apps to help you monitor your progress. My favourite tracking software by far is a free web-based application called Dan's Plan (DansPlan.com). The purpose of Dan's Plan is to bring more attention to your lifestyle habits and encourage daily actions that support health. It combines several variables (for example, sleep, physical activity and weight) into a 'Health Zone Score', which gives you a quick visual indicator of whether you're reaching your daily health goals. Dan's Plan integrates with several popular hardware tracking tools, such as the FitBit (for sleep, step and weight data). But Dan's Plan also helps you track the kind of daily movement practice we've been discussing in this chapter. Exercise is measured in a simple, flexible way so that you get credit for any type that you do. Your total physical activity is also tracked and reported, so you can be sure you're getting enough overall activity to promote health. Dan's Plan is simple to use and takes only a few minutes of your time each day, but it provides powerful feedback that quickly tells you whether you're living in your 'Health Zone'. I use Dan's Plan myself and I recommend it to all of my patients.

Are you overtraining?

Most of my patients know when they're not getting enough exercise. They're less likely to be aware that they're overtraining.

Competitive athletes who specialise in endurance sports, as well as any person who performs intense, strenuous exercise several times a week, are at the highest risk of overtraining. You may be at risk too, even if you don't put yourself into those categories, because if you're chronically ill, injured, sleep deprived, or restricting calories, it's possible to be overtrained at much lower levels of physical activity. This is why it's so important to customise your exercise and other activities to your unique circumstances and needs — which often change over time. (I also recommend you work with a qualified trainer who can monitor if you're overdoing it.)

How do you know if you're overtrained? Typically you'll experience one or more of the following signs and symptoms:

Decreased performance

Increased recovery time

Fatigue or lethargy

Insomnia

Brain fog

Muscle and joint pain

Low libido

Amenorrhoea in women

Anxiety or depression

The longer you overtrain, the more severe these symptoms become — and the more difficult it is to recover. Remember: sometimes less is more. You don't have to train like an Olympic athlete to stay fit. In fact, unless you actually are an Olympic athlete, training like one is likely to cause more harm than good.

If you think you're overtrained, here are some suggestions for recovery:

Reduce, or even stop, anything more than moderate physical activity for a while. How long depends upon how severe your symptoms are and how long you've been overtraining. Most people benefit from at least a month of reduced activity, but some will need three months or even longer.

Focus on gentle, nourishing activities like walking, gardening, leisurely hiking, and so on. Low-level physical activity is unlikely to exacerbate the problem and will protect against too much sedentary time.

Spend time outdoors Spending time in nature and getting exposure to sunlight seems to be particularly helpful for recovery.

Get plenty of sleep and rest At least eight hours a night, but preferably ten or even more if you're significantly overtrained. If you're tired during the day, take a nap.

Eat! Do not diet or restrict calories when you're overtrained. Your body needs an adequate supply of macronutrients (especially protein) and micronutrients to repair itself.

Read the bonus chapter on adrenal fatigue syndrome (available on my website) and follow the suggestions on treatment. The brain–adrenal axis is typically most affected by overtraining.

I know scaling back might be difficult for you. But consider this: the more you rest and take care of yourself, the faster you'll recover and be able to resume a more normal level of activity. I've seen people string their recovery out for years by not taking the necessary time to rest or going back to their high-intensity routine too quickly. That just deepens the hole they're already in and makes it harder to ever get out.

GO BARE: WHY BAREFOOT IS BEST

Our ancestors walked, ran and performed other physical activities barefoot or in simple leather shoes. I recommend you do the same.

Today's running and fitness shoes are often highly cushioned with elevated heels and other features that impair range of motion and create an unnatural gait. Studies have shown that most athletic shoes increase the risk of overuse walking and running injuries, such as plantar fasciitis, ankle sprain, Achilles tendonitis, hamstring tears and lower back pain. Likewise, studies have also shown that simpler shoes that don't restrict range of motion or change natural foot-strike dynamics are less likely to cause injury and are better for long-term orthopaedic health than typical fitness or running shoes.

For these reasons, walking, running and exercising barefoot or with minimalist footwear have become increasingly popular. Some of the more popular minimalist footwear brands include Vibram, VivoBarefoot and Innov-8. Brands like New Balance, Merrell and Patagonia also offer minimalist options. (Some of these companies also make shoes with flat, thin soles for work and casual wear.) I go barefoot or wear minimalist shoes almost exclusively at this point (including while I'm walking at my treadmill desk).

Barefoot running is not without controversy, however. Some recent studies suggest that runners who go barefoot or wear minimalist shoes are prone to injuries – they're just prone to different injuries than runners who wear traditional running shoes. That said, most experts in barefoot or minimalist running believe that the injuries associated with it are primarily due to poor technique and making the transition from traditional to minimalist footwear too quickly.

If you decide to give this a try, it's crucial to focus on proper biomechanics and make the transition slowly – especially if you're a runner. Here are a few tips for making the switch:

- Go slowly. Don't expect to be able to run your typical mileage when you first move to barefoot or minimalist shoes.

- Run on a hard surface to begin with. This allows you to determine if you're heel striking and it provides more immediate feedback on your form. (Heel striking means that you're striking the ground with your heel first, rather than your forefoot. This generates a much greater force upon impact and is harder on the body than a forefoot strike.) We evolved to run lightly on the balls of our feet, not hitting the ground hard with our heels, as we do when we wear typical running shoes.

- Try alternating running and walking at 200m intervals. This can help you make the transition to barefoot/minimalist training.

- Do most of your barefoot/minimalist running on level ground to begin with – for at least the first month, if not longer. Running uphill or downhill places additional stress on your body.

- Pay extra attention to good biomechanics. Christopher McDougall, author of *Born to Run: The Hidden Tribe, the Ultra-runners and the Greatest Race the World Has Never Seen*, has some instructional videos on his site. See my website for links.

Once you're accustomed to going barefoot or wearing minimalist footwear, consider doing your walking or running on soft, natural surfaces such as grass and dirt and over uneven terrain. This was the norm for humans until very recently. It's difficult to imagine a situation in our past where we would have walked for miles on a solid, flat, hard surface – yet this is exactly what most modern runners do. No wonder we get so many injuries! A preliminary study reported that some runners that transitioned from typical running shoes to minimalist footwear developed the stress injury called 'bone marrow oedema'. It's unclear whether this injury developed because the runners were putting in miles on unforgiving pavement, or because they transitioned too quickly from highly cushioned footwear to un-cushioned footwear, or for some other reason. The authors of the original study suggested that runners should transition 'very slowly and gradually in order to avoid potential stress injury', which makes good sense to me.

Go barefoot and you'll never go back.

Move: it will change your life

I've told you about how my back pain and fatigue dissipated once I began to SWAP. Given my profession, I was naturally open to the benefits of exercising this way, but even I was amazed at my improved physical and mental state – and I'll never work 'the old way' again. For my patient, Terry, the benefits of SWAP improved his quality of life tremendously

When 35-year-old Terry came to see me, he had a laundry list of complaints: metabolic syndrome/pre-diabetes, very high cholesterol and obesity, as a start. 'I'm tired all the time,' he told me. 'My back's so bad I've got to take painkillers just to get to sleep.'

A computer programmer, Terry sat for eight to 12 hours a day, five or six days a week. He was on metformin for his blood sugar and statins for his cholesterol. 'Time to get moving, Terry,' I told him. Since he worked from home, I suggested he get a treadmill desk for his office along with TRX straps, Powerblocks, kettle bells, an abdominal wheel and push-up bars. I set Terry a goal of walking at least 10,000 steps a day each day (which he built up to slowly). I also had him sprinkle higher-intensity strength-training exercises throughout his working day.

Terry lost 1 stone 6lb (9.3kg) in the first 30 days and 4 stone 4lb (27.2kg) over the first six months. 'I can't believe it!' he told me. 'My back pain disappeared! My blood sugar and cholesterol are back to normal! I haven't had this much energy in years!' His doctor even stopped his medications.

Like me, like Terry, and like our Paleo ancestors who walked, ran and simply moved throughout their day for basic survival, you can easily incorporate movement into your daily routine. It will make your life better – and probably longer.

Summary: move like your ancestors

- Stand for half your day.
- Take a standing break every 30–45 minutes.
- Aim for walking 10,000 steps a day.
- Integrate as much light activity into your day as possible.
- Aim for 150 minutes of moderate-intensity activity per week, or 75 minutes of vigorous activity per week, or 30 sets of highest-intensity activity per week, or some combination of the above.

CHAPTER 13

Sleep More Deeply

Questionnaire: Sleep

Complete the questionnaire below and add up the total of points for those questions you answered 'yes' to, then use the answer key to determine your sleep score.

	Points
I have not been diagnosed with a sleep disorder, such as sleep apnoea.	1
I regularly sleep for more than eight hours per night.	2
I rarely feel sleepy or struggle to remain alert during the day.	1
I rarely have difficulty falling asleep.	2
I rarely wake up earlier in the morning than I would like to.	1
I never have thoughts racing through my mind, preventing me from getting to sleep.	1
I rarely have trouble concentrating at work or school.	1
I have never fallen asleep while driving.	1
I almost never doze off while watching TV, reading, or sitting in a car.	1
I have never been told that I snore.	1
I do not expect to have a problem with sleep during the week.	1
I feel full of energy.	1

Notes for this chapter may be found at ChrisKresser.com/ppcnotes/#ch13

It is easy for me to get up in the morning.   2

I do not experience vivid dreams or hallucinations upon
falling asleep or awakening.   1

After taking a nap, I feel refreshed.   1

I have never worked in a job that involves shift work or
night work.   1

I rarely travel across times zones (east–west travel).   1

I rarely use an electronic device with a screen (TV, laptop,
mobile phone, iPad, and so on) within one hour of
going to sleep.   1

My sleep environment is quiet and/or completely dark.   1

I feel that the quality of my sleep is satisfactory.   1

TOTAL

Answer key:

Total points	What your points mean	Your aim
7+	You are probably getting an adequate amount of sleep during the week	Complete Your Personal Paleo Diet 3-Step programme. No additional personalisation is required
4–6	You're probably not getting enough sleep, or the quality of your sleep is poor	Complete Your Personal Paleo Diet 3-Step programme and add the recommendations in this chapter
0–3	You may be experiencing a sleep disorder or very low-quality sleep	Complete both steps above and see a health-care provider for additional assistance. This should be a major focus for you, and ignoring this area may stand in the way of improvement elsewhere

There are few things more important to health than a good night's sleep. A large body of evidence suggests that most people require seven to nine hours of sleep each night for optimal function and prevention of disease. But an increasing number of people in industrialised countries are falling far short of this ideal. According to data from the National Health Interview Survey, approximately one-third (35 per cent) of US adults sleep fewer than six hours a night. This may not seem unusual today, but it's a relatively recent phenomenon: just 50 years ago only 2 per cent of Americans averaged fewer than six hours of sleep a night. During that period American adults and adolescents lost between one and a half to two hours sleep a night, and chronic sleep loss and sleep disorders are now estimated to affect 70 million Americans.

The consequences of chronic sleep deprivation are nothing short of catastrophic. The sleep–wake cycle – an important part of our 24-hour biological clock, known as the 'circadian rhythm' – affects nearly every aspect of our physiology, including brainwave patterns, hormone production, cell regulation, immune function and metabolism. In fact, studies suggest that the circadian cycle controls from 10 to 15 per cent of our genes. This may explain why disruption of the sleep–wake cycle is associated with numerous conditions such as depression, obesity, memory loss, type-2 diabetes and cardiovascular disease, as well as an increased risk of death.

Perhaps not surprisingly, our understanding of the negative impacts of sleep deprivation has increased during the very time period that sleep duration has decreased so precipitously. We're effectively engaged in a giant, society-wide experiment using ourselves and our children as test subjects, and so far the results are not encouraging. Despite current attitudes ('I'll sleep when I'm dead'), sleep is not optional. It's crucial to the proper function of every system of our bodies, and we can't escape the consequences of getting too little of it. Likewise, improving the quality, duration and timing of your sleep is one of the single most powerful interventions you can make to improve your health.

MODERN THREATS TO SLEEP

The prevailing theme of this book is that human beings are biologically and genetically adapted to a particular diet and lifestyle and that we are 'mismatched' with our current environment. This is as true for sleep behaviour as it is for diet and physical activity. For the vast majority of our evolutionary history, we lived in harmony with the natural rhythms of day and night, without exposure to artificial light. We were active during the day and rested at night, we did not have ready access to stimulants such as caffeine and tobacco and we didn't have mobile phones, computers, tablets, video games and other electronic devices. Today, these influences are ubiquitous – and their effects are profound. They include:

Light pollution (excess artificial light) Artificial light has many benefits – such as increasing our productivity and making recreational activities possible at night – but it hasn't come without a cost. Exposure to artificial light at night affects our circadian system (along with nearly every other aspect of our physiology) and shifts our natural biological clock. It does this primarily by suppressing the production of melatonin, an important hormone that helps regulate our sleep–wake cycle and plays a role in numerous other biological functions.

Electronic media use – including television, computers, tablets, mobile phones and video games – is another relatively new phenomenon that has become ubiquitous in modern society. Too much electronic media use at night has been shown to interfere with getting a good night's sleep.

Changes in work habits Work is the primary activity exchanged for sleep, and work hours in the US have been steadily increasing over the past several decades. But it's not just how much we work that is eating into our sleep time; it's also the way we work. Twenty per cent of the population in industrialised countries now works beyond the normal day shift in various types of shift work or flexible work schedules and, thanks to mobile phones, laptops and the internet, the barriers that previously separated work and leisure time have dissolved.

Jet lag is another modern phenomenon that affects the natural rhythms of the circadian clock. Chronic jet lag – which is associated with regular travel across time zones – has been shown to decrease sleep quality, reduce cognitive function, raise cortisol levels (a sign of stress) and even increase the risk of cancer (due to disturbance of melatonin levels).

Other aspects of the 'modern lifestyle' Physical inactivity, excess alcohol consumption, illicit drug use, cigarette smoking and caffeine are all associated with decreased sleep duration and quality.

Now you know how much less we're sleeping and why, but what, exactly, does chronic sleep deprivation do to us?

HOW SLEEP LOSS DESTROYS YOUR HEALTH

Changes in sleep duration and quality increase the risk of everything from heart disease to diabetes to overall mortality; there's little doubt that sleep loss is directly contributing to the modern epidemic of chronic, inflammatory disease.

Let's examine the effects of poor sleep on three particular areas in more detail.

Cardiometabolic disease

The term 'cardiometabolic disease' refers collectively to diabetes, cardiovascular disease and obesity. It is by far the most common cause of death and disability worldwide. Although most people are aware of the connection between other lifestyle factors such as diet and physical activity and cardiometabolic disease, the contribution of chronic sleep deprivation is less well known.

This is already changing, though, since numerous scientific studies have shown that sleep loss directly affects cardio-vascular and metabolic function in several ways:

- A single night of partial sleep deprivation causes insulin resistance even in healthy subjects with no pre-existing metabolic disease.

- Exposure to even low levels of artificial light at night may contribute to weight gain by promoting late-night snacking and disrupting metabolic signals.

- A randomised, controlled trial with 225 participants found that restricting sleep over five consecutive nights led to increased calorie intake (especially late at night) and weight gain when compared to control subjects whose sleep wasn't restricted.

The effects of sleep deprivation on food intake alone could almost single-handedly explain the connection observed between obesity and impaired sleep. One study showed that restricting sleep for eight consecutive days increased calorie intake by 566 calories per day, with no changes in energy expenditure. Imagine this pattern over the long term: eating an extra 500 calories a day with no changes in how many calories you burn is equivalent to gaining a pound (450g) a week, or 3 stone 10lb (23.5kg) in one year! But the connection between sleep and obesity goes both ways: obesity has been shown to worsen sleep quality, usually due to a higher prevalence of sleep disorders such as central sleep apnoea.

How better sleep helped Jen shed the final 5 pounds (2.25kg)

Jen, aged 28, came to see me complaining of difficulty reaching her target weight. She had started a Paleo diet nine months prior to her visit and she lost 1 stone 11lb (11.3kg) – almost all of the 2 stone 2lb (13.6kg) she wanted to lose – over the first five months. But no matter what dietary modifications she made, Jen couldn't lose those final 5 pounds (2.25kg). 'It's so frustrating,' she told me. 'I'm eating perfectly and exercising every day, but nothing changes. I'm completely stuck.'

As I reviewed Jen's case history, I noticed that she had a habit of staying up until midnight or later. She often used her laptop or iPad at night to check email or chat with her friends on Facebook. She woke up frequently throughout the night and sometimes had trouble falling back to sleep. And although she was often in bed for eight hours, she woke up feeling unrefreshed. I suggested to Jen that inadequate sleep and too much exposure to artificial light at night might be disrupting her metabolism and preventing her from losing those last 5 pounds (2.25kg). I suggested she try:

- Getting to bed by 10.00 or 10.30pm each night.
- Stopping electronic media use at least two (and preferably three) hours before bedtime.
- Wearing orange glasses that filter out melatonin-suppressing blue light after dark (see page 268).
- Making her sleep environment pitch dark, cool, quiet and free of electronic devices (Jen had a habit of leaving her phone on the bedside table).

- Getting exposure to natural light first thing in the morning by taking a 15–20-minute walk outside.

After making these simple changes, the quality of Jen's sleep improved dramatically and she was finally able to lose those last 5 pounds (2.25kg). 'I have so much more energy when I wake up,' she reported, 'and I feel much calmer throughout the day. But the best part is that I don't feel hungry all the time anymore and I've lost the extra weight without even trying.'

Immune dysfunction

Disrupted circadian rhythms and chronic sleep loss alter immune responses, leading to an increased risk of cancer, greater susceptibility to infection and more inflammation. Melatonin plays a key role in the inhibition of cancer development and growth, and the enhancement of immune function. In a remarkable study at Johns Hopkins University, researchers injected two groups of mice with a known cancer-causing agent. Then they exposed one group to 16 hours of daylight and the other to 16 hours of darkness. In the group that experienced darkness, melatonin levels were significantly higher and not a single animal developed cancer; however, in the group that was exposed to light, 90 per cent of the animals developed cancerous tumours. The authors of the study speculated that adequate periods of darkness each day and seasonally throughout the year are necessary for proper immune function. Human studies have found similar results. People who are exposed to light at night on a regular basis (such as shift workers, or those who stay up late using the computer or playing games) experience melatonin suppression and are at higher risk of developing several different types of cancer, including breast, colon, prostate and endometrial cancer, as well as influenza and chronic infections.

Stress tolerance, cognitive function and mood

Perhaps the most immediately noticeable effects of sleep loss are the changes that occur in mood, cognitive function and stress tolerance. If you have children, you might recall how you felt during those early months when your baby wasn't sleeping through the night. You may have been more emotionally reactive, less tolerant of stress and less able to focus and think clearly than you would normally be. Numerous studies support this connection between sleep loss and emotional, cognitive and neurological function:

- When compared to people sleeping normally, sleep-deprived people report significantly greater subjective stress, anger and anxiety in response to low-grade stress.

- Sleep loss increases cortisol levels. High cortisol levels are a sign of stress and are associated with several diseases.

- Poor sleep has multiple effects on cognitive function, ranging from decreased short-term memory, reduced learning capacity, a decline in mental stamina and an inability to sustain attention, and a decrease in performance in tasks requiring complex thinking.

Perhaps the best way to think about sleep loss in this context is as a chronic stressor. The body is constantly working to maintain a state of internal balance, or homeostasis, in which it functions optimally. Sleep deprivation overloads the body's capacity to maintain homeostasis, which results in the numerous changes and increased risk of disease and death we've reviewed in this section. This is why getting a good night's sleep is so crucial to maintaining health.

HOW TO SLEEP LIKE A PRO

Now that we understand why sleep is so important, let's take a look at what to do if you're not getting enough.

Make sleep a priority

If you don't allow adequate time for sleep, the rest of the suggestions I'm going to make below won't help much. The amount of sleep that's required for optimal function varies from person to person, and even throughout a given individual's life, but research suggests that most adults need between seven and nine hours each night.

As a starting place, I recommend allowing eight hours for sleep. For many of you, this will mean going to bed earlier, as you may have less control over when you wake up due to your work schedule. Patients often tell me they're 'naturally' night owls and they've always preferred to stay up late and sleep in. But, in truth, there's nothing natural about this. For millions of years of human history, sleep patterns probably remained in sync with the daily variation in exposure to daylight and darkness. This is what our bodies are adapted for. Having a lot of energy late at night and being excessively tired in the morning is often a sign that your circadian rhythm is out of whack. In most cases, if you follow the suggestions here, you'll start to get tired earlier and wake up with more energy.

Control your exposure to light

Light is the primary determinant of our circadian rhythm and sleep–wake cycles. Exposure to light at night suppresses melatonin production (which impairs sleep), and exposure to light in the morning resets the internal biological clock and improves sleep at night. It follows, then, that controlling exposure to light is a powerful tool for regulating sleep. The first step would be to reduce your exposure to artificial light at night. This can be done by:

- Avoiding or minimising the use of computers and tablets within three hours of your bedtime.

- Dimming, covering or removing anything that emits light in your bedroom, such as an alarm clock.

- Using blackout curtains to make your bedroom as dark as possible.

- Wearing a face mask when you sleep to further block any light you might be exposed to.

Of course, unless you want to go back to living by candlelight, most of us will inevitably be exposed to some artificial light at night. One way to mitigate the impact of that is to wear special orange-tinted glasses that block out the spectrum of light that suppresses melatonin. These glasses have been shown to be remarkably effective in reversing artificial light's melatonin-suppressing effects in clinical studies and to improve sleep quality as well as mood. My patients with sleep difficulties have had great improvements in sleep from wearing them after dark. Simply put them on after the sun goes down and wear them until you go to bed. They're especially important to wear if you're using electronic media (such as computers, tablets, smartphones or the TV) after dark. See my website for more on this.

The next step would be to increase your exposure to light in the morning and during the day. Again, this mimics our natural evolutionary pattern and has been shown in studies to regulate the circadian rhythm and sleep–wake cycle. The circadian system evolved in order to synchronise our physiology and behaviour to the natural periods of day and night imposed by the earth's rotation. Because the cycle length of the earth's rotation is close to – but not exactly – 24 hours, the circadian rhythm must be 're-trained' to the 24-hour day on a regular basis. This would have happened without conscious effort in our ancestors, who lived outdoors and in harmony with the natural cycles of light and darkness; however, in modern society, our exposure to light and darkness can be much less regular.

In these circumstances, purposely exposing yourself to bright light first thing in the morning can help reset your circadian rhythm and thus improve your sleep at night. If it's bright outside in the morning where you live, going outside (without sunglasses) and perhaps taking a walk for 15–30 minutes is the best choice. If it's dark outside where you live in the morning, or you have to rise before it gets light, another option is to buy a light machine that emits 10,000 lux of light and sit in front of it for 15–20 minutes after rising. These machines have been studied extensively for seasonal affective disorder and depression, but research also suggests they can be effective in resetting the circadian rhythm. Please see my website for a specific recommendation.

Move your body

Physical activity is positively associated with sufficient sleep, as extensive research shows. In one study of roughly 15,000 ninth- to twelfth-grade students in the US, students who engaged in more than 60 minutes of daily physical activity had significantly higher odds of getting adequate sleep than students who got less than 60 minutes of daily activity. Studies also suggest that too much sedentary time (in other words, sitting) may decrease the quality and duration of sleep. For optimal sleep, follow the recommendations I made in Chapter 12 for movement. This means not only getting enough exercise but also, and even more importantly, reducing sedentary time and increasing non-exercise physical activity.

Optimise your sleep nutrition

Some people sleep better after eating a light dinner. This is especially true for those with digestive issues. Others – such as people with a tendency towards hypoglycaemia – do better with a snack before bed (and possibly even during the night). In general, it's best to be neither overly full nor hungry when you go to bed.

I haven't seen any research on this, but in my experience working with patients I've found that both low-fat and low-carbohydrate diets can cause insomnia. Long-chain saturated and monounsaturated fats such as butter, lard, tallow, olive oil and palm oil contribute to satiety and help prevent hunger throughout the night. Carbohydrates increase the ability of the amino acid tryptophan to enter the pineal gland or cross the blood–brain barrier; tryptophan is the precursor to serotonin and melatonin, both of which are crucial for sleep. If you're on a low-carb diet and you're experiencing insomnia, try adding a little carbohydrate back in – especially at night.

Certain amino acids that are found in muscle meats and eggs compete with tryptophan for transport across the blood–brain barrier and entry into the pineal gland; however, gelatinous animal products such as skin, cartilage and bones don't have this effect because they aren't rich in the amino acids that compete with tryptophan. Balancing your intake of muscle meats and eggs with fattier cuts of meat and bone broth can promote the uptake of tryptophan and the production of serotonin and melatonin in your brain.

Ditch the stimulants

Many people can drink a cup of coffee or two a day without any adverse effects on their sleep. But if you're having trouble sleeping, one of the first things you should do is stop all caffeine intake for at least 30 days. In some cases this single change alone can completely cure insomnia; however, if your sleep doesn't improve while you're off it and doesn't worsen when you start again, it's probably safe to assume that caffeine isn't an issue for you.

Remember, caffeine is a drug, and like all drugs, stopping cold turkey is not easy. If you've been consuming large amounts of caffeine for many years, you may need to cut back slowly instead of stopping all at once to reduce the potential for withdrawal symptoms; for example, you might reduce your intake by 25 per cent each week over four weeks so that it takes you a month to stop entirely.

Regulate your nervous system throughout the day

Many of us run around like chickens with their heads cut off all day and then wonder why we can't fall right asleep as soon as our head hits the pillow. If our nervous system has been in overdrive for 16 hours, it's unrealistic to assume that it can switch into low gear in a matter of minutes simply because we want it to. Of course this is why sleeping pills are growing in popularity each year.

One of the keys to getting a good night's sleep is managing your stress levels throughout the day. See Chapter 14 for specific tips on how to do that.

Create an environment that is conducive to sleep

In addition to the steps above aimed at optimising your physiology for sleep, it's important to optimise your environment for sleep. This includes adopting 'sleep hygiene' recommendations:

- Using your bed (and preferably bedroom) only for sleep and sex. Avoid working and using electronic media in the bedroom – especially near bedtime. Do not bring your phone into the bedroom. (Be aware that if you like to read in bed, sometimes a good book with a gripping plotline can hook you in – and prevent you from sleeping – as easily as more high-tech forms of entertainment!)

- Creating a pleasant and relaxing environment. Make your bed as comfortable as possible, control the temperature (most people sleep better in a slightly cool room) and create an ambience that is conducive to sleep and rest.

- Avoiding emotionally upsetting conversations or activities. Just before bed is not the time to get into a heated discussion with your partner or a family member, or review your stock portfolio after a bad day in the markets. Create an emotional 'buffer' between the rest of your day and the 30–45 minutes prior to bedtime.

- Using blackout curtains and a face mask, if necessary, to darken the room and decrease your exposure to light.

- Reducing the noise level. If there's a lot of noise outside your bedroom, use earplugs and/or a white-noise machine to block it out.

WHEN SLEEP HYGIENE ISN'T ENOUGH

Let's say you've incorporated all of the sleep hygiene tips in the last section, but you're still having trouble sleeping. Perhaps you toss and turn for hours before you fall asleep, or perhaps you have no trouble falling asleep but you wake frequently through the night or don't feel refreshed when you get up in the morning. In these cases you may need some additional support. See Chapter 14 for tips on managing stress (a key step towards improving sleep) and visit my website for a list of natural supplements and stress-management techniques that are especially helpful for sleep.

Summary: sleep more deeply

- Make sleep a priority. Individual sleep needs vary, but as a starting place aim for spending at least eight hours in bed per night.
- Control your exposure to artificial light at night by minimising the use of electronic devices before bed, dimming or covering anything that emits light in your bedroom, using blackout curtains to darken your bedroom and wearing orange-tinted glasses that filter out blue light.
- Get plenty of exercise and physical activity during the day.
- Optimise your sleep nutrition: find your optimal ratio of carbohydrates and fats and make sure you consume bone broth and gelatinous cuts of meat in addition to lean meats.
- Create an environment that is conducive to sleep: use your bedroom only for sleep and sex, keep it slightly cool and use white noise or earplugs to reduce outside noise.
- If you're having sleep difficulties, avoid caffeine, chocolate, tobacco and other stimulants.

CHAPTER 14

Manage Your Stress

Questionnaire: Stress

Complete the quiz below and add up the total of points for those questions you answered 'yes' to, then use the answer key to determine your stress score.

	Points
I actively pursue a hobby.	1
I belong to a social or activity group that meets at least twice a month.	1
I practise some form of relaxation exercise at least five times a week.	1
I have a place in my home to which I can go to relax or be by myself.	1
I practise time-management techniques daily.	1
I do not bring work home with me.	1
I know exactly which situations make me feel stressed.	1
My average day always includes time for exercise and fun.	1

Notes for this chapter may be found at ChrisKresser.com/ppcnotes/#ch14

I rarely have a hard time coping with stress.   I

I feel that I'm able to control my anger.   I

I can forgive people after they've hurt or angered me.   I

I have an activity, hobby or routine I use to release my
feelings of stress.   2

I avoid unnecessary conflict and stress (for example,
internet debating with strangers)   I

I get seven to eight hours of sleep every night.   I

I have an income adequate to meet basic expenses.   2

TOTAL

Answer key:

Total points	What your points mean	Your aim
10+	You are probably controlling your stress well	Complete Your Personal Paleo Diet 3-Step programme. No additional personalisation is required
4–9	You may benefit from additional stress-relieving efforts/ activities	Complete the Your Personal Paleo Diet 3-Step programme and add the recommendations in this chapter
0–3	You may be dealing with serious or uncontrolled stress	Complete both steps above and see a health-care provider for additional assistance. This should be a major focus for you, and ignoring this area may stand in the way of improvement elsewhere

I believe stress management is one of the most important – yet also most neglected – steps you can take to improve your health. Why? Because no matter what diet you follow, how much you exercise and what supplements you take, if you're not managing your stress you will still be at risk of modern degenerative conditions like heart disease, diabetes, hypo-thyroidism and autoimmunity.

I see this every day in my practice. I have a lot of patients who are following a 'perfect' diet and yet they are still sick. Stress is often the cause. (I'll define stress more clearly in a moment.) Yet as pervasive as stress is, many people don't do anything to mitigate its harmful effects. The truth is, it's a lot easier to make dietary changes and pop some pills – whether drugs or supplements – than it is to manage our stress. Stress management bumps us up against core pat-terns of belief and behaviour that are difficult to change. It also forces us to slow down, to step back, to disengage – if only for a brief time – from the electric current of modern life and to prioritise self-care in a culture that does not value it.

Not surprisingly, those who are the most stressed out and in the greatest need of stress management are also the least likely to carve out the time for it. Although I empathise with the difficulty of managing stress in such a hectic and crazy world, and I still struggle to find the time for it myself occa-sionally, I won't sugar-coat this: if you're not doing some form of regular stress management, you will sabotage all of your best efforts with diet, exercise and supplements.

In this chapter I'm going to teach you how to effectively manage stress and reduce its harmful effects. Before I do that, though, I'm going to define stress more clearly, discuss its evo-lutionary purpose and describe how too much of the wrong type of stress causes disease.

WHAT IS STRESS?

Stress isn't all bad. In fact, we couldn't survive without it. Stress helps us adapt to our environment and meet and overcome challenges. When the body experiences acute stress, a range of physiological responses occur to prepare us for 'fight or flight': heart rate and respiration increase, nutrients are mobilised, the immune system is activated and awareness heightens. At the same time, resources are diverted from processes that aren't needed for immediate survival, such as digestion and reproduction. This exquisitely regulated response to stress provided our ancestors with the energy and wherewithal they needed to survive in a dangerous natural environment.

Exercise is another example of the adaptive effects of stress. During exercise you stress your muscles and cardiovascular system. In response, your body will build larger muscles and increase the capacity of your heart and lungs so that you can meet the same challenge (that is, the same distance on a run, or the same amount of weight lifted) more effectively in the future.

This beneficial type of stress, referred to as 'eustress', or positive stress by some researchers, is not harmful. It motivates us and focuses our energy, improves performance and enhances our ability to thrive in whatever environment we live in. It is typically short term and perceived to be within our coping abilities. But what happens when stress exceeds our capacity to adapt successfully? It becomes 'distress', or negative stress. In contrast to eustress, distress feels unpleasant, decreases performance and can lead to mental, emotional and physical problems. It can be both short and long term, but it is more commonly chronic stress that causes distress.

Why does distress cause disease? The human body is constantly working to keep critical physiological variables like blood pressure, glucose, pH and hormones within the narrow range required for optimal health. This delicate and dynamic state of internal balance is called homeostasis. Under conditions of eustress, the body is able to maintain homeostasis – or return to homeostasis fairly quickly if it's disturbed. For example, if you go to the gym and lift weights, you're placing stress on your muscles and cardiovascular system, but your body will recover fairly quickly after you finish your workout (assuming you're not overtraining; see pages 251–253 in Chapter 12). With distress, your body cannot maintain homeostasis because the intensity or frequency of the stressor exceeds its capacity to cope. This might occur with the death of a loved one, a divorce, legal or financial problems or chronic injury or illness. In these cases stress is no longer adaptive – it's destructive.

What determines whether you experience something as distress? What makes stress 'stressful'? When we're faced with a potential stressor, we (consciously or unconsciously) ask ourselves the following questions:

- Does this matter to me?

- Do I have the resources to cope with this?

A stressor that is important to us and exceeds our capacity to cope will be perceived as negative, whereas a stressor that is relatively trivial and is well within our capacity to cope may be experienced as positive or not experienced as stress at all. This suggests that the same stressor could be perceived differently depending on the person or circumstance – or the meaning assigned to it; for example, a flood would be a direct threat (and therefore stressor) for a human being, but not necessarily for a bird. The loss of a job for a single, young professional who was ready to quit is much less a stressor than for a salaried employee whose family depends upon his or her income. A pregnancy for a woman in her mid-thirties with a strong social and financial support system would be far less stressful than for a teenager with limited resources and no desire to have a child. In other words, how we experience stress is subjective and depends a lot on our internal resources and perspective. This is important to understand, because it suggests that strengthening those resources and changing our perspective can buffer us against the effects of stressors that we can't avoid. (I'll discuss this in more detail shortly.)

HOW STRESS WREAKS HAVOC ON YOUR HEALTH

When the body perceives a stressor, the hypothalamic–pituitary–adrenal (HPA) axis is activated. This axis consists of the hypothalamus and the pituitary gland, both located in the brain, and the adrenal glands, located on top of the kidneys. This axis releases several different hormones, such as cortisol and epinephrine (aka adrenalin) that orchestrate and govern the stress response.

The first stage of the stress response is called the 'alarm reaction'. It includes the following changes:

- Heart rate, respiration and blood pressure increase to supply more oxygen to the muscles and brain.

- Blood flow is shunted to the brain and skeletal muscles, and diverted from the gut, kidneys, liver and skin.

- Reproductive and immune functions are suppressed.

- Natural painkillers are released into the bloodstream.

- Stored fats and sugars – the body's primary fuel sources – are mobilised to provide energy.

- Senses such as vision and hearing become sharper and awareness heightens.

Cortisol is the hormone responsible for many of these changes. It's a diurnal hormone, which means it is not secreted uniformly throughout the day. Cortisol levels are highest at about 8.00am and then decline throughout the rest of the day and into the evening. When cortisol is produced in appropriate amounts at the right times, it protects the body from excessive stress; however, when cortisol production is too high for too long, or when it is secreted at the wrong time (like at night), numerous problems ensue. These include:

- High blood sugar

- Depressed immunity

- Intestinal permeability (aka 'leaky gut')

- Increased craving for 'comfort' and junk foods

- Poor cognitive function and memory

- Poor thyroid function

- Increased fat storage in the liver and abdominal area

- Anxiety and depression

As you can see, the negative effects of stress impact nearly every system of the body. This explains why chronic stress is associated with a wide range of diseases and health conditions. Chronic stress has been shown to:

- Contribute to both type-1 and type-2 diabetes by reducing blood sugar control.

- Play a role in weight gain by promoting overeating, snacking and consumption of junk food. (Conversely, studies have shown that managing stress facilitates weight loss.)

- Increase circulating inflammatory markers such as C-reactive protein, which are associated with many chronic diseases.

- Play an important role in both the onset and exacerbation of asthma and allergies.

- Impair cognitive function and mental health via cortisol's direct effects on the brain.

- Trigger or worsen numerous autoimmune diseases, including multiple sclerosis, Crohn's disease, psoriasis and rheumatoid arthritis.

This is by no means a complete list. In fact, there are few chronic, inflammatory diseases that stress is not associated with.

'Managing my stress finally cleared up my skin'

Celeste, aged 43, came to see me complaining about persistent acne. 'It's so embarrassing,' she said, 'I'm 43 years old, but I look like a teenager.' Celeste was under a lot of stress. She worked long hours as the vice president of a large company; she had two young children; she was concerned about her mother, who was beginning to show early signs of dementia; and she was struggling in her relationship with her husband.

I told Celeste about the relationship between stress and the skin and suggested that she incorporate some stress-management practices into her routine. Initially she was resistant. 'I don't have time for stress management!' she told me. 'I can barely fit everything in as it is.' Of course people in such situations are the ones who need stress management the most, and Celeste was no exception. After trying a few other treatments with limited success, Celeste agreed to commit to a short daily meditation practice and a weekly yoga class. She also started getting acupuncture once a week.

After about six weeks on this regimen, Celeste's skin had improved significantly. After three months, her skin was almost entirely clear. She also noticed other benefits, such as improved sleep, better digestion and more stable moods. 'At first I couldn't imagine how I'd find the time for stress management,' she told me. 'Now I can't imagine my life without it.'

MINIMISING THE IMPACT OF STRESS

There are two different approaches to minimising the impact of stress, and both are important.

1 Reducing the amount of stress you experience

Reducing stress means just what it sounds like: reducing your total exposure to all forms of stress, whether psychological or physiological. Of course, it's never possible (or even desirable) to completely remove stress from our lives, but even in the most pressure-packed circumstances, it's still possible to reduce it.

The first step is to avoid unnecessary stress. Obvious – but it's a challenge for most of us because it's easy to overlook habitual patterns of thought and behaviour that cause unnecessary stress. Here are a few guidelines for how to avoid this kind of stress:

Learn to say no Know your limits, and don't take on projects or commitments you can't handle.

Avoid people who stress you out You know the kind of person I'm talking about: drama kings and queens. People who are constantly taking and never giving. Limit your time with these people or avoid them entirely.

Turn off the news (or at least limit your exposure to it) If watching the world go up in flames stresses you out, limit your exposure to the news, especially the sensationalistic nature of so much of today's news coverage. You'll still know what's going on in the world, but you'll be in control of what you're exposed to.

Give up pointless arguments There is obviously a place for discussion and debate and working towards change. But have you noticed that heated, highly emotional arguments don't lead to real change? In fact, they tend to have the opposite effect – each side becomes more defensive and entrenched in their world view. Find other ways to get your point across, learn to listen with empathy and know when it's time to walk away.

Escape the tyranny of your to-do list Each day, spend some time in the morning really considering what needs to be done that day. Drop unimportant tasks to the bottom of the list. Better yet, cross them off entirely. The world will go on.

Reduce your exposure to online stress Social media can be a fun way to connect, but it's truly a mixed bag, peppered as it is with strangers primed for endless arguments (not to mention those Facebook 'friends' from college who want to debate your political views). Pay attention to how much energy you expend tweeting, texting, emailing and commenting – do you really need to respond to everything? Trying to do so is quite stressful – and you can never really have the last word when it comes to online exchanges.

The second step in reducing the amount of stress you experience is to address any physiological problems that are taxing your adrenal glands. These can include anaemia, thyroid issues, blood sugar swings, gut inflammation, food intolerances (especially gluten), essential fatty acid deficiencies and environmental toxins. The basic 3-step Reset, Rebuild and Revive approach will help with many of these condition. I discuss more specific strategies for addressing some of them throughout the book and in the bonus chapters on my website.

2 Mitigating the harmful effects of stress you can't avoid

Obviously there are times when we just can't avoid stress. Perhaps we have a high-stress job, or we're caring for an ailing parent, or we're having difficulty with our partner or spouse. In these situations it's not about reducing stress itself, but about reducing its harmful effects.

How do you do that? There are several different strategies:

Reframe the situation We experience stress because of the meaning we assign to certain events or situations. Sometimes changing our perspective is enough to relieve the stress; for example, being stuck in traffic can be a 'disaster' or it could be an opportunity for contemplation and solitude.

Lower your standards This is especially important for you perfectionists out there. Don't let the perfect be the enemy of the good. Let good enough be good enough.

Practise acceptance One of my meditation teachers used to say, 'All suffering is caused by wishing the moment to be other than it is.' Many things in life are beyond our control. Learn to accept the things you can't change.

Be grateful Simply shifting your focus from what is not OK or not enough to what you're grateful for or appreciative of can completely change your perspective – and relieve stress.

Cultivate empathy When you're in a conflict with another person, make an effort to connect with their feelings and needs. If you understand where they're coming from, you'll be less likely to react and take it personally.

Manage your time Poor time management is a major cause of stress. When you're overwhelmed with commitments and stretched too thin, it's difficult to stay present and relaxed. Careful planning and establishing boundaries with your time can help.

In addition to everything I've listed above, other important ways to mitigate the harmful effects of stress include cultivating more pleasure and play in your life and spending more time outdoors. I will cover these in more detail in Chapters 15 and 16, respectively.

In the next section, we'll discuss specific strategies for managing stress that I've found to be helpful in my own life and in my work with patients.

STRATEGIES FOR STRESS MANAGEMENT

There are many different clinically proven ways to manage stress, from yoga to deep breathing to biofeedback to acupuncture. Now I'm going to share the practices I've found to be the most helpful for myself and my patients over the years. This isn't meant to be an exhaustive list, and if you're drawn to something else that I haven't mentioned here, don't let that stop you! The important thing is not what type of stress-management practice you do, but that you commit to doing it on a regular basis. By 'regular' I mean every day or as close to that as possible.

Here are a few general tips for incorporating a stress-management practice into your life:

Start small Instead of committing to one hour of meditation each day, which will be hard to follow through if you're new to it, start with just five minutes. Then gradually increase the time as you become accustomed to the practice.

Make it a priority I ask my patients to schedule stress management into their calendar in the same way they would an important appointment.

Choose a mix of practices Some days you might be so wound up that doing a movement-based stress-management technique, such as yoga or t'ai chi, would be preferable. On the other hand, if you're exhausted, a more sedentary technique like mindfulness-based stress reduction or deep breathing might be better.

Be gentle with yourself Don't beat yourself up if you miss a session, and don't treat this as another thing you have to be good at. Stress management should feel like a peaceful and restorative break from your normal routine.

Find a teacher Many of these practices can be learned at home with books or recordings, but there's something to be said for finding an experienced instructor to work with.

Finally, a note about exercise. Although it's true that exercise relieves stress, I'm purposely not including it here. The techniques I mention below induce a particular pattern of brainwave activity that exercise does not. I view exercise and stress management as complementary, not as substitutes for one another.

Mindfulness-Based Stress Reduction

MBSR, or Mindfulness-Based Stress Reduction, combines mindfulness meditation and yoga to cultivate greater awareness of the unity of mind and body, as well as of the ways unconscious thoughts, feelings and behaviours can undermine emotional, physical and spiritual health. It was developed by Dr Jon Kabat-Zinn at the Stress Reduction Clinic at the University of Massachusetts Medical Center in 1979.

Through clinical research at the University of Massachusetts and elsewhere, MBSR has been shown to effect a range of autonomic physiological processes, such as lowering blood pressure and reducing overall arousal and emotional reactivity. Mindfulness meditation has been found to improve sleep – particularly slow-wave sleep – in several studies. MBSR is offered as an eight-week intensive training in hospitals and medical centres around the world. It is also offered as an online course, and can be done via home study with books and audio recordings.

MBSR is particularly effective for anyone struggling with chronic illness or pain. I've found it to be particularly helpful in my own life and in my work with patients.

Meditation

In spite of the fact that I'm listing it here, I don't consider meditation as a 'stress-management' technique – although it can certainly have that effect. Meditation is an awareness practice. Through meditation we learn to witness our thoughts, feelings and sensations and dis-identify with the story we tell ourselves about them. We learn to stay present to our lives even in the face of great difficulty or pain.

Contrary to popular belief, you don't have to be able to 'relax' to meditate. Sometimes we are relaxed during meditation; sometimes we are quite agitated. We don't meditate to manipulate our feelings, but to learn to observe them without reacting to or 'becoming' them.

One of the books I often recommend to people who'd like to learn more about meditation practice is *Opening the Hand of*

Thought, by Kosho Uchiyama. Another excellent resource is *Meditation for Beginners*, by Jack Kornfield. If you do pursue meditation, I recommend working with an experienced teacher. You might consider doing a beginner's meditation course at a retreat centre, finding a local teacher in your area or doing an email class. See my website for links to specific resources.

Finding joy in the heart of pain

In her book *Finding Joy in the Heart of Pain*, my late Zen teacher, Darlene Cohen, posed a number of questions. How do we live through unbearable situations like a catastrophic disease without being destroyed? How do we deal with the mundane anguish of our everyday lives? How do we continue to live under crushing stress? And even further, how do we not just get through these things but have rich, full and worthwhile lives that we actually want to live – under any circumstances?

For me, and for many others in similar circumstances, meditation is the answer. As I explained at the start of this book, I was seriously ill for several years. I was scared, exhausted and in great pain during this period. I had tried so many things and seen so many doctors – it was hard not to lose hope. Yet my meditation practice taught me how to find 'joy in the heart of pain', how to stay present in circumstances that felt unbearable, and how to love and forgive myself through it all – whether I felt sick or well, sad or happy, frustrated or at peace.

Have you ever taken a walk in the woods or on the beach, only to realise that you've been completely lost in your thoughts for the past ten minutes and have hardly experienced your surroundings? Compare that with a time when you were completely present to what was happening around you: the feeling of the breeze against your skin and the sand between your toes, the sound of the waves crashing against the shore and the taste of salt in the air. When you are fully present and aware, your experience of life becomes far more rich and full. Your senses are heightened, your heart is opened and your connection to the world around you deepens.

Meditation practice taught me how to slow down, remain present and experience these moments of joy, peace and connection even in the midst of severe illness and unrelenting pain. Those moments are what made my life worth living and prevented me from succumbing to darkness and despair.

Yoga

The word 'yoga' comes from the Sanskrit root *yuj*, which means 'to unite'. Today, yoga is used as a general term to refer to physical, mental and spiritual disciplines, which originated in ancient India. Yoga has been shown to reduce stress and improve cardiovascular and respiratory health, flexibility, cognitive performance and overall well-being. It is particularly effective in relieving stress-induced disorders, such as insomnia, anxiety, depression, hypertension and asthma.

Yoga is a great choice for stress management for several reasons. First, it's a movement-based practice, which is often suitable for people who are new to stress management or who have very busy minds and find it difficult to sit still. Second, yoga is often practised in a group or class setting, which has additional benefits. Third, because of its popularity, it's now easy to find a teacher or class in most places.

Massage

Touch is vital to human health. In fact, touch is so important that infants deprived of it are unlikely to survive. Human beings are highly social creatures and touch is part of the way we relate to and communicate with others. This is one reason that massage can be such an effective stress-management strategy.

Massage has also been shown to cause hormonal shifts, such as an increase in oxytocin and a decrease in the hormone ACTH, which help regulate the HPA axis and decrease stress. I will discuss the benefits of touch and massage in more detail, along with specific recommendations for how to incorporate it into your life, in Chapter 15.

Feldenkrais (Awareness through Movement)

As the name implies, Feldenkrais (Awareness through Movement) classes are movement lessons that bring awareness to our everyday actions. They help people to become aware of tension patterns that have become unconscious and cause stress, fatigue and pain. Through this awareness, and through learning new patterns of movement, people report feeling more relaxed and at ease moving through their day, which often leads to better sleep at night. People also notice an improvement in how they do everyday activities from sweeping the floor to working out. Although Feldenkrais isn't as well-known as yoga, acupuncture, massage or other stress-management modalities, I've found it to have more profound and long-lasting results in many cases.

Biofeedback

Biofeedback is a process of becoming aware of the body's physiological functions. Specialised sensors deliver information about blood pressure, heart rate, skin temperature and muscle tension, which the participant uses to learn to modify their physiological response to stress.

Biofeedback has been shown to significantly reduce stress and anxiety among high-stress groups such as nursing students and doctors. It has also been shown to reduce chronic pain associated with stress, and to improve sleep in soldiers in combat zones and lessen pre-operative anxiety in children with cancer.

In the past few years, low-cost, portable biofeedback devices have been developed that work with smartphones and tablets. (Emwave2, BioZen and Quantum Life are examples.) This is perhaps the easiest and most accessible way to learn biofeedback.

SUPPLEMENTS FOR STRESS MANAGEMENT

There are a number of supplements that support the HPA axis and help with stress management; however, don't be tempted to think that you can simply take the supplements and ignore all of the behavioural and lifestyle changes I've discussed in this chapter. That won't work. Supplements can be an important part of a stress-management programme, but they should never be seen as a substitute for making the necessary changes to reduce the amount of stress you experience and reduce its harmful effects.

Please see my website for additional stress-management techniques, including links to free instructional audio recordings that you can download.

Summary: manage your stress

- Reduce the amount of stress you experience by learning to say 'no', avoiding people who stress you out (when possible), turning off the news, giving up pointless arguments, escaping the tyranny of your to-do list and addressing any physiological problems (for example, blood sugar swings, gut infections, chronic inflammation, and so on) that are taxing your adrenals.

- Reduce the impact of stress you can't avoid by reframing the situation, lowering your standards, practising acceptance, cultivating gratitude and empathy, and managing your time.
- Make stress management a priority. Give it as much attention as you give other aspects of staying healthy, such as diet, exercise and sleep.
- Commit to a regular stress-management practice. Choose a mix of techniques that suit your temperament and lifestyle, including meditation, yoga, massage, Feldenkrais, mindfulness-based stress reduction, acupuncture and biofeedback.
- If you're new to stress-management practices, start small and be gentle with yourself. Consider finding a skilled teacher who can help you get started and deepen your practice.

CHAPTER 15

Cultivate Pleasure and Connection

Questionnaire: Pleasure and Connection

Complete the quiz below and add up the total of points for those questions you answered 'yes' to, then use the answer key to determine your pleasure and connection score.

	Points
I have a close friend or confidant that I regularly confide in.	1
I am in a committed, loving relationship.	2
I have a strong social support network.	2
I enjoy regular touch and physical contact (that is, massage, sex, partner dancing, and so on).	1
I listen to music that inspires or relaxes me on a daily basis.	1
I have supportive family around me.	1
I play an instrument and practise or make music at least twice a week.	1

Notes for this chapter may be found at ChrisKresser.com/ppcnotes/#ch15

I engage in activities that make me laugh out loud at least
three times a week.   I

I have a good sense of humour and tend not to take
life too seriously.   I

I volunteer for an organisation or cause I believe in.   I

I have a dog, cat or other pet.   I

I have one or more friends to confide in about
personal matters.   I

I set time aside to play, exercise and interact with my
pet at least three times a week.   I

TOTAL

Answer key:

Total points	What your points mean	Your aim
6+	You're probably doing well with pleasure and connection	Complete Your Personal Paleo Diet 3-Step programme. No additional personalisation is required
3–5	You may benefit from more focus on pleasure and connection	Complete Your Personal Paleo Diet 3-Step programme and add the recommendations in this chapter
0–2	You are likely suffering from a lack of pleasure and connection	Complete Your Personal Paleo Diet 3-Step programme and add the recommendations in this chapter. This should be a major focus for you, and ignoring this area may stand in the way of improvement elsewhere

For the vast majority of our history, humans lived in tight-knit, extended family or kin groups with regular social contact. Like all other primate species, we're inherently social animals: we thrive when we feel a sense of connection and belonging, and we suffer when we feel isolated and alone.

Socially isolated people have a higher risk of disease and death, even after controlling for traditional risk factors such as physical health, smoking and alcohol consumption. On the other hand, having a positive social support system has been shown to extend lifespan and improve cardiovascular, endocrine, immune and mental health.

Unfortunately, both the quality and quantity of our social relationships in the industrialised world are decreasing. We've gone from living primarily in extended family or tribal units to living in single family or even individual units; we're more mobile and thus less likely to put down roots; we get married later; and we have more dual-career families. Perhaps most disturbingly, over the past two decades the number of Americans who report having no close confidant has increased threefold and it is now the rule rather than the exception.

This is ironic in a world characterised by electronic hyper-connectivity. Never before have we been able to communicate with such speed and ease. A written message that used to take weeks, if not months, to travel from one end of the world to the other can now be sent in less than a second, and social media has allowed us to interface with more people in a month than we would have met in an entire lifetime just a few hundred years ago. Yet the findings above suggest that, despite these increases in technology and global connectivity, people are becoming more – rather than less – socially isolated.

Like social connection, pleasure is not only part of our cultural heritage; it's also essential to health. The experience of pleasure releases powerful chemicals that promote health and prevent disease. Pleasure protects against the harmful effects of stress, strengthens and regulates the immune system and improves mood. In many ways, pleasure is the antithesis of stress.

Yet in our increasingly busy and hectic world, many people have difficulty finding time for pleasure. Although leisure time has actually increased over the past 40 years, much of that time is devoted to distraction, not pleasure. Distraction and pleasure might seem similar on the surface, but they're fundamentally different. Distraction is something that prevents us from giving full attention to ourselves and our lives. Pleasure is almost exactly the opposite. When we experience pleasure we are more fully present to life, more grounded in our bodies, more alive and aware. Although there's a time and a place for distraction, it shouldn't replace pleasure in our lives. Unfortunately, statistics suggest that this is happening today. The average American now devotes half of his or her leisure time each day to watching television, and computer activities such as checking email and using social media are also on the rise.

Social connection and pleasure are vital to our health and well-being, and we'll benefit from bringing more of each into our lives.

WHY WE NEED PLEASURE AND CONNECTION

In Chapter 14 we talked about how chronic stress contributes to everything from insomnia and anxiety to obesity and heart disease. Scientists have devoted vast amounts of attention to understanding the mechanisms of the 'fight or flight' response. We know that when we're faced with stress, a cascade of physiological changes occurs, triggered by stimulation of the sympathetic nervous system, from increased blood flow to spikes in adrenalin levels.

There's also another nervous-system response that's just as important as fight or flight to our survival that's often ignored in the scientific literature and in mainstream articles about stress. We're not only set up to deal with stress or challenges but also to enjoy life, to relax, to bond and to heal. This is the parasympathetic state, often referred to as the 'rest and digest' or 'calm and connect' response. It has the opposite biochemical effects on our body to fight or flight. Our heart rate and respiration slow down, our blood pressure drops, our blood flow increases to the digestive tract, our skin and reproductive organs, and our stress hormones decrease.

Both fight or flight and calm and connect are essential to life. We need the ability to meet challenges and mobilise our physical and mental resources to take action. But we also need to digest food, replenish our energy stores and heal ourselves. It's likely that these different systems were in a state of relative balance in our distant ancestors. Imagine a day of mostly relaxing, interacting with others, gathering food or building shelters. This might be punctuated by an acutely stressful event, such as a hunt or an encounter with a predator. But it would probably be followed again by more 'rest and digest' or 'calm and connect' time, such as gathering around a fire and feasting on the day's hunt. Human beings are adapted to this balance between pressure and calm, stress and relaxation, sympathetic versus parasympathetic stimulation.

Unfortunately, most of us today have lost touch with this balance. Fight or flight isn't usually a temporary situation – such as warding off immediate physical danger or engaging in a hunt – that quickly passes. Instead, it's an almost continuous reaction to the excessive demands placed on us by modern life. Worrying about money, watching the news, being skipped over for a promotion and driving in traffic may not literally threaten our survival but our bodies react as if they do. We have the exact same physiological response – only to a lesser degree.

PLEASURE: THE ANTIDOTE
TO CHRONIC STRESS

Stress is the antithesis of pleasure: it feels unpleasant, raises our heart rate and blood pressure, weakens our immune system and makes us sick. And if stress is the antithesis of pleasure, it follows that one of the best ways to fight stress is with pleasure.

Our nervous system is relatively black or white. Either we're experiencing stress and the sympathetic nervous system (fight or flight) is activated, or we're in a state of relative ease and the parasympathetic nervous system (rest and digest) is activated. This suggests that if we're experiencing pleasure, we're not experiencing stress – and it explains why pleasure is such a powerful antidote to stress.

Endorphins are the body's 'feel good' chemicals. They look and act just like opium, the poppy-derived narcotic that has been used for thousands of years to induce euphoria and reduce pain. Endorphins are responsible for intensely pleasurable experiences such as orgasm and the 'runner's high' some people experience with exercise. In fact, animal research has shown that endorphin levels are up to 86 times higher after animals experience multiple orgasms. But endorphins are also released, albeit at lower levels, in more mundane daily activities such as playing with a pet, watching a funny film, listening to our favourite music, visiting a favourite place or connecting with loved ones. In addition to counteracting stress hormones and improving mood, endorphins:

- Improve immune function by producing anti-bacterial substances.

- Enhance the 'killer instincts' of various white blood cells that help to fight infection, including B cells, T cells and natural killer (NK) cells.

- Enable certain immune cells to secrete their own endorphins as a way of improving their disease-fighting capacity.

In other words, endorphins don't just make us feel good but also improve our health and protect us from disease. This explains why experiences that bring us pleasure, such as warm, caring touch, listening to music and interacting with pets, are associated with a greater sense of well-being and even longer lifespans.

SOCIAL CONNECTION: NO MAN (OR WOMAN) IS AN ISLAND

For almost two million years humans lived in tight-knit extended family or tribal groups. We had regular, daily contact with family members and others we were close to and an inherent sense of community and belonging. Yet today, most people in the industrialised world live either alone or with their immediate family.

Throughout this book we've discussed the idea that there's a 'mismatch' between our current diet and lifestyle and the one we're adapted to. The decline in the quality and quantity of close relationships and social connection is yet another way that this mismatch manifests in the modern, industrialised world. And although you might suspect that diet and other lifestyle factors like sleep and exercise would have a far greater impact on our health than social support, research suggests otherwise. A landmark study published in 2010 involving over 300,000 participants found that social support was a stronger predictor of survival than physical activity, body mass index, hypertension, air pollution, alcohol consumption and even smoking 15 cigarettes a day! The researchers found that people with adequate social relationships have up to a 90 per cent greater likelihood of survival than those with poor or insufficient relationships.

This is probably a conservative estimate, because this study didn't take the quality of relationships into account, and previous studies have shown that negative relationships actually increase the risk of death. Had the researchers examined the effect of positive relationships separately, it almost certainly would have been higher.

There are several theories to explain why social support is so important to health. One theory is that social relationships help buffer the effects of chronic stress by providing emotional and other forms of support. Another theory holds that social relationships more directly influence our health through their effect on our physiology, behaviour and mood. In either case, it's likely that a hormone called oxytocin plays a strong role.

Oxytocin plays a critical role in both the causes and effects of positive social interaction and is associated with a general feeling of mental and physical well-being. Oxytocin stimulates a sense of calm, improves trust, reduces fear and enhances our desire to connect with others. (Some even refer to it as the 'tend-and-befriend' hormone.) It is secreted during sex, caring touch, non-verbal expressions of love, eye contact and mother–infant bonding, including breast-feeding. Studies have shown that oxytocin levels are higher in men and women who report greater support from their partners and that administering oxytocin encourages close and intimate contact. On the other hand, low levels of oxytocin are associated with social isolation, cardiovascular disease, psychiatric problems and decreased quality of life.

A lack of social support also causes harm in ways that don't directly involve oxytocin; for example, lonely people have higher blood pressure and heart rate, and greater amounts of atherosclerosis, than people with adequate social support. They also suffer from more inflammation, insomnia, infectious disease, cancer, depression and stress. Conversely, people who are more socially integrated have lower serum levels of inflammatory substances like C-reactive protein (CRP) and interleukin-6

(IL-6), are less likely to experience cardiovascular disease and infection and have longer lifespans.

Although most people recognise the inherent value of pleasure and social connection, my guess is that few realise how important they are to physical health and longevity. Yet the studies we've covered in this chapter suggest that together pleasure and social connection may have as much of an influence on our well-being as the food we eat, how much exercise we get and how well we sleep. With this in mind, let's explore some ideas for how to bring more pleasure and connection into your life.

SIX WAYS TO BRING MORE PLEASURE AND CONNECTION INTO YOUR LIFE

1 Touch

The sense of touch is the first to develop in the womb, and it's the most fundamental means of relating to the world around us. It plays an important role in our social interactions, governs our emotional well-being, stimulates the release of potent chemicals that influence all aspects of our health, and serves as a clear – but often overlooked – channel of communication.

Unfortunately, touch is often actively discouraged in the US and UK and some other industrialised societies, because of concerns about litigation and changes in public attitudes. This has led some experts, such as Dr Tiffany Field (who has published over 100 research articles documenting the beneficial effects of touch) to speculate that many people living in modern societies are suffering from what she calls 'touch hunger'. And despite the increasing availability of long-distance forms of communication such as phone calls, text messaging, email and social media, these cannot compensate for a lack of flesh-to-flesh contact. Electronic communication simply does not have the same impact on the body and the mind that physical touch has.

Numerous studies have documented the beneficial health effects of touch. For example:

- A study of 59 women found that more frequent hugs with their partner increased oxytocin levels and decreased blood pressure.

- A study of 95 students at UCLA found that massage was associated with an increase in oxytocin and reductions in hormones associated with stress.

- A study of 183 men and women found that brief episodes of warm, physical contact prior to a stressful event significantly reduced blood pressure and heart rate increases upon exposure to that event when compared to a control group.

If you're suffering from 'touch hunger', here are some suggestions for bringing more nurturing physical contact into your life:

Be a hugger Hug your spouse, your kids, your friends and those you love and see the most. You might even consider hugging people you don't know as well. (In European cultures, the default greeting for strangers of both genders is often a kiss on each cheek.)

Receive or give bodywork or massage If you can get a professional massage or other form of bodywork on a regular basis, that's fantastic. But another option is to take a massage class with your partner, spouse or a close friend and then trade off giving and receiving massages. This is a great way to cultivate intimacy in addition to experiencing more touch.

Have sex Sex releases more oxytocin than any other form of physical contact.

Take a yoga class where you sometimes work with partners
Partner yoga, which is a growing trend in the US, is a non-sexual form of yoga where two people rely on each other's support to keep correct body alignment, balance and focus in a posture. In Iyengar yoga you sometimes work with a partner in this way, so you will get the benefit of working with others as well as working on your own.

Take a dance class Ballroom dancing, tango, contact improvisation and other dance forms that involve partner-to-partner contact are also a great non-sexual way to experience more touch.

2 Intimate relationships

We've known for decades that married people in general have greater life satisfaction, happiness, mental health and life expectancy, and lower rates of disease, when compared to single people. (This is also true for people living together in committed relationships, but who aren't married.) Conversely, single adults without a close confidant have three times the risk of premature death than singles with a confidant or married people.

Recent research has provided deeper insight into exactly which relationships are most beneficial and what it is about relationships in general that promotes health and protects against disease; for example, we know that poor-quality marriages don't carry the same benefit as higher-quality marriages. Chronic relationship stress – characterised by mistrust, conflict and instability – has been tied to greater levels of inflammatory chemicals over time. Hostile married couples have higher levels of these chemicals when compared to couples with a supportive relationship, and married women with rheumatoid arthritis who experienced more criticism from their spouse had higher markers of disease activity.

We also know that of all the types of social support studied, emotional support is the most consistent predictor of better health. More specifically, social support must engender feelings of intimacy and belonging to have the greatest health benefits. One study examining the effect of social support on blood pressure found that support in general did not change blood pressure one way or the other; however, emotional support was significantly associated with lower blood pressure. Other studies have shown that trusting and satisfying relationships are associated with lower levels of inflammatory cytokines such as interleukin-6 and C-reactive protein and lower levels of stress hormones like cortisol. The beneficial effects of emotional support are especially pronounced in women, perhaps because oxytocin appears to have a stronger impact on the female nervous system.

Here are some suggestions for cultivating intimacy in your current relationships and creating new supportive connections with others:

Be honest, open and vulnerable Intimacy is based on mutual trust, and mutual trust is based on honesty, full disclosure and a willingness to let your guard down. Sharing heartfelt feelings can be difficult and scary, especially for men, but true intimacy isn't possible without such open communication.

Schedule regular time for intimacy In today's busy and hectic world, many couples have trouble finding time for intimate contact. Try scheduling regular dates and times to be alone with each other and stick to them just like you would any other appointment. You could do a monthly romantic dinner, a weekly massage, a short walk in the morning before work, or perhaps a shared activity that you both enjoy.

Get professional help If you're struggling in your relationship, seek out professional help. Plodding along in a toxic, hurtful relationship is not only alienating and painful but harmful to your health. You might also consider peer-to-peer counselling methods such as 'co-counselling'.

Don't be a martyr If your relationship is not meeting your needs and you've done everything you can to make it work (including getting help), consider a separation or divorce. This can be terrifying for many people, but ultimately it may not only save your sanity; it may also save your life.

Put yourself out there If you're looking for a partner, online dating is a great option. But another way to increase the chances of meeting that special someone is to surround your-self with people who share your interests and values. Volunteer for a cause you support, join a book club or other activity group, play tennis or football, learn ballroom dancing, go to parties and get out and about!

3 Pets

Pets – especially dogs – have been part of human culture for a long time. Most scientists believe that dogs were first domes-ticated about 10,000 years ago, right when humans shifted from nomadic, hunter-gatherer lifestyles to agriculture; how-ever, some recent archaeological findings suggest that dogs may have been human companions as early as 33,000 years ago. Why such a strong mutual attraction? Although there are probably many answers to this question, one of the most sig-nificant reasons is our need for companionship and to give and receive affection. Pets aren't just pets – they're our friends and family members. We love them, play with them, touch them, care for them and grow old with them. In return, they love us unconditionally, make us laugh and are always there when we need them.

On top of all that, pets make us healthier:

- Pets improve physical fitness by encouraging exercise.

- Pets decrease anxiety and the fight or flight response.

- Pets decrease loneliness and depression by providing companionship.

A study of roughly 480 people who had previously suffered a heart attack found that those with pets were more likely to be alive one year later. Other studies have shown that pet owners have lower blood pressure and triglycerides, greater stress tolerance, improved immune health and fewer minor health problems than non-pet owners. These beneficial effects aren't limited to owning a dog; caring for a cat or a bird, or even watching fish in an aquarium, appears to promote relaxation.

Here are some tips for benefiting from pet ownership:

Choose the right pet Most of the research on the benefits of pet ownership has involved dogs. But if you're not a dog person, don't get a dog! Get a pet that you and your family members can all agree on and will be a good fit for your temperament and lifestyle.

Choose the right breed If you're a runner, don't get a bulldog. If your mobility is limited and you can't take your dog for long walks (or runs) every day, you should probably think twice about a vizsla or border collie.

Train your dog A trained dog means a happier dog – and a happier guardian. An untrained dog can be a source of stress and frustration – and that's not the point! I think positive training methods are more likely to increase pleasure and connection, and they're very effective.

Make time to play Once you have your pet, be sure to carve out time in your schedule to play together. That's one of the best ways to connect with your pet, and play has its own benefits, as I'll explain in the next chapter.

Volunteer at a local shelter If pet ownership isn't for you right now, volunteering at a shelter will give you the opportunity to connect and interact with many different animals while supporting a good cause. And, as you'll see, volunteering is one of the six ways to bring more pleasure and connection into your life.

4 Music

Listening to, and making, music has been part of human experience for thousands of years – and perhaps much longer. In traditional hunter-gatherer groups, such as the Aboriginal Australians, music was an important part of ceremonial and cultural life. In the 6th century BC, the Greek philosopher Pythagoras wrote about music's contribution to health. He prescribed music and a specific diet to restore the harmony of the body and soul. In the mid-1800s, the now-renowned nurse Florence Nightingale used music in hospital wards to accelerate the healing process for soldiers injured in the Crimean War.

Today, we know that music affects us by engaging specific brain functions involved in memory, learning and multiple motivational and emotional states. Music can enhance positive and calming emotions and is used therapeutically in everything from surgery to intensive care to pain relief.

It's important to note that not all music has a relaxing effect, however. Some music is calming and reduces blood pressure and other parameters associated with stress, whereas other music can be stimulating and actually increase blood pressure, heart rate and markers for stress. It appears that the tempo of music is the most important factor, with slow and flowing music that has 60–80 beats per minute showing the most positive outcomes on relaxation and pain relief. Research also suggests that music intended for relaxation should be non-lyrical (without words), consist predominantly of low tones, comprise mostly strings with minimal brass or percussion and have a maximum volume of 60 decibels.

Of course, this doesn't mean you shouldn't listen to faster-tempo, more upbeat music; it just means that that kind of music will have a different physiological effect. Faster, more rhythmic music – especially when you dance to it – is more likely to release endorphins and other feel-good chemicals associated with pleasure, play and celebration. This is great, and it also has a healing effect. It's just not calming and relaxing. The important thing is to know what you need in a given moment and to choose the right music for the job.

Here are some tips for using music to bring more pleasure and connection into your life:

Build playlists for specific purposes Make a playlist with slow, flowing, melodic and meditative music for listening to while working or at other times when you need to take the edge off. Make a playlist with faster, more upbeat music for when you need to get the endorphins and feel-good chemicals flowing.

Be selective Why listen to the radio with a lot of intrusive advertisements and music you don't like, when you can build your own 'smart' radio station that learns about your preferences with services like Pandora in Australia or Spotify in the UK. Music that appeals to you is more likely to boost chemicals associated with pleasure and stress reduction, so don't settle for music you don't like.

Expand your horizons We have more access to a wider variety of music than ever before. Perhaps you'd like to try Afro-Cuban, Gregorian chant, Tibetan throat singing or classical? Whatever your taste, there's something out there for you and, thanks to the internet, you can add it to your playlist.

Ask friends for recommendations and search out new music that makes you happy.

Start or join a music exchange Consider starting or joining a group of friends who share music with one another. This is a great way to get exposed to new music.

Learn how to play and sing Even if you never received music instruction as a child, it's never too late to learn. Making music has additional benefits above and beyond listening to it. We all have music in us, and there's an instrument out there for everyone. Playing music in groups – like in a drum circle or a band – is especially beneficial.

5 Humour

The idea that humour can heal can be traced at least as far back as biblical times, with the maxim that 'a merry heart doeth good like a medicine' (Proverbs 17:22). More recently, physicians like Norman Cousins and Patch Adams have advocated for the use of humour in medicine, and some researchers have argued that humour may have evolved specifically as a strategy for coping with stress. The US psychologist Rollo May believed that humour allows us to distance ourselves from our problems, view them from a different perspective and thus reduce the feelings of anxiety and helplessness we might experience in the face of them. And the British philosopher Bertrand Russell once said that 'Laughter is the most inexpensive and most effective wonder drug. Laughter is a universal medicine.'

Humour has been shown to reduce stress, relieve pain and improve the overall quality of life. Laughter can lead to changes in heart rate, skin temperature, blood pressure, pulmonary ventilation, skeletal muscle activity and brain activity. It also may improve immune function by blocking the production of stress hormones (such as cortisol, ACTH – adrenocorticotropic hormone – and adrenalin) and by stimulating the production of feel-good chemicals (such as endorphins). Laughter may increase the activity of natural-killer cells, which help fight infection and keep cancer at bay.

Here are some tips for benefiting from humour and laughter:

Lighten up Learn not to take yourself and your life so seriously. Take a step back, get some perspective and remember that 'this too shall pass'.

Watch a funny film (or TV programme) If you watch TV, you might as well watch shows that are funny and improve your health. Just don't watch too much, or the benefits of laughter might be outweighed by the harm of sitting on your butt for too long.

Go to a live comedy show Watching a live stand-up comic or improvisation performance has the added benefit of laughing with a group of people. Watch for listings in your area and make this a regular event.

Go on a news diet Let's face it: the news is often depressing. Although I believe it's important to stay informed and not to avoid or deny tragedy when it occurs, your life will not be enriched by hearing about every murder, car crash or catastrophic event that happens in the world. Consider limiting your news consumption to 15 minutes per day on most days, with perhaps a longer read of the Sunday paper, for example.

Avoid people who bring you down This isn't always possible, and there's a certain amount of interpersonal struggle we all have to face in life. But there's no reason to go looking for it, or to invest your limited time and energy into relationships that are a constant drain on you.

Play with your kids and pets Kids and animals are specialists in the art of humour, play and fun. Learn from them.

6 Volunteering

Whether as a parent, spouse, partner, parishioner or friend, we've all experienced the joy of giving. Giving and receiving are essential to who we are and how we relate to others, as necessary to our survival in the modern world as breathing, eating and sleeping. Perhaps it won't surprise you, then, to learn that research on giving has shown that people who help others experience satisfaction, happiness and self-esteem from giving. People who volunteer have longer lifespans than people who do not, and they're less likely to suffer from disease.

There are a number of reasons why volunteering might yield both mental and physical health benefits, but one of the strongest is that it increases meaningful social connection; for example, people who give social support have lower blood pressure. They're also more likely to report greater received social support (what goes around comes around!), greater self-efficacy, less depression and less stress than people with a lower tendency to give support to others. As I'm sure many of you have experienced, giving increases our sense of value and purpose and makes life more meaningful.

Here are some tips for volunteering and giving:

Find a cause you believe in Volunteering for a cause you believe in will be even more meaningful, since you'll be working towards a world more in line with your values and ideals. It's also a great way to meet like-minded people and to expand your social network.

Volunteer at your church, temple, mosque or religious organisation Some of the research on volunteering suggests that those with the strongest faith receive the greatest benefits.

Volunteer in person Volunteering remotely (that is, doing computer work for an organisation across the country) is still worth doing, but research suggests that volunteer work that involves live contact with other people is likely to be more beneficial.

Don't over-extend yourself Informal giving and volunteer work have been shown to benefit health, but extreme giving (such as caregiving for a disabled or very sick person) is detrimental to health. Of course there are times when that is necessary and unavoidable, but don't over-extend yourself if you don't have a compelling reason to do so.

The healing power of pleasure and connection

I'd like to finish this chapter by sharing a personal story. At one point in my long struggle with illness I felt I had reached the end of my tether. I was demoralised, discouraged and exhausted. I had tried at least six special diets, I had a cupboard full of supplements that had done nothing for me (and even made me worse) and I'd seen at least 15 specialists in all different fields without much, if anything, to show for it. I came to a place where I simply didn't know what to do and I didn't have the energy or will to focus on yet another diet or supplement programme.

So I did something radical – or at least it seemed that way at the time. I decided to focus almost exclusively on cultivating more pleasure and connection in my life and not to worry much about diet or supplements. I was feeling isolated and somewhat disconnected from my life after being sick for so long, and intuitively I knew that I had to nourish myself on a deeper level than food or supplements could achieve in order to regain my strength. I created a weekly 'pleasure and connection' programme that involved a massage trade, acting/improvisation classes, regular social visits with friends, dancing at least once a week and volunteering as a teacher of meditation to inmates at San Francisco County Jail. During this time I continued to eat an overall healthy diet, but I resolved not to be overly restrictive or think too much about what I was eating. In fact, I made sure to eat plenty of things that brought me pleasure – even if they didn't fit my concept of 'healthy' food.

After about three months on this programme I felt like a different person. I was more calm, relaxed and happy. I didn't feel so alienated and alone. But the benefits weren't just psychological and emotional: I felt more energetic, my digestion improved, I gained about 10 pounds (4.5kg) that I had lost during my illness, and my sleep became more restorative. In fact, nearly everyone that knew me remarked on how much more vital and healthy I looked.

There's no question that diet and exercise are crucial to health, but experiencing pleasure and feeling connected to others are also important and, in certain circumstances, perhaps even more so than diet. You may not need to go to the lengths I did to reap the benefits of pleasure and connection, but I hope this story inspires an appreciation of just how powerful they can be.

Summary: pleasure and connection

- Make pleasure and connection as much a priority as eating well, managing stress and getting enough sleep and exercise.
- Get plenty of physical contact and touch from hugs, massage, sex, partner dancing and partner yoga.
- Cultivate intimate relationships and expand your social support network by being open and honest, scheduling time with loved ones, joining a friendship group and putting yourself in situations where you're likely to meet people you'll connect with.

- Get a dog, cat or other pet, or if you already have one, set aside time to play and interact with it.
- Listen to music that makes you feel alive, happy, relaxed and at peace. Use software or music-exchange groups to discover new music and expand your horizons.
- Volunteer for a cause you believe in and focus on giving more to the people in your life.

CHAPTER 16

Go Outside

Questionnaire: Nature and Sunlight

Complete the questionnaire below and add up the total of points for those questions you answered 'yes' to, then use the answer key to determine your nature and sunlight score.

	Points
I often spend a large portion of my day outside.	2
I am outside for more than 30 minutes daily.	2
I frequently walk or bike to work or to do errands.	2
I don't always cover my skin with sunblock or clothing when I go outside.	1
I live in an environment with a lot of green space, parks and/or natural attractions.	1
My office or place of work has many windows.	1
I spend less than 8 hours looking at a screen daily (computer, television, phone, and so on).	1
Most of my physical activity takes place outdoors.	1
I have frequent interaction with nature (trees, water, plants, animals, and so on).	1
TOTAL	

Notes for this chapter may be found at ChrisKresser.com/ppcnotes/#ch16

Answer key:

Total points	What your points mean	Your aim
6+	You are probably spending adequate time outside	Complete Your Personal Paleo Diet 3-Step programme. No additional personalisation is required
3–5	You may benefit from more focus on time outside	Complete Your Personal Paleo Diet 3-Step programme and read this chapter for additional tips on how to bring more outside time into your life
0–2	You are likely not spending enough time outside	Complete both steps above. This should be a major focus for you and ignoring this area may stand in the way of improvement elsewhere

Most people intuitively know that spending time outdoors is good for them. But we're now beginning to understand that nature may be as essential to health as sleeping enough, getting adequate exercise or eating a healthy diet.

We evolved over hundreds of thousands of generations in a natural, outdoor environment rich with sunlight (in what is now modern-day Africa) and we've inhabited urban environments for only a few hundred years. Human beings have never before spent as little time in contact with plants and animals as we do today. And although the consequences of this profound separation are not yet entirely clear, recent evidence suggests that too much artificial stimulation and time

spent in purely human-made environments may cause everything from fatigue and a loss of vitality to a decline in health.
Just as we're not adapted to an industrialised diet full of
processed and refined foods, we're not adapted to a life with
little to no contact with nature. This disconnection from the
natural world is yet another way that humans are 'mismatched' with our current environment and is probably
contributing to the epidemic of modern disease.

There are three features unique to spending time outdoors,
each essential to health: sunlight, contact with nature and the
unique benefits of outdoor exercise. Let's look at them in more
detail.

SUNLIGHT IS NOT OPTIONAL

Our distant ancestors spent about half their days in the light of
the sun. But today, sun exposure is actively discouraged because
of fears that it will cause skin cancer, and modern lifestyles often
involve long hours spent indoors under artificial light. Although
there's no doubt that too much ultraviolet radiation in the form
of sunlight can increase the risk of skin cancer in fair-skinned
people, not enough sunlight can also cause problems.

One of the primary benefits of sunlight is its ability to stimulate vitamin D production. Vitamin D is formed when a
particular type of ultraviolet light (ultraviolet 'B') interacts
with 7-dehydrocholesterol in our skin. Fair skin produces
about 10,000 to 25,000iu of vitamin D in response to 20–30
minutes of summer skin exposure, whereas those with darker
skin may need to spend up to two hours in the sun to obtain
the same amount.

We now know that vitamin D deficiency is a major predis-
posing factor for at least 17 varieties of cancer, as well as heart
disease, stroke, hypertension, autoimmune disease, type-2 diabetes, depression, birth defects, infectious disease and more.

Yet as important as vitamin D is, exposure to sunlight isn't absolutely necessary to obtain it, and it's possible to use supplements and lab testing to ensure an optimal vitamin D level and avoid toxicity. Does that mean we don't really need sun exposure for optimal health? No. A growing body of evidence suggests that sunlight has additional benefits above and beyond its capacity to stimulate vitamin D production, including reducing the risk of cardiovascular disease and regulating the immune system.

Scientists observed a connection between sunlight and cardiovascular disease as far back as the 1970s, when clinical trials on hypertension showed that blood pressure was consistently lower in summer than winter. Later studies showed that both the prevalence of hypertension and average blood pressure are directly correlated with latitude; in other words, those living at northern and southern latitudes (with less sunlight) had more hypertension and higher average blood pressure, whereas those living closer to the equator had less hypertension and lower average blood pressure. Although some have argued that this variation may be due to genetic differences, when people migrate from one place to another their risk of death changes to that of their new place of residence – which of course suggests that latitude and sun exposure, and not genetics, are to blame. In the UK the risk of death from heart disease is directly correlated with latitude, with more deaths at higher latitudes even after taking all other known risk factors (such as obesity, family history, and so on) and possible protective factors (such as fruit and vegetable consumption, physical activity, and so on) into account. Finally, clinical experiments have provided direct evidence that ultraviolet light reduces blood pressure. In one study, researchers exposed one group of people to lamps that gave off ultraviolet light as well as heat and another group to lamps that gave off only heat. In the group that received both heat and ultraviolet light, blood pressure dropped significantly after just one hour of exposure, whereas those that received heat alone experienced no change in blood pressure.

How does sunlight lower blood pressure and reduce the risk of cardiovascular disease? Sunlight stimulates the production of a chemical called nitric oxide in our skin. Nitric oxide helps our blood vessels to relax and expand, which in turn reduces blood pressure. This is important because high blood pressure is one of the strongest risk factors for cardiovascular disease, and even relatively small reductions in blood pressure can dramatically reduce the deaths from both heart attack and stroke; for example, a drop of 20mmHg in systolic blood pressure (blood pressure is expressed in terms of variations of pressure – for example, 120/80 – and systolic refers to the first number) leads to a twofold reduction in the overall risk of death in both men and women between the ages of 40 and 69. Sunlight may also reduce the risk of cardiovascular disease by putting the brakes on inflammation. These beneficial effects of sunlight are likely to extend to other organs and tissues as well, since both blood pressure and inflammation have widespread effects in the body.

Another effect of sunlight that isn't mediated by vitamin D is its ability to regulate immune function. Studies have shown that the more hours of sun there are where you were born, the lower the risk you'll develop multiple sclerosis. Along the same lines, the more exposure to sun people have where they work and live as adults, the lower their rates of MS, and relapse rates for MS are higher in winter than in summer. Evidence for benefit from sunlight is strong for other autoimmune diseases as well, such as type-1 diabetes. Finally, exposure to sunlight may improve endocrine function, elevate mood (via its effects on certain brain chemicals like serotonin), increase DNA repair capacity and reduce skin lesions in psoriasis, eczema and vitiligo.

Researchers aren't entirely clear on how sunlight protects against autoimmune disease, but one possibility is that ultraviolet radiation suppresses the immune system. This explains why too much sun exposure can cause skin cancer: excessive ultraviolet radiation overwhelms the natural defence mechanisms in our bodies that keep the growth of cancer cells in check. But it also suggests that not enough sunlight could lead to an overactive immune system that starts attacking its own organs and tissues. Importantly, these immune-suppressing effects of sunlight appear to be completely independent of vitamin D.

With all of this in mind, how much sun exposure is 'just right'? How can we minimise our risk of skin cancer while optimising vitamin D levels and getting the additional cardiovascular and immune benefits of sunlight? Just follow these guidelines for you and your family members:

- If you have fair skin, aim to spend about half the amount of time in the sun that it takes for your skin to turn pink (without sunscreen) two to three days a week. This could be as little as ten minutes for those with very fair skin. If you have dark skin, you may need up to two hours per day to generate the same amount of vitamin D (which is why supplementation may be necessary for those with darker skin).

- Never burn yourself in the sun. Cover yourself with light clothing, wear a hat, shade yourself with an umbrella, tree or canopy, wear sunglasses and/or use a safe sunscreen (see 'Not all sunscreens are created equal' on page 321) to prevent sunburn if you're going to be exposed to sunlight for a prolonged period.

- Pay attention to the time of day, latitude and season. This probably goes without saying, but you need less sun exposure at midday during the summer on the equator to generate a given amount of vitamin D than in the late afternoon during the winter in London or Melbourne. Vary your exposure accordingly.

- Infants under six months old don't have much of the protective pigment (melanin) in their skin. It's best to avoid direct sun exposure at midday, use protective clothing and a hat, and limit exposure to the morning or late afternoon hours. Infants may be particularly susceptible to the toxic effects of some sunscreen ingredients, so use clothing or shade when possible and closely follow the recommendations in the box below.

Not all sunscreens are created equal

According to a report from the Environmental Working Group, only 25 per cent of 800 sunscreens that were tested are effective at protecting your skin without the use of potentially harmful ingredients.

The report made the following recommendations for choosing a safe and effective sunscreen:

- Look for zinc oxide, titanium oxide, Mexoryl SX or avobenzone (3 per cent) as active ingredients.
- Use lotions, not sprays or powders. Many sunscreens contain tiny nanoparticles of zinc oxide and titanium dioxide. Although these don't generally penetrate the skin, they can be inhaled from sprays or powders – with unknown health consequences.
- Don't be fooled by artificially high SPF ratings. If you buy higher than SPF 50, you may think you have a free pass to stay in the sun for as long as you'd like without skin damage. But research suggests that SPF ratings higher than 50 are a hoax. Stick with SPF 15–50, depending on your skin tone and sun intensity.
- Avoid sunscreens with vitamin A (retinyl palmitate). Although vitamin A is beneficial when consumed in the diet, some

studies suggest that rubbing it on the skin may increase the risk of skin cancer.

- Avoid oxybenzone, a synthetic oestrogen that can penetrate the skin and disrupt hormone regulation.
- See my website for a link to the Environmental Working Group's Sunscreen Guide, which has a list of recommended products that meet these criteria.

HOW NATURE SOOTHES YOUR BODY AND MIND

For as long as civilisation has existed, humans have sought out nature as a refuge from the business, noise and pollution of urban environments. More than 2,000 years ago, Taoists in China created gardens and greenhouses that they believed promoted health. At the end of the 17th century, the book *English Gardener* suggested that readers 'spare time in the garden, either digging, setting out, or weeding; there is no better way to preserve your health'. By the 1890s, landscape architects and park planners were developing large urban parks for health purposes. Parks were considered the 'lungs of the city' and the health benefits of exposure to nature were an unquestioned article of faith.

Without nature, there would be no life. Humans are entirely dependent upon the natural environment for food, water and shelter. But nature is more than just a source of raw materials; it's necessary to our psychological, emotional and spiritual well-being. Frederick Law Olmsted, the famous 19th-century US landscape architect, believed that nature 'operates by unconscious process to relax and relieve tensions created by the artificial surroundings of urban life'. Yet over the last few hundred years, we've become profoundly disconnected from the natural world. As we moved from rural areas to the city and transitioned from working primarily outdoors (for example, as farmers) to working indoors (for example, in offices), we have lost our vital contact with nature and our health has suffered as a result. A recent review of studies found that people living in the US, Japan and Spain are spending on average between 18 and 25 per cent less time in wilderness or natural environments today than they were in 1981.

In his book *Last Child in the Woods: Saving Our Children from Nature Deficit Disorder*, Richard Louv refers to this disconnection from nature and its effects as 'Nature Deficit Disorder'. It affects both children and adults of all economic, social and cultural backgrounds and leads to 'diminished use of the senses, attention difficulties and higher rates of physical and emotional illnesses'. According to Louv, the disorder can affect individuals, families and communities, perhaps even changing human behaviour in cities, since the absence of parks and open space has long been associated with high crime rates, depression and other urban maladies.

Louv and other commentators point to a growing body of evidence suggesting that regular contact with nature is important to health, and a lack of such contact contributes to both physical and mental health problems; for example:

- Natural environments have restorative and rejuvenating effects, reduce stress and blood pressure and improve our outlook on life.

- Patients in hospital rooms recover faster when they're exposed to plants or nature, prison inmates whose cell windows face nature have fewer illnesses than those whose cell windows face the prison courtyard, and office workers with views of trees and flowers felt that their jobs were less stressful and more satisfying than those with windowless offices.

- Spending even a little time outdoors can reduce the symptoms of ADHD – even among kids that failed to respond to medication.

- Nature can improve our capacity to tolerate stress and reverse mental and physical fatigue.

What's happening here? Why is contact with nature so essential to health? The simplest answer is that nature is in our DNA. For hundreds of thousands of generations, we lived, worked, ate, played and slept outside in undeveloped, natural environments. Living indoors with artificial light, air conditioning and central heating has been common only for a few generations, and we're still biologically adapted to life on the savannah. This concept – that humans have an innate affinity to the natural world – was called the 'biophilia hypothesis' by Harvard University scientist and Pulitzer Prize-winning author E.O. Wilson. It's supported by more than a decade of research demonstrating how strongly people respond to open, grassy landscapes, scattered stands of trees, meadows, water, winding trails and elevated views – exactly the environment that humans evolved in.

There are also other reasons contact with nature improves our health. Studies using geographic information databases have found a strong correlation between greater amounts of parks and open, green spaces in an area and increasing levels of cycling, walking and other forms of physical activity. In pre-school children, time spent outdoors is the single most predictive factor in how physically active they will be. In addition to encouraging activity, nature protects against the harmful effects of air pollution. According to the California Air Resources Board, indoor air-pollutant levels are 25–62 per cent greater than outside levels, and this difference poses a serious risk to our health. And while crowding, high temperatures and noise have all been linked to increases in aggression and violence, natural settings appear to have the opposite effect.

Here are a few tips to increase your exposure to nature:

Put plants in your home and office Studies have shown that caring for, and seeing, plants in your home and work space has beneficial effects on health.

Get to know your local parks Many urban environments have great parks and open green spaces you can take advantage of without leaving town. Studies have found associations between the use of urban green spaces and stress reduction, regardless of age, sex or socio-economic status.

Limit your screen time (and your children's) Studies consistently show that increased screen time leads to less time spent outdoors.

Exercise outdoors Outdoor exercise has some unique benefits, which I'll cover in the next section.

Go camping Camping is a great way to get out of the city and to interact with nature.

Get a dog Dog-owners are more likely to be physically active, and having a dog may make you more likely to visit nature – especially if you have good walks where the dog can be off the lead where you live.

Get closer to nature People who live and work closer to nature – including urban parks and green spaces – tend to be healthier overall than people who don't have access to nature. This is true even for people with offices and homes with views of nature, rather than those that look out on completely human-made environments.

'I lost touch with nature – and myself'

Rich, aged 28, came to see me complaining of brain fog, mental fatigue, depression and malaise. 'I used to have such a zest for life,' he told me. 'Now I just feel like I'm going through the motions.'

Rich worked for a high-tech company – and that's about all he did. On most days he'd arrive at the office at 8.30am and wouldn't leave until after 9.00pm. He worked weekends and also on holidays, when he got around to taking them (which wasn't very often). I asked Rich more about his childhood and what he loved to do. I noticed that almost everything he mentioned involved contact with nature: camping, going to the beach, surfing, snowboarding and hill-walking.

I suspected Rich was suffering from 'Nature Deficit Disorder', so I prescribed a regular programme of getting outside and interacting with the natural world. At lunch he drove to a hiking track not far from his office and went for a walk. He cut back on his work schedule and started surfing again a few days a week. He enrolled in an outdoor t'ai chi class, and he scheduled a regular camping trip once every three months. Over the course of a year Rich gradually regained his enthusiasm for life. 'I don't dread getting out of bed like I used to. In fact, I look forward to my days now,' he told me. 'And the best part is, I'm getting even more done at work in less time.'

A little bit of nature can go a long way!

WHY OUTDOOR EXERCISE BEATS INDOOR EXERCISE

Outdoor exercise provides more exposure to beneficial sunlight and contact with nature, but there are additional advantages. Running outdoors, for example, tends to impact your muscles differently than if you run inside on a treadmill: you flex your ankles more and, since you'll probably end up running downhill at some point, different muscles in your legs will be used than would be used when running exclusively on a flat surface. Outdoor exercise in general is often more strenuous than indoor exercise, in part because of wind resistance and changes in terrain. (Think of cycling, where wind resistance can cause significant drag and thus much higher energy expenditure.)

There are also less tangible benefits of outdoor exercise. Compared with exercising indoors, outdoor exercise is associated with greater feelings of revitalisation and positive engagement, decreases in tension, confusion, anger and depression, and increased energy. Joggers who exercise in a natural, green setting with trees, foliage and landscape views feel more restored than people who burn the same number of calories in gyms or other human-made settings.

Those who exercise outdoors are also more likely to exercise longer and more often than those who exercise indoors. One study outfitted men and women over 66 years of age with a device that measured their activity levels for a week. Those who exercised outside got about 30 minutes more exercise during the week than those who walked or did other forms of exercise indoors.

Exercise in natural (rather than human-made) environments appears to have benefits above and beyond simply exercising outdoors, especially for children. Research in Norway and Sweden compared preschool children who played on flat playgrounds to children who played for an equivalent amount of time on varied, natural terrain. At the end of the one-year study period, the kids who played among the trees, rocks and uneven natural surfaces tested better for balance, agility and other markers of motor fitness.

Here are some suggestions for boosting your outdoor exercise:

- Choose sports and hobbies that encourage outdoor activity, such as hiking, trail running, surfing, rock climbing or snowboarding. If you swim or play tennis all year round, do it outside as much as possible.

- Consider a morning or evening walk with your partner, dog or children as a daily ritual. This will not only get you moving outside; it's also a good opportunity to connect and play with those you love.

- Do your own gardening.

- Join an activity group that involves outdoor exercise, such as a running, cycling or walking club.

- Buy some high-quality all-weather gear, so that you won't be deterred from going outside when the weather is bad. You won't get the benefits of sunshine in these cases, but all of the other advantages of outdoor exercise still apply.

Summary: go outside

- Get approximately 15–20 minutes of midday sun exposure without sunblock two to three days a week. Actual exposure time should vary based on skin tone, sun intensity, latitude and the time of year.
- Avoid sunburn by using safe, effective sunscreens, covering up with clothing and hats, or shading yourself with an umbrella or canopy.
- Spend as much time in contact with nature as your schedule and lifestyle permit. At a minimum, aim for two excursions into nature (urban parks and green spaces included) each week.

- Put plants in your home and workplace. If you have outdoor space, plant a simple garden (a container garden is one easy option) and sit outside. If you have a choice, live in close proximity to (and preferably in sight of) natural environments.
- Exercise outdoors whenever possible on varied terrain that includes hills, footpaths, rocks and other natural features.

CHAPTER 17

Get Serious About Play

Questionnaire: Play

Complete the questionnaire below and add up the total of points for those questions you answered 'yes' to, then use the answer key to determine your play score.

	Points
I am a playful person.	1
I play with pets or children at least three times a week.	1
I play individual or group sports at least once a week.	2
I engage in playful/fun physical activity (that is, surfing, snowboarding, and so on) at least once a week.	2
I play board games or other games at least once a week.	1
My work involves creativity and innovation.	1
I have a playful relationship with my spouse or partner.	1
I make time for play and consider it a priority.	2
I make a point of learning new skills and participating in activities that I think would be fun.	1
TOTAL	

Notes for this chapter may be found at ChrisKresser.com/ppcnotes/#ch17

Answer key:

Total points	What your points mean	Your aim
6+	You are probably getting adequate amounts of play	Complete Your Personal Paleo Diet 3-Step programme. No additional personalisation is required
3–5	You may benefit from more focus in this area	Complete Your Personal Paleo Diet 3-Step programme and read this chapter for additional tips on how to bring even more play into your life
0–2	You are probably not playing enough	Complete both steps above. This should be a major focus for you and ignoring this area may stand in the way of improvement elsewhere

Imagine a life without play: no games, sports, films, art, music, jokes, stories, daydreaming, flirting or make-believe. Such a life would hardly be worth living. 'If you think of all the things we do that are play-related and erase those,' says play expert Dr Stuart Brown, 'it's pretty hard to keep going. Without play, there's a sense of dullness, lassitude and pessimism, which doesn't work well in the world we live in.'

We all start out playing naturally as kids; no one needs to teach us how to do it. It is effortless, spontaneous and universal. As we grow older, though, we're often made to feel guilty for playing. Play is seen as a waste of time and, since 'time is money', play is almost like throwing money down the drain. Yet despite these cultural attitudes, a growing body of evidence suggests that play is as fundamental to life as sleep, dreams, pleasure and connection. Play is not simply a frivolous luxury; it's necessary for the development of empathy, social altruism and other behaviours needed to handle stress. It keeps our minds and brains flexible and it helps us to adapt to a changing and unpredictable world.

WHY WE NEED PLAY

Play is part of our evolutionary heritage. It emerged and became more prevalent in warm-blooded animals with larger brains. In fact, the smarter an animal is, the more it plays. Dogs, snow leopards, dolphins, otters, killer whales, grizzly bears, and even ravens and ants, devote time to play. They even have special play signals, such as a relaxed, open-mouthed expression (the 'play face'), that are recognised across species lines.

Why would this be? Evolution favours behaviour that improves a species' chance of surviving and reproducing. On the surface, play appears to be a waste of time – and if there's anything nature doesn't tolerate, it's waste. But scientists now believe that play is 'training for the unexpected': it encourages flexibility and variability in behaviour and adaptation to a changing environment. And in an unpredictable world that presents constant challenges and obstacles, anything that helps a species to adapt will also help it to survive and reproduce.

This may explain the findings of ethologist Robert Fagen, a professor at the University of Alaska, who spent 15 years studying the behaviour of bears in the wild. He discovered that the bears who played the most often throughout their childhood lived longer and healthier lives and thus left more offspring behind.

Other studies of animals suggest that play may directly

contribute to the growth of regions of the brain responsible for motor control, balance and coordination. Professor John Byers, a zoologist at the University of Idaho, found a strong correlation between how often an animal plays and the growth of its cerebellum during childhood. Along the same lines, Canadian neuroscientist Sergio Pellis showed that rats that are deprived of play develop abnormalities in their brains. This research suggests that play is particularly crucial during the period of rapid brain development that occurs during childhood in both animals and adults.

In adults, playfulness is associated with several positive behaviours, such as creativity, productivity, flexibility, optimism, empathy, social altruism and the capacity to handle stress. It encourages cooperation, promotes problem-solving and fosters a sense of community and belonging. Perhaps above all, play helps us to face what play scholar Brian Sutton-Smith refers to as our 'existential dread' – it opens us to possibilities and gives us hope for the future. This may explain why the human drive towards play exists even under horrific circumstances: children continued to play in concentration camps during the Holocaust.

On the other hand, play does diminish when basic needs are unmet, or when children suffer long-term, chronic deprivation or abuse. The absence of play in these situations may have catastrophic consequences. Dr Stuart Brown, a psychiatrist and author of the book *Play: How it Shapes the Brain, Opens the Imagination and Invigorates the Soul*, studied a group of 26 young murderers in the Texas prison system. He found that 90 per cent of the murderers he interviewed had been deprived of play or had major 'play abnormalities' as children. Less than 10 per cent of the non-violent comparison group in the study had suffered play deprivation or abnormalities. In Dr Brown's clinical psychiatry practice, playless lives were characterised by depression, over-control, driven ambition, envy and, eventually, personal breakdown.

HOW TO BRING MORE PLAY
INTO YOUR LIFE

Before we talk about how to bring more play back into our lives, we have to define what it is. It may seem that play is unnecessary – and perhaps even impossible – to define, but having a better understanding of what play is (and isn't) may help us to see more opportunities for cultivating it in all aspects of our lives. According to Dr Brown, play is:

- **Apparently purposeless** Play is done for its own sake, not to achieve a goal.

- **Voluntary** Play is not a requirement or an obligation.

- **Inherently attractive** Play is fun and feels good.

- **Outside time** When fully engaged in play, we lose a sense of the passage of time.

- **Outside self** When fully engaged in play, we become less self-conscious. We don't worry about whether we look good or awkward or stupid.

- **Improvisational** Play is spontaneous and doesn't lock us into a rigid way of doing things.

- **Mildly addictive** Play makes us want to do more of it.

As you can see from this list, play isn't limited to games or sports. Art, music and all forms of creative expression can be play. Cooking a meal for your family can be play. Even work can be play. Conversely, activities that are often considered play may not truly be experienced as play, if they don't meet the criteria above; for example, if you're frustrated, miserable and completely preoccupied with winning during a round of golf or a tennis match, that's not play.

Are video and computer games play?

We live in an era where there seems to be less and less time for play – especially among children. Many young children have a schedule at school that would put a busy CEO to shame, with little time for idle, creative and unstructured play. And parents mourn that their kids don't play the way they themselves used to: spontaneously, out on the street, with whatever neighbourhood kids happened to be around.

One form of play that has increased over the past two decades is playing computer and video games. According to a poll by the Kaiser Foundation, children in the US play an average of eight hours of video games per week, an increase of over 400 per cent from 1999. A staggering 99 per cent of American boys play video games, as do 94 per cent of girls.

Are video games truly play, though? Although they do satisfy many of the criteria of play, they lack the 'interpersonal nuance' that can be achieved only by play that engages all five senses in the three-dimensional world. This doesn't mean that video games should be avoided entirely; in fact, some studies have shown that playing video games can improve coordination, increase social behaviour and promote some kinds of learning. But it does suggest that they shouldn't be the sole means of play in a child's (or adult's) life.

With this in mind, here's a list of tips for encouraging more play in your life:

Look back at your play history Think about the things you loved to do as a child or when you had more play in your life. What got you excited? What gave you the most joy? What activities did you lose yourself in?

Make a list of play activities Using the results of your play history above, make a list of ways you love to play and put it somewhere you will see it every day. It's easy to get wrapped up in the hustle and bustle of life, and sometimes a quick glance at this list will be enough to remind you to do something playful.

Create opportunities for play Play is all about perspective. If you look for chances to play, they're everywhere: throw a ball for a dog, play hide-and-seek with your kids, improvise on the piano, have a board-game night, carry a sketchbook with you or simply go on an aimless walk in the woods.

Embrace 'beginner's mind' In Zen practice, the phrase 'beginner's mind' refers to an attitude of openness, curiosity and humility, and a lack of preconceived notions. This is an excellent mental state to cultivate for play, since fear of looking silly, awkward or unskilled is one of the biggest obstacles to play for adults.

Follow your bliss – but don't mistake play for fun Play can be fun, but it can also be absorbing, challenging and demanding; for example, if you've always dreamed of building your own sailing boat and sailing it on a long journey, much of that process may not be 'fun', but it can still be play.

Make play a priority If you're busy with work, family and other obligations, it can be difficult to find time for play. Schedule time for play just as you schedule time for other necessities in your life. If this seems daunting, start small – perhaps just 30 minutes a week. After you experience the benefits, my guess is that you'll naturally find time for more.

Summary: play

- Think like a child – kids are the experts at play.
- Pick activities that bring you joy – repainting the bathroom may not sound like play, but if it meets the criteria (it feels good, you are fully engaged, you're doing it voluntarily, and so on), then go for it. Remember: one person's work can be another person's idea of play.
- Look for opportunities everywhere to play.

Revive Your Health

CHAPTER 18

Fine-Tuning Your Personal Paleo Diet

Now that you've developed Your Personal Paleo Diet through beneficial changes to your diet and your lifestyle, let's focus on four areas where you can fine-tune your diet even further. You feel great now, but you'll feel (and look) even better once you zero in on personalised answers to these questions:

- **Macronutrient ratios** How much carbohydrate, fat and protein should you eat?

- **Calorie intake and meal frequency, timing and size** How often, and how much, should you eat?

- **High activity level** What changes should athletes and highly active people make?

- **Super-foods** Which foods are highest in essential nutrients? How can you further optimise your health and prevent disease?

Notes for this chapter may be found at ChrisKresser.com/ppcnotes/#ch18

- **Supplementation** Which supplements should you take, and which should you avoid?

MACRONUTRIENT RATIOS

Protein, carbohydrate and fat – macronutrients – are the nutrients that humans consume in the largest quantity and comprise the bulk of our calorific intake. In Step 1 we discussed macronutrient quality: which *types* of fat, protein and carbohydrate are optimal for human health. In this section, we're going to discuss macronutrient ratios: *how much* protein, fat and carbohydrate you should eat, and in what proportion to each other.

Despite the recommendations from mainstream health organisations, nutrition experts and diet gurus to go low fat, low carb or high protein (or some magic combination of all three), the truth is that there's no one-size-fits-all approach when it comes to macronutrient ratios. We share a lot in common as human beings, but we're not robots; we have different genetics, lifestyles, health statuses, activity levels and goals, and all of these factors will influence what an optimal macronutrient ratio is for each of us. And since these factors can change over time (for example, if we develop a chronic illness, or significantly reduce our activity because of an injury, or move to a new climate, or start training for an athletic competition), our own ideal macronutrient ratio can also change over time – and even seasonally throughout the year. The key is to learn how to listen to your own body to determine what it needs, and follow that, rather than jumping from one fashionable diet trend to the next.

For most people, the *quality* of macronutrients that we eat has a much more significant impact on health and well-being than the *quantity* or *ratio*. The fact that hunter-gatherers, free of modern diseases, thrived on a variety of diets, as we've seen throughout this book, and macronutrient ratios supports this idea.

If the low-fat diet gurus are correct, then we'd expect the Inuit and Masai, with their extremely high-fat diets (up to 90 per cent of their calories from fat for the Inuit), to be obese and dropping dead left and right of heart attacks. But if the low-carb gurus are correct, then we'd expect to see a lot of overweight and metabolically dysfunctional Kitavans, whose diet averages 70–90 per cent carbohydrate, or even higher! In fact, we see neither. All of these populations are virtually free of the modern diseases that are killing Westerners in spades every year, such as obesity, diabetes, heart disease and autoimmunity. They also tend to be lean and muscular – without spending hours on the treadmill at the local gym.

What factors determine the ideal macronutrient ratio for you?

Humans can thrive on a wide range of macronutrient ratios. Let's take a closer look at the factors that determine what specific mix of fat, carbohydrates and protein is right for you:

Constitution (genetics, physiology, biology) Modern studies have shown that some people have genes that predispose them to problems metabolising glucose (sugar), whereas others may have genes that make it more likely that they will have problems burning fat. There is still much we don't understand about the contribution of genetics to diet and the relationship between genes and environmental factors.

Season During the summer your body will naturally crave different foods than it does during the winter. It's also true that our ancestors had access to only certain foods at certain times of the year. If they lived in Northern Europe, they weren't eating mangoes from Thailand in the winter.

Geography/climate If you've ever been to the tropics, you've probably found yourself craving lighter foods with a higher water content, such as fruit and vegetables, more than you do at home. Likewise, in cold climates you probably gravitate towards eating more protein and fat-rich foods like meat stews. There's a reason for this.

Health status Have you ever noticed that you crave different foods when you're coming down with a cold or the flu? The body has different needs in different physiological states. Women often crave more carbohydrates during pregnancy, because the developing foetus has a need for glucose, and women naturally become somewhat insulin resistant as a result. People with thyroid problems may suffer on very low-carb diets, because insulin is required for proper thyroid hormone conversion. As people age and become less active, they often find that they need less food than they did when they were younger, or perhaps less of a particular macronutrient.

Activity level A construction worker doing manual labour for eight hours a day or a high-level athlete in training will have different dietary and macronutrient needs than someone who works at a desk. This should go without saying but, amazingly, it is often ignored in the discussion about macronutrients.

Goals If you're training for the next bodybuilding competition, you will very probably eat different foods than an obese person wishing to lose weight.

Before we move on, keep these numbers in mind:

- 1g of carbohydrate has 4 calories
- 1g of protein has 4 calories
- 1g of fat has 9 calories

You'll use these numbers to do some quick maths when you calculate your own ratios. You can use one of the nutrition-counting websites, such as nutritiondata.com, to calculate this for you.

Carbohydrates: starting points for experimentation

The average carbohydrate intake in the US is about 45–65 per cent of total calories. For a moderately active man eating 2,600 calories a day, this works out to between 290g and 420g a day (using the numbers in the box on page 344, that's approximately 1,200–1,700 calories from carbohydrate). For a moderately active woman eating 2,000 calories a day, it's about 225–325g a day (about 900–1,300 calories from carbohydrate). On a typical Paleo diet that includes starchy vegetables, fruit, some dairy products and perhaps white rice (if tolerated), carbohydrate intake tends to range between 15–30 per cent of total calories a day. A low-carbohydrate Paleo diet ranges between 10–15 per cent of total calories as carbohydrate, and a very low-carbohydrate Paleo diet would be anything lower than 10 per cent. On a high-carbohydrate Paleo diet, carbohydrate intake would be somewhere between 30–45 per cent (or higher) of total calories.

We're only counting carbs from starchy plants and fruit. That means if you're eating a meal with meat, broccoli, sweet potatoes and fruit for dessert, to calculate the carb content for that meal you'd only look up sweet potatoes and fruit on nutritiondata.com. There's no difference between starchy carbs and any other carbs.

Carbohydrate quantities on low-carb diets

Paleo diet	Carbohydrates (% of total calories)
Very low carb	<10
Low carb	10–15
Moderate carb	15–30
High carb	30–45+

Although many health experts include non-starchy vegetables (such as green vegetables, carrots, peppers, and so on) when counting carbohydrates, I do not. Although these foods do contain carbohydrates (primarily glucose), they are difficult to break down and our bodies actually expend glucose in the process of digesting them. Therefore, I only count carbohydrates from starchy plants (sweet potatoes, potatoes, taro, yuca, plantains, white rice, buckwheat, and so on), fruit, dairy products and sweeteners.

Ultimately, the only way to determine your optimal macronutrient ratio is to experiment. Most of my patients do best with a standard, moderate-carbohydrate Paleo approach with between 15–30 per cent of total calories of carbohydrate per day, which I'll explain in a moment. First, however, here are some situations that may call for a carbohydrate intake that is either lower or higher than standard:

Low carbohydrate

(10–15 per cent of total calories – roughly 65–100g daily on a 2,600 calorie diet and 50–75g daily on a 2,000 calorie diet.)

- Those who need to lose weight and who have not tried low carb before.

- Anyone with metabolic problems, such as insulin or leptin resistance.

- Those with high blood sugar (hyperglycaemia) or low blood sugar (hypoglycaemia, often seen as reactive hypoglycaemia, which occurs after meals).

- Those with mood disturbances (although mood disturbances can sometimes be helped with higher carbohydrate intake, especially if sleep problems are involved).

Very low carbohydrate

(Less than 10 per cent of total calories – roughly less than 65g daily on a 2,600 calorie diet and less than 50g daily on a 2,000 calorie diet.)

- Those who have significant weight to lose or metabolic issues whose blood sugar responds very poorly to dietary carbohydrate.

- Those with neurological or cognitive problems.

- Those who have tried a low-carbohydrate diet with some success (who may find added benefit from trying a very low-carbohydrate diet).

High carbohydrate

(30–45+ per cent of total calories – roughly 200–300g+ daily on a 2,600 calorie diet and 150–225g+ daily on a 2,000 calorie diet.)

- Those who are highly active or training hard.

- Those who are lean and have trouble maintaining their weight on low-carb diets.

If none of the above applies to you, **begin with a moderate-carbohydrate Paleo diet** (that is, 15–30 per cent of calories from carbohydrate). This amounts to roughly 100–200g per day on a 2,600 calorie diet (400–800 carbohydrate calories) or 75–150g per day on a 2,000 calorie diet (300–600 carbohydrate calories). (See 'High activity level' on pages 359–362 for information on how many calories a day you should aim for if you're exercising regularly.)

Try eating at the lower end of the range for two weeks and then the higher end of the range for the following two weeks. Performing this experiment is valuable, because you'll get a first-hand sense of how changing the ratio of carbs to fat affects you personally, and you can use that information to fine-tune your macronutrient intake right down to the daily, or even hourly, level; for example, I've found that eating fewer carbohydrates helps me to focus mentally. On the other hand, if I eat low carb on a regular basis, my energy flags and I don't sleep well. So I will often eat a relatively low-carb breakfast and lunch, to support mental clarity throughout the day, and a higher-carb dinner, to support sleep and energy levels.

If you have any of the conditions I listed above, try the low-carbohydrate or very low-carbohydrate approach as indicated. But remember: some people on low-carbohydrate diets find more benefit from adding carbohydrates back into their diet, rather than reducing them further. This is where your personal experience should guide you. Pay attention to all of the variables I listed above and adjust your ratios accordingly. As a general rule, as your activity level increases you will want to increase your carbohydrate intake commensurately. If it's wintertime and you're living in a cold climate, you may find that eating extra fat helps keep you warm (although others get that effect from eating more carbohydrate, possibly because of the effects of carbohydrate intake on thyroid hormone). In addition, following very low-carb diets over a long period may adversely affect the gut flora, leading to digestive symptoms like constipation or diarrhoea, halitosis (bad breath), gas, bloating or abdominal pain. If you experience these changes on a very low-carb diet, I'd suggest increasing your intake of fermentable fibre and fermented foods, and/or taking prebiotic and probiotic supplements. See Chapter 10 and the bonus chapter on digestive disorders on my website for more information.

The point is this: you need to experiment. Nobody (including me) can tell you what your ideal ratio is. But by following these basic guidelines and keeping track of your symptoms, you should have no trouble working it out.

When to think twice about a very low-carb diet

There's no doubt that very low-carb diets are beneficial in certain situations; however, in other cases, they may actually be harmful. These include:

Hypothyroidism Some evidence suggests that very low-carb diets may contribute to poor thyroid function. Insulin is required to convert T4, the inactive form of thyroid hormone, into T3, the active form. Insulin levels are chronically low on a very low-carb diet, which in turn can lead to low levels of T3 and hypothyroid symptoms. This doesn't happen for everyone on a very low-carb diet, but I've seen it often in my practice. If you develop cold hands and feet, fatigue, brain fog, hair loss and other symptoms of poor thyroid function while on a very low-carb diet, try increasing your carbohydrate intake until they resolve.

Pregnancy Carbohydrate needs may be slightly higher during pregnancy, due to the growing baby's need for glucose. I've noticed that most pregnant women tend to do better with moderate carbohydrate intake (that is, 15–30 per cent of calories), rather than low carb or very low carb. The exception would be women with type-1 or type-2 diabetes, who may need lower-carb approaches to avoid hyperglycaemia, which can harm the growing baby.

Adrenal fatigue I've found that most of my patients with adrenal fatigue syndrome (described in more detail in the bonus chapter on this subject on my website) don't do well on a very low-carb diet.

Insomnia If you find yourself waking up frequently throughout the night and you're on a very low-carb diet, try increasing your carbohydrate intake slightly. In some cases this single change can resolve the insomnia.

High levels of physical activity If you're highly active and training hard, you're going to be burning a lot more fuel. Although some athletes seem to do well on very low-carb diets, most do better with a significantly higher carbohydrate intake – as high as 50–60 per cent of calories (roughly 325–400g per day on a 2,600 calorie diet and 250–300g on a 2,000 calorie diet) in some cases. See the section below on how to modify your diet if you're highly active for more information.

As always, you'll have to experiment to see what works for you. But if you have hypothyroidism, are pregnant, or are training hard, I'd suggest beginning with a more moderate (that is, 100–200g per day) intake of carbohydrates.

Summary of carbohydrate intake

Goal/population	Carb intake (% of total calories)	Carb intake (g per day on a 2,600 calorie diet)	Carb intake (g per day on a 2,000 calorie diet)
For significant weight loss, where there are severe blood sugar issues, neurological and cognitive problems	<10	<65	<50
For weight loss, blood sugar regulation, and where there are mood disturbances	10–15	65–100	50–75
General health and maintenance	15–30	100–200	75–150
Athletes, people who are highly active and/or lean with a fast metabolism	30–45	200–300	150–225

Protein

Most people naturally eat the right amount of protein for their needs. Protein is such a crucial nutrient that our brain has specific mechanisms that increase our desire for it if we need more and decrease our desire for it if we're getting too much; these mechanisms are difficult to override through conscious willpower alone. For this reason, my general recommendation is to simply eat as much protein as you crave. In most cases, this will be about 10–20 per cent of calories, or roughly 65–130g per day on a 2,600 calorie diet (260–520 protein calories) and 50–100g per day on a 2,000 calorie diet (200–300 protein calories).

This recommended range is supported by observing protein intakes (as a percentage of total calories) in healthy, pre-industrial cultures around the world:

- Masai (Kenya and northern Tanzania): 19 per cent protein

- Kitava (Trobriand Islands, Papua New Guinea): 10 per cent protein

- Tokelau (Pacific island territory of New Zealand): 12 per cent protein

- Inuit (Arctic): 20 per cent protein

- Kuna (Panama): 12 per cent protein

Interestingly, it's also supported by what is consumed in the US, where the average protein intake is 15 per cent of calories. (As a comparison for another Western country, in Sweden it is 12 per cent.)

It's rarely a good idea to decrease protein intake to below 10 per cent of total calories. However, there are some situations where it may be advantageous to increase protein intake to 20–30 per cent, or even as high as 35 per cent, of total calories (that is, 100–175g per day on a 2,000 calorie diet) – at least for a temporary period:

Weight loss Protein is one of the most satiating (that is, satisfying) macronutrients, and higher-protein diets can spontaneously reduce appetite and calorie intake, and increase metabolic rate, all of which contribute to weight loss.

Blood sugar problems Higher protein intakes tend to have a stabilising effect on blood sugar – whether it's high or low.

Muscle mass Protein is the nutrient required to build and rebuild muscle. Those who want to add or maintain muscle mass (for example, endurance athletes, weightlifters, the elderly or the chronically ill) should consume more protein.

Why stop at 35 per cent? Studies suggest that the ability of humans to metabolise protein tops out at 35 per cent of total calories. The body releases nitrogen in the process of metabolising protein. Nitrogen forms toxic ammonia, which is then converted to urea, a safe, non-toxic compound. But conversion of ammonia to urea is limited when protein intake exceeds 35 per cent of calories. Eating more protein than this for an extended period can lead to a toxic build-up of ammonia in the body, which may have serious consequences (including nausea, diarrhoea and death) if protein intake exceeds 45 per cent of total calories consumed.

This threshold may be significantly lower in pregnant women. During pregnancy, the conversion of ammonia to urea appears to peak at a protein intake of 25 per cent of total calories. Some studies suggest that protein intakes above this level may lead to poor pregnancy outcomes, such as decreased birth weight and increased risk of disease and death for the baby. For these reasons, I recommend that pregnant women limit protein intake to 15–20 per cent of calories, regardless of whether they are overweight or have a blood sugar problem.

There is some research surrounding protein restriction and longevity. To read more about these studies and the link between protein intake and increased lifespan, please visit my website.

Summary of protein intake

Goal/population	Protein intake (% of total calories)	Protein intake (g per day on a 2,600 calorie diet)	Protein intake (g per day on a 2,000 calorie diet)
Pregnancy	10–15	65–100	50–75
General health	10–20	65–130	50–100
For weight loss, blood sugar regulation and to gain muscle mass	20–35*	130–230	100–175

*Once weight loss, blood sugar regulation and muscle gain goals have been reached, I suggest decreasing protein intake into the 'general health' range listed above, or perhaps slightly higher (that is, 25 per cent).

Fat

Once you've determined your optimal carbohydrate and protein intakes, the remainder of your calories will come from fat. This can range from as high as 80–85 per cent on a very low-carb, relatively low-protein diet, to as low as 10–15 per cent on a high-protein, high-carb diet. Fortunately, as I mentioned above, studies of traditional diets indicate that humans can thrive and remain free of modern disease on a wide range of fat intakes – provided it's the right mix of fats (that is, mostly saturated and monounsaturated with a much smaller amount of polyunsaturated fat).

CALORIE INTAKE AND MEAL FREQUENCY, TIMING AND SIZE

It's not just what we eat that affects our health, but how much and how often, although I don't think it's necessary for most people to count calories. Once you determine Your Personal Paleo Diet and identify your optimal mix of protein, carbohydrate and fat, you should simply eat to satisfy your appetite.

What if you're trying to lose weight? Although it's true that eating fewer calories will lead to weight loss, it's also true that consciously restricting calories often fails as a weight-loss strategy. See Chapter 20, page 391, where I outline a basic weight-loss strategy, and also look at the bonus chapter on weight loss on my website where I introduce an approach that leads to a spontaneous reduction (without voluntary or conscious effort) in calorie intake. But also bear in mind that the basic 30-Day Reset Diet will lead to weight loss in the vast majority of cases.

Meal frequency and size are more variable. You'll hear some people claim that we should eat only one huge meal at night and fast for the entire day. Others will suggest eating six small meals throughout the day. And then you have the conventional approach of three square meals a day.

What about snacking? Again, some insist that snacking between meals will make you fat and should be strictly avoided. Others say there's no problem with snacking as long as you're eating the right kind of foods.

My experience tells me that everybody (and every body!) is different. Some people do better with smaller meals spaced more frequently throughout the day (and/or snacking between meals) and others will do better with larger meals eaten less frequently with no snacks. The key, as always, is to choose an approach based on your health status and goals and to experiment and see what works for you.

With this in mind, I can give you some general guidelines:

If you're trying to lose weight or have high blood sugar, insulin resistance or diabetes, you'll probably have more success by not snacking between meals. Avoiding snacks may have a beneficial effect on the hormones that regulate fat storage. Some people with digestive problems also feel better when they don't snack, because it gives their digestive system a chance to rest between meals.

If you have low blood sugar, you'll likely feel better eating small meals every two to three hours throughout the day. This can prevent your blood sugar from dropping too low which can lead to symptoms like lightheadedness, agitation, brain fog and sugar cravings. And although some people with digestive problems do better when they don't snack, others do better eating frequent, small meals, because they can't tolerate large amounts of food at one sitting. (See how individual this is?)

If you're generally healthy, are not overweight and don't have blood sugar or immune problems, then three meals a day, with or without snacks (depending on your appetite), is a good approach. You may want to experiment with the other strategies above just to see if they make you feel better, but they're not necessary.

If you're fighting a chronic infection or have a weak immune system, are trying to optimise longevity, are overweight, or have high blood sugar and metabolic problems, you may find that restricting your food intake to an eight-hour window each day ('intermittent fasting') is helpful. See the section below for details.

Intermittent fasting

Intermittent fasting is a pattern of eating that alternates between periods of fasting and non-fasting. Studies suggest that intermittent fasting may be as effective (and easier to stick to) than voluntary calorie restricting for weight loss. It has also been shown to improve insulin sensitivity and other indicators of metabolic function, reduce inflammation and oxidative stress, decrease seizures, protect brain cells and promote healthy brain function.

There are several theories about why intermittent fasting provides health benefits. One is that intermittent fasting causes positive stress. As you may recall from Chapter 14, not all stress is harmful; when cells in the body are under mild stress, they adapt by enhancing their own ability to fight that stress and protect against disease. Another related theory is that intermittent fasting promotes a cellular clean-up and repair process called autophagy, which may protect against degeneration of brain cells, infections and cancer.

There are many ways to do intermittent fasting, but the method that I recommend involves restricting your food intake to an eight-hour window each day; for example, you would eat only between the hours of 12.00pm and 8.00pm. During the fasting period, you may have some coconut oil (by itself, or perhaps added to coffee – don't knock it until you try it!) if you feel hungry or 'spaced out'. This will not interfere with the benefits of the fast. During the feeding period, you simply eat as your hunger dictates: there's no need to purposely restrict calorie intake, nor should you try to overeat to make up for the meal you skipped. You might have two meals only, two meals and a snack, or three meals. If you're trying to aggressively lose weight or you have very high blood sugar, eating two meals without a snack in between is probably the best strategy – but since you're already getting the benefits of a 16-hour fast, snacking during the feeding window of an intermittent fast is less likely to impede your progress than it is while eating normally.

If you do well with the method I've described above and you want to benefit further from fasting, you can add an extended (40-hour) fast once or twice a month (or as often as once a week, if you're highly motivated). This involves fasting for an additional 24-hour period above and beyond your daily 16-hour fast; for example, on Tuesday you would eat between 12.00 and 8.00pm as usual, but instead of your next meal coming at midday on Wednesday, it would be midday on Thursday.

On the other hand, you might discover that intermittent fasting every day is too much for you, but doing it three to four days a week is just right. This is what I find myself doing most of the time. I will typically skip breakfast about four days a week and then eat normally on the other three days. I don't plan in advance; I let my schedule and my body tell me what to do. If I wake up feeling very hungry and I have a long and active day ahead, I will probably eat breakfast. If I wake up feeling less hungry and/or I have a less active day, I might skip breakfast. (I'm aware of the research surrounding the link between skipping breakfast and overeating at lunch, but I am doing this in the context of intermittent fasting and what works for me; you should do the same.) The point is that there's no right or wrong way to do this – there's just the way that works best for your needs and goals.

Although intermittent fasting is a good approach for many people, there are some situations where I don't recommend it:

- **Pregnancy** Although occasional intermittent fast days may be fine for some women during pregnancy (be sure to check with your doctor first), I don't recommend 16-hour fasts daily, nor do I recommend extended 40-hour fasts.

- **Adrenal fatigue** In my clinical experience, intermittent fasting often worsens adrenal fatigue conditions. These patients usually do better with several small meals throughout the day, or with three normal meals and snacks in between. See Chapter 20 for more on adrenal fatigue syndrome.

- **Hypothyroidism** Although there's some evidence that suggests intermittent fasting can be helpful for hypothyroidism, most of my patients with this condition do better eating regular meals.

- **Eating disorders** If you have a history of anorexia, bulimia or any other eating disorder, please check with your health-care provider before embarking on an intermittent fasting programme.

- **Kids** Growing children and young adults need to eat regular meals for physical and cognitive 'fuel' and shouldn't go for long stretches without healthy foods.

High activity level

I often see patients who are competitive athletes, CrossFit enthusiasts (CrossFit is a popular strength-conditioning programme in the US which is just taking off in the UK and Australia), or just very active physically and suffering from fatigue, hair loss, low libido and other problems. Almost inevitably they are on a low-carb diet. Back in the 1980s, fat phobia was the norm. Athletes who wanted to stay lean and competitive adopted the low-fat dogma just as most other health-conscious people did. Unfortunately, many found that dramatically restricting fat intake – particularly healthy traditional fats like butter, coconut oil and lard – had a negative impact on their health. Rates of obesity, metabolic disease and other problems continued to rise as unsuspecting people trying to do the right thing switched their steak-and-eggs breakfast for cold cereal, dry wheat toast and orange juice. Then in the mid-1990s, the pendulum swung back in the other direction, as people realised the folly of avoiding dietary fat and the perils of processed carbohydrate. Suddenly, low-carb diets were all the rage and the athletic community, which is often at the forefront of nutritional changes, began to shun all carbohydrates (not just processed, refined carbs) with the same zeal with which it had previously shunned fat.

Although some people are able to thrive for long periods, and even indefinitely, on a very low-carb diet, serious competitive athletes, martial artists, cyclists, runners, boxers and high-intensity trainers almost always begin to experience problems when they dramatically restrict carbohydrate. Why? Because intense physical activity is dependent on a steady supply of glucose to replace the muscle glycogen that would otherwise be depleted during glucose-dependent activity. And studies have consistently shown that low-carbohydrate diets are not capable of maintaining optimal glycogen levels during intense exercise.

Lack of carbohydrate during this type of exercise causes glycogen depletion, which in turn leaves muscles unable to get the glucose they need to produce ATP (adenosine triphosphate), the fundamental energy unit of the cell. Glycogen depletion can be a good thing in certain circumstances – such as when you have diabetes or are trying to lose weight. But this is another example of the no-one-size-fits-all approach and the key principle behind the Personal Paleo Diet. Just because something is appropriate for treating a disease or a specific problem, that doesn't mean it's appropriate for healthy people, and it especially doesn't mean it's appropriate for serious athletes.

It's interesting to note that very low-carb diets (under 10 per cent of calories) never caught on among professional athletes whose livelihoods depended on consistently high performance. And although very low-carb diets were adopted by top-flight bodybuilders for a period of time, the trend has recently switched back in the other direction. A recent article in *Muscle Development* magazine chronicled this change, pointing out that Jay Cutler and Branch Warren, the number-one and number-two finishers in the 2009 Mr Olympia, ate 700g and 1,000g of carbohydrate per day respectively! I'd say that's a pretty far cry from a low-carb diet.

Here's the bottom line: very low-carb diets are usually not a good idea for people who regularly perform strenuous exercise. That said, in keeping with the principle of this programme, I don't want you to take my word for this. I want you to experiment and see what is true for you. Even the best theories are useless if they don't produce practical results. I'd recommend 25 per cent of calories as carbohydrate as an absolute minimum for anyone doing frequent, intense exercise. If you're training at a very high level, you may need much more than this. Keep in mind that the Mr Olympia bodybuilders got up to 700g and 1,000g per day, which accounted for 50–60 per cent of total calorie intake. Granted, few people are competing at that level and few people will need that much, but I mention it simply to illustrate the range.

Another important consideration when you're highly active is making sure you're eating enough overall. I often see patients in my practice that are doing intense physical activity but are simply not eating enough calories to sustain their activity level. This is a great formula for fat loss, but once your body fat reaches a low level, muscle will be broken down in order to provide the fuel your body needs to function properly.

With all of this in mind, here are some guidelines for highly active people (that is, training at least three to five times a week at moderate-to-high intensity), broken down into three goals: fat loss, maintenance or muscle gain.

Guidelines for highly active people

Goal	Carbohydrate* (% of total calories)	Calories (per lb of bodyweight)	Protein (g per lb of bodyweight)
For fat loss	7–20	15–16	0.8–1.0
Maintenance	25–60	17–18	0.8–1.0
For muscle gain	25–60	19–21	1.0–1.25

*Remember: when I refer to a number of grams of carbohydrates, I'm only referring to carbs from starchy vegetables, dairy products and fruit, not non-starchy vegetables such as broccoli or carrots.

Let's look at two examples of how this might work out in practice:

1 An 8 stone 13lb (56.7kg) lean female cyclist wants to increase muscle mass and performance. At 20 calories per pound (450g) of body weight, she'll require 2,500 calories a day to meet her goal. She should eat 125–156g of protein per day (20–25 per cent of total calories on her 2,500 calorie diet) and between 156–375g of carbohydrate per day (25–60 per cent of total calories), depending on her activity level and individual preference/tolerance to carbs.

2 A 16 stone 6lb (104kg) male athlete wants to lose 1 stone 11lb (11.3kg) and lean out. At 15 calories per pound (450g) of body weight, his target calorie intake will be 3,450 per day. He should eat 184–230g of protein per day (21–27 per cent of total calories on his 3,450 calorie diet) and between 60 and 170g of carbohydrate (7–20 per cent of total calories), depending on activity level and individual preference/tolerance to carbs.

Carbohydrate timing

In addition to matching your overall carbohydrate intake with your activity level and goals, eating your carbs at specific times may provide additional benefit. After a workout is an ideal time to eat more carbohydrates, and carbohydrate intake should be higher on workout days than on non-workout days. This will help with recovery and preserving (or adding) muscle mass, if that's your goal.

Some recent studies suggest that eating the majority (that is, 60–80 per cent) of your carbohydrates at dinner leads to hormonal changes that promote fat loss and improve metabolic function; however, this can be difficult to do if you're eating a large amount of carbohydrate. For example, if you're eating

300g of carbohydrate a day and you aim to eat 60 per cent at dinner, you'd have to eat three large baked potatoes! In practice, if you aim to eat a larger percentage of your carbohydrates after workouts, on workout days and in the later part of the day, you'll get most of the benefit of carbohydrate timing.

SUPER-FOODS

You hear a lot these days about 'super-foods' that promise to boost vitality, improve mood, increase libido, burn fat, lengthen your life and turn you into a millionaire. OK, perhaps they don't make that last claim, but just about. I'm talking about protein powders, green drinks, energy bars, sports goo, bee pollen, maca root, acai berries and all kinds of other stuff you've probably never heard of, or if you have heard of it, you probably have no idea what it is.

In some cases I think these products make legitimate claims. Maca root does have a history of medicinal use (primarily to increase libido and improve sperm quality) in South America, where it is native; however, it contains glucosinolates, which, in combination with a diet low in iodine, can cause thyroid problems. It suppresses the function of the thyroid gland by interfering with iodine uptake, possibly leading to the development of a swelling of the thyroid gland called a goitre.

This single example highlights one of the problems I have with most so-called 'super-foods'. In general, they are at least one of the following:

- Powerful botanicals (herbal medicine) that can cause potentially serious side effects and complications when used improperly.

- Highly processed and refined isolated nutrients that don't share the beneficial qualities of the whole food they were extracted from (protein powder falls into this category, in my opinion).

- Surrounded by misinformation and misconceptions; for example, vegetarians and vegans have been led to believe that spirulina and brewer's yeast contain vitamin B_{12}, a nutrient that both populations are often deficient in. But spirulina and brewer's yeast contain B_{12} analogues called cobamides, which actually block the uptake and absorption of true B_{12}.

You might not be surprised, then, to learn that I'm not generally a fan of these super-foods. Some of them, such as protein powder and spirulina, probably won't hurt when used in moderate amounts in the context of an overall nutrient-dense diet. This is especially true for bodybuilders who are trying to put on significant amounts of muscle and are having trouble getting enough protein in their diets. However, I am a big fan of nature's own super-foods and I believe they should be incorporated into every diet.

Another way of thinking of them is as nature's multi-vitamins. These are the foods that are densely packed with micronutrients that fuel all of our cellular machinery, keeping us healthy and strong. I've mentioned these foods and their benefits throughout this book, but here's an all-in-one listing.

- Organ meats (nutrient dense)
- Eggs (including the yolk with its essential micronutrients)
- Cold-water, oily fish (salmon, mackerel, sardines, herring)
- Traditional fats (such as ghee, butter and duck fat)
- Pastured, full-fat dairy (preferably raw)
- Bone broths (rich in all-important glycine)
- Tougher cuts of meat, skin and cartilage (for the same reasons as bone broth)

- Dark, leafy greens (kale, spring greens, spinach, rocket, mustard greens and more)

- Fermented foods (vegetables, dairy and beverages, such as kombucha)

- Seaweed (loaded with minerals and nutrients that are difficult to obtain elsewhere in the diet)

SUPPLEMENT WISELY

The best way to obtain nutrients is from food. That's how we're naturally adapted to getting them. Most nutrients require enzymes, synergistic co-factors and organic mineral-activators to be properly absorbed. Although these are naturally present in foods, they are often not included in synthetic vitamins with isolated nutrients.

That said, no matter how well we eat, some nutrients are difficult to obtain in significant quantities from food alone; for example, magnesium is found in many foods, but as soil quality has declined over the past several decades, so have magnesium levels in fresh produce. And with the exception of cold-water, oily fish, food has never been a primary source of vitamin D; our ancestors produced it from exposure to sunlight. In addition, our modern eating habits impact our consumption of valuable nutrients. Vitamin A (retinol) is only present in high amounts in organ meats, which our Palaeolithic ancestors and many traditional cultures considered superior to muscle meats (which they are, from a nutritional perspective); however, organ meats have fallen out of favour and few people eat them today.

The chart on pages 366–367 lists the nutrients that are not abundant even in a 'typical' Paleo diet that doesn't include organ meats, fish liver oils, seaweed and grass-fed dairy, along with my recommendations for how to obtain them (from either special foods or supplements). Please see the website for a bonus chapter on supplementation with more detailed information about these nutrients, including quizzes to help you determine which of them you may need to supplement. I also include specific, up-to-date brand recommendations for the supplements listed below.

Recommended supplements

Nutrient	Recommendation
Vitamin A	10,000–15,000iu per day. Best obtained from ½–1 teaspoon per day of high-vitamin cod liver oil.
Vitamin D	It is difficult to make a blanket recommendation for vitamin D, because the optimal dose for a given individual depends on so many factors. That said, ½–1 teaspoon per day of high-vitamin cod liver oil is often sufficient to meet vitamin D needs and it's an excellent choice since it also contains vitamin A, which works synergistically with vitamin D.
Magnesium	Most people following a Western diet are deficient in magnesium and most benefit from supplementing it, because it's difficult to obtain from food. I suggest a dose of 300–500mg per day in either malate or glycinate form.
Vitamin K_2	Vitamin K_2 improves bone health and protects against cardiovascular disease, among other benefits. Many people don't get enough of this important vitamin. You can meet vitamin K_2 needs by eating foods that are rich in it, such as natto, eggs and cheese from grass-fed animals and fermented foods. See Chapter 9 for a complete list. If you don't eat these foods, if you have low bone density, or if you are at risk of or have cardiovascular disease, I suggest taking 100–1,000mcg per day of vitamin K_2 in MK-7 or MK-4 form. Doses as high as 45mg per day have been used for osteoporosis, and vitamin K_2 appears to be safe and well tolerated even at that amount.

Nutrient	Recommendation
Iodine	Iodine is another important nutrient that can be difficult to obtain even in the context of a healthy diet. I suggest getting iodine from seaweed (kelp, kombu, wakame, hijiki, arame, dulse), fish (especially cod, prawns and tuna) and dairy products, if you tolerate them. See the bonus chapter on thyroid disorders on the website for a chart of iodine-rich foods. If these foods aren't an option for you, you should supplement iodine at a dose of 800mcg per day. Kelp tablets are a good option.
Selenium	Selenium plays an important role in thyroid and immune health. Most people get enough selenium from food, but people with thyroid or immune-related issues may benefit from supplementation. The recommended dose is 200mcg per day. This can be obtained by taking a selenium supplement, or by eating 2–3 Brazil nuts per day. See the bonus chapter on thyroid disorders on the website for a chart of selenium-rich foods.
Vitamin C	A nutrient-dense Paleo diet with a wide spectrum of fruits and vegetables should provide sufficient levels of vitamin C. However, vitamin C deficiency is common: 34 per cent of men and 27 per cent of women don't get enough. If you're dealing with a chronic health challenge, fighting an infection, or just need immune support, I suggest supplementing 500–1,000mg per day of vitamin C. The liposomal form is best.

Five nutrients to be cautious with

We've talked about the four micronutrients I generally recommend supplementing – via either super-foods such as cod liver oil or supplements – as well as other micronutrients people with specific health conditions or goals may also wish to supplement. But there are some micronutrients that I don't recommend, unless you have a specific reason to do so: iron, calcium, vitamin E, beta-carotene and folic acid.

1 Iron is essential for life, but too much iron causes inflammation and oxidative damage; excess iron can cause everything from blood sugar problems, to depression, to fatigue, to hypogonadism and hormonal imbalance.

2 Calcium is popular as a preventive measure against osteoporosis, but the newest research shows that calcium supplements don't reduce fracture rates in older women and may even increase the risk of hip fractures. Studies on the relationship between cardiovascular disease and calcium suggest that dietary intake of calcium protects against heart disease, but supplementation my increase the risk.

3 Vitamin E (alpha-tocopherol) Some authorities recommend supplementing vitamin E to protect against heart disease, but studies show no real benefit and some have demonstrated potential harm.

4 Beta-carotene can be converted into retinol (the active form of vitamin A) but it can also be converted into potentially harmful substances that increase the risk of oxidative damage and interfere with active vitamin A metabolism.

5 Folic acid By this, I mean the synthetic compound used in dietary supplements and food fortification; folate refers to the forms of the vitamin found in food and in natural folate supplements such as 5-methyl-tetrahydrofolate (5-MTHF). Folic acid can be converted to folate, but this conversion is limited in humans. High levels of unmetabolised folic acid in the blood can mask B_{12} deficiency, speed the progression of certain cancers and depress immune function. Natural folate supplements such as 5-MTHF do not have these effects, and should be used instead of folic acid for protecting against neural-tube defects during pregnancy and in other situations where additional folate is indicated. See the bonus chapter on supplementation on the website for more on this topic.

For more information on why to exercise caution with these micronutrients, please visit ChrisKresser.com/PPC.

CHAPTER 19

'Lifehacking' Your Personal Paleo Diet

In the US the word 'lifehacking' is used to describe any trick, shortcut or skill to get things done. Here are some final strategies for integrating Your Personal Paleo Diet into your life. Think of these techniques as ways to 'hack' your diet and lifestyle changes – and therefore to make them sustainable for years to come. You'll also find some information and support on what to do when you're not having as much success as you'd hoped.

STAYING FLEXIBLE: THE 80/20 RULE

There's no doubt in my mind that optimal nutrition is the key to health. Yet, as you know from working through Step 2 (and as I've said all along), there's more to health – and to life – than food. As you also learned in Step 2, social connection is

Notes for this chapter may be found at ChrisKresser.com/ppcnotes/#ch19

a fundamental human need. Extreme dietary restriction can lead to social isolation, which in turn can cause illness and disease. I'd like to tell you a story that illustrates this.

When I began my medical studies, I interned for a holistic physician who specialised in treating people with chronic illnesses. We had a patient – I'll call him Sam – who was only 24 years old but very sick. He was skinny as a rail, with dark circles under his eyes, severe fatigue, terrible digestion, depression, skin problems, a dysfunctional immune system and several other problems.

Both the doctor I was working with and Sam were convinced his problems were food-related, so he was on a very restrictive diet, but he just kept getting worse. The worse he felt, the more foods he removed from his diet. At one point Sam was eating only steamed broccoli, quinoa and lamb. That's it – nothing else. He stopped coming in for treatment after a while and we lost track of him, but about six months later he returned for a visit. He looked like a different person. He had gained about 2 stone 2lb (13.6kg), his colour was good, digestion improved, mood lifted, skin clear. It was an incredible transformation.

The doctor and I were of course keen to know what had happened. We asked him, 'Was it diet?'

Sam said, 'Yep.'

'Well, which diet?' we asked. 'The candida diet? Macrobiotics?' (This was 15 years ago and I didn't know about the Paleo diet yet!) He shook his head at each question we asked. Finally, we said, 'Tell us what it was then!'

And here's what he told us: 'It was the beer and pizza diet.'

Sam made sure he went out to eat beer and pizza with his friends twice a week, and the rest of the week he ate a fairly healthy diet of the foods he liked.

Previously, during his period of increasing food restriction, he had become more and more socially isolated. He couldn't eat out with friends. His girlfriend broke up with him because he never wanted to leave the house, eat out or travel anywhere for fear of being exposed to 'toxic foods'. And the more socially isolated he was, the more depressed he became. At some point he decided that life really wasn't worth living the way he was living it.

Therefore, he didn't have anything to lose by abandoning his rigid diet and focusing instead on having fun, connecting with his friends and eating the foods that brought him pleasure. It only took a few months of that to completely change his life. His health improved, he had friends again, he started a new relationship and he shifted to a new job that suited him much better than the old one.

I hope you understand that I'm not suggesting you go out and eat beer and pizza twice a week. That's not the point. The point of this story is that there's more to life than food, and that social engagement and pleasure are very important to health. There's a saying in Chinese medicine – the oldest continuous medical tradition in the world – that reflects this point: 'It's better to eat the wrong food with the right attitude than the right food with the wrong attitude.'

This is why I advise most people to follow something I call the '80/20 rule'. It suggests that 80 per cent of the time you should follow the guidelines I've outlined in this book closely and 20 per cent of the time you're free to loosen up and just eat what you want to eat. That might mean having beer and pizza once a week for you (although gluten-free pizza and beer would probably be a better choice). Or it might mean going out for ice cream with your kids on Saturday nights. Or perhaps it means grabbing something quick that isn't 100 per cent Paleo when you're close to missing your flight.

In reality, most of my patients feel so much better when they follow their Personal Paleo Diet that the 80/20 rule becomes something more like the 95/5 rule, or the 90/10 rule. Often the foods they thought they'd miss so much when they first started (like beer and pizza!) are no longer as appealing as they once were, or perhaps the pleasure of eating them isn't worth the price that's paid the following day. The point of the 80/20 rule isn't the exact ratio; that's for you to determine, based on your particular health circumstances, preference and goals. Instead, the purpose of the 80/20 rule is to make your approach to nutrition more flexible and adaptable, so that it simply becomes the way you eat rather than a 'diet' that you follow.

This is one reason why on my US site I refer to Paleo as a code rather than a diet, and I don't refer to eating non-Paleo foods as 'cheating'. Conceptualising Paleo as a 'diet' that you 'cheat' on almost inevitably leads to either additional stress (from struggling to perfectly adhere to the diet), or a yo-yo relationship with food. For example, before they started working with me, some of my patients had a history of doing 30-Day Resets interspersed with periods of almost complete return to poor eating habits. Instead of transitioning to a more flexible approach after the 30-Day Reset, they tried to adhere to guidelines that were unnecessarily strict for them, which was unstainable.

There may be something fundamental about human psychology at work here. I've noticed – and perhaps you have too – that most people don't like to be told what to do. This is true even when they're the ones telling themselves what to do! If you say to yourself, 'You can never eat ice cream again', that can create a dynamic where you eat ice cream just to set yourself free of that sense of overbearing control. The choice is often not completely conscious and may have little to do with actually craving that food. But what if you say, 'I can have ice cream occasionally if I feel like it, but I choose not to eat it every day because I don't feel good when I do'? That shifts the dynamic. It's no longer about autonomy and control; it's about what makes you feel healthy and vibrant.

Unfortunately, the 80/20 rule doesn't always apply to those dealing with serious health challenges or allergies, or intolerances to specific foods. It's never a good idea for someone with gluten intolerance or coeliac disease, for example, to throw caution to the wind and eat half a loaf of wheat bread. That could trigger an immune reaction lasting up to several weeks. Those who are allergic to certain foods or nutrients will have to avoid them 100 per cent of the time, but they may employ the 80/20 rule for other foods that aren't part of their Personal Paleo Diet, but won't cause serious harm. Those with serious, chronic illness may be better off with a 90/10 or a 95/5 rule and still avoid the most serious potential offenders, such as gluten, refined sugar, or whatever it is that triggers a negative reaction. After all, the point of the 80/20 rule isn't to hurt yourself; it's to make you feel good.

TIPS FOR EATING IN RESTAURANTS

One of the biggest challenges to adopting a Paleo-type diet, especially at the start, is what to do when you're eating in a restaurant or travelling and trying to find good food. Enjoying a meal away from home should be a pleasurable and low-stress experience. Here are some ideas for how to make sure that it is:

- If you're eating out with friends, take control (in a friendly, helpful way!) and suggest a restaurant that you've researched and you know will be safe for you – and enjoyable for everyone else.

- If you don't have control of where you're eating, go online and check out the menu so that you aren't surprised when you get there. Call ahead and see if they can accommodate special requests, or if they have special gluten-free options that may not be listed on the menu.

- If you're in an unfamiliar city, ask the reception desk at your hotel, or friends, family and colleagues familiar with that city, for suggestions. If you use it, social media can be a big help. Whenever I'm in a city I don't know well, I'll write a quick tweet asking for restaurant recommendations, and I always get great responses.

- Search Google using keywords like 'local', 'foodie', 'gluten-free', 'grass-fed', 'organic', or 'pasture-raised' together with 'restaurants'. Those searches usually turn-up some good prospects, including places that will often feature locally grown produce and meats, and wild fish. At such establishments, the waiting staff is also more likely to know what's in the food and more willing (and accustomed) to accommodate special requests.

- Use online review sites like Yelp, Chowhound, TripAdvisor and Urbanspoon to read legitimate reviews of restaurants from people like you.

- Don't show up starving at a restaurant. That's a really good way to put yourself in a situation where you are likely to make bad choices (the 80/20 rule notwithstanding). Eat a healthy snack before you leave for the restaurant, especially if it's a place that won't have much that you can eat.

- Be a pain in the butt. When you go out to restaurants, don't be afraid to be the person who asks the waiter a million questions. Yes, they might think you're a pain, and it might be a little embarrassing if you're out on a date. But think of it this way: you'll probably never see the waiter again, and if your date is really annoyed by your food intolerances, is that someone you want to spend a lot of time with? If you're gluten intolerant, always ask if there is gluten in a dish you're ordering, even when it seems like there isn't. Restaurants use hidden ingredients all the time. And if the waiter seems not to know, insist that they ask the chef.

- Avoid sauces. Sauces are likely to contain sugar, gluten, soya and other ingredients you're trying to avoid. That's why eating out at Thai and Chinese places can be a bit of a challenge. If you're doing that as part of your 80/20 allowance, that's fine. But otherwise, it's best to stick with grilled, steamed or roasted meats, steamed or baked vegetables and simple starches such as potatoes or white rice. They're less likely to have sauces – and you can ask for them as a side dish.

- Ask for the dressing separately. Salad dressings, like sauces, often have a lot of undesirable ingredients in them. In particular, they tend to contain industrial seed oils. If you order a salad at a restaurant, which is otherwise a safe choice, ask for some olive oil and balsamic vinegar instead of the dressing that comes with it.

The charts below list some considerations for the different foods and types of cuisines you're likely to encounter when you eat out.

Accompaniments to choose or be careful of

Food	Follow Your Personal Paleo Diet
Meat, fish, poultry	Try to avoid sauces, because they often contain industrial seed oils, gluten, soya and/or sugar; grilled, steamed or poached are usually the safest cooking methods
White rice	If you tolerate white rice, many Asian restaurants can serve a simple dish with meat, vegetables and white rice
Vegetables	Be careful with sauces, which may contain undesirable ingredients
Starchy plants	Baked or boiled new potatoes are a good choice and are available in steakhouses and other restaurants
Salad	A salad with fish, beef or chicken is available in some form at most restaurants; if in doubt about the dressing, ask for oil and vinegar instead

Which foods to choose from different cuisines

Type of cuisine	Follow Your Personal Paleo Diet
Mexican	Order a tostada and don't eat the tortilla, or a fish/chicken/beef plate with rice, vegetables, salsa and guacamole
Chinese/Thai/ Korean/ Vietnamese	Meat/fish, rice, vegetables or rice noodle soups with meat, fish and vegetables; be careful with sauces
Japanese/sushi	Bring your own wheat-free tamari to the restaurant and avoid soya sauce
Italian	Italian food is one of the most challenging types of cuisine, because of its heavy focus on pasta and bread. Choose a fish or meat dish with a vegetable or salad and be careful of cross-contamination with gluten
Indian	Somewhat difficult because of sauces, but tandoori meat with rice and a vegetable curry might work; ask about gluten in food/sauces
Continental	Often the safest choice; order grilled meat, vegetables, potato and/or salad
Seafood	A good choice. Order fish, vegetables or salad and potato

SMART SNACKING

Most typical snack foods – including so-called 'healthy snacks', such as energy or granola bars, not to mention all the 'healthy whole-grain' foods that jam the supermarket aisles, washed down with 'energy drinks' and 'juice beverages' that are loaded with added sugars – are loaded with ingredients that you've eliminated from your diet. Fortunately, you can avoid eating those foods if you follow some simple advice:

Plan ahead Most people slip up because they haven't planned ahead. They get in the car and head out (whether it's a few hours of local errands or on a longer road journey) only to realise they're starving three hours later and have forgotten to bring any food. They're stuck in a shopping centre or on a motorway and the only choices are fast-food eating places or the petrol station shop or motorway services. Avoid this by referring to the chart on page 379 and stocking up on some safe travel foods, whether you'll be gone for a few hours or a few weeks.

Make big batches of snacks Let's say you're going to soak and dehydrate some nuts to eat. Instead of doing just a few servings, why not do 900g? That way you'll have nuts to hand for a couple of weeks – and they're one of the quickest and easiest snack foods available.

Eat before you go If possible, eat a substantial meal before you leave the house for an extended period. If you're starving when you leave the house and you only brought a small snack, it's more likely that you'll end up eating something you'll regret while you're out.

The following is a list of foods that are great for snacking and travel. See my website for a printable version of this chart.

Snacks

Food	Follow Your Personal Paleo Diet
Grass-fed beef jerky	Buy soya/gluten/sugar-free varieties locally or online
Prepared meats	Salami, pepperoni and other prepared meats, preferably grass-fed
Smoked salmon	Make sure it's soya-free
Nuts and seeds	Soaked and dehydrated to improve digestibility and absorption
Raw vegetables or fruit with nut butter	Macadamia, almond and hazelnut butter are best
Cheese	If you tolerate dairy products
Hard-boiled eggs	Eat with cherry tomatoes and avocados for a hearty snack
Kale crisps	See recipe on page 445
Plantain/taro/sweet potato crisps	Thinly slice and roast at 200°C/Gas 6 in duck fat or lard for 10–13 minutes until crisp
Fruit smoothie	Make with coconut milk, almond milk, kefir or yoghurt as a base, depending on your preference or tolerance
Olives	Eat with nuts, cheese or prepared meats
Thinly sliced leftover meat	Enjoy with mustard or Paleo mayonnaise (see page 450 for recipe)
Canned salmon or tuna	Eat with avocado or shredded lettuce
Lettuce wraps	Make with leftover meats, fish, avocado, shredded veggies or other fillings
Full-fat yoghurt or kefir	If you tolerate dairy (cow or goat), consume alone or with fruit and/or nuts

EATING PALEO ON A BUDGET

Making the switch from a standard Western diet to a nutrient-dense, Personal Paleo approach to eating can initially be a shock at the supermarket checkout. This is especially true for people accustomed to buying cheap grain products such as bread and pasta, canned beans, or conventionally raised animal products. That first big trip to the supermarket to prepare for your 30-Day Reset might produce a terrifying bill compared to what you're used to spending – and it might even be enough to deter some from sticking with their new, healthier diet.

Fortunately, with a little planning and some smart shopping techniques, there's no reason why eating Paleo should cost significantly more than your old way of eating. Granted, there may always be a slightly higher cost associated with eating high-quality, real foods (isn't your health worth it?), but there are several ways to keep your grocery bills from getting out of control. Here are seven tips for eating Paleo on a budget.

1 Buy ingredients, not products

It's cheaper to buy raw ingredients and cook food yourself than buying pre-packaged meals, snacks and other food items. A lot of people who are new to Paleo tend to be overwhelmed at the supermarket and look for 'Paleo-friendly' products like nut milks and beef jerky and other items that can be easily made at home but are tempting to buy when just starting out. Also, some end up buying one or more of the many pre-made meals, sold online, that have been designed to be compliant with the Paleo diet and often cost an arm and a leg.

The more food you cook from scratch, the more money you'll save. You'll find some fantastic recipes (for meals and snacks) in Chapter 21, plus there are countless recipes online (at ChrisKresser.com and on other websites). Another major advantage to preparing your own food is that you know what all of the ingredients are and you avoid mystery additives, preservatives and artificial sweeteners.

2 Buy in bulk and share

Buying in bulk (online or at your local shop) can significantly reduce your food expenses, particularly for storecupboard items such as coconut oil, olive oil, ghee, canned tomatoes, and so on. You can buy grass-fed/organic meat in bulk direct from some farms (or online), so you could get together with a group of health-minded friends and share it. The more people involved, the lower the cost and the less need for extra freezer space. Joining a community-supported agriculture (CSA) farm allows you access to local farm crops for less than you'd pay at most shops. Try the US idea of having 'potlucks' with friends, where each person (or couple) cooks a dish to share, rather than going out to eat; it's a great way to save money on social dining occasions while still eating well. The more food you share with neighbours, friends and extended family, the more money you'll save.

3 Get down to basics

Buy ingredients that are versatile and can be used for a wide variety of dishes. Instead of buying expensive spices that you might use only once, get the basics like fresh garlic, onion powder, Italian/Mexican/Cajun (or the ethnic food of your choice!) seasoning, curry paste and anything else that can be used for a multitude of dishes. Choose a couple of useful fats such as olive oil, coconut oil or butter and use them for all your dishes. Don't be afraid to use frozen vegetables, as they're just as nutritious as fresh and can be used in many different dishes, plus they have a much longer shelf life than fresh veggies. For those who tolerate starches, white potatoes and sweet potatoes are cheap and filling, and can be used at any meal. Avoid buying speciality items such as gluten-free flours or other ingredients that sit in your cupboard uneaten for months because you don't know what to use them for.

4 Cook in bulk

Making large batches of meals (you can double up many of the recipes you'll find in Chapter 21) yields tasty leftovers that save both time and money. As those living on their own know, it gets expensive trying to buy single-serve food items, and food waste can be a huge problem when buying in bulk. That's why cooking large meals and saving the leftovers can be especially helpful for those cooking for just themselves or perhaps one other person. Try making multiple servings of an all-in-one meal such as a soup or stew and freezing them for later in the week. Not only will you save cooking time but you'll also be able to use ingredients bought in bulk and not have to worry about spoilage when you can't eat all the meat or vegetables you've purchased.

5 Choose your battles

Not everything you buy has to be organic, grass-fed, free-range and local. There are many food items that are fine to buy from a conventional supermarket on a regular basis. Although you always want to buy organic celery and strawberries, it might not be so important to look for organic onions or mangoes. See the Environmental Working Group's 'Dirty Dozen Plus' and 'Clean Fifteen' lists (page 160) for what to focus on. The same goes for animal products. Although you would probably want to avoid conventionally raised chicken, pork and organ meats, you may be fine buying lamb, eggs and some natural cheeses that aren't from 100 per cent grass-fed and organic sources.

Canned fish such as salmon, skipjack tuna, sardines and herrings or mackerel are far less expensive than fresh, wild fish and are extremely nutrient-dense choices. Of course, you should always get the highest-quality animal foods you can afford, but not everyone has access to ideal sources of meat. It's better to eat non-organic eggs than organic cereal for breakfast, and it's better to have a dinner of conventionally raised beef and non-organic asparagus than a plate of organic pasta. If you're unable to buy the best-quality meats and produce, it's a good idea to do your homework and work out which items are worth the splurge and which might be all right to spend less money on.

6 Cut out the extras

Write a list of those 'luxury items' you buy – coffee-shop coffees, bottled water, fancy ingredients you use once for an extravagant recipe, protein powders, and so on – and cut them out. Yes, high-quality eggs do cost more per dozen than conventional eggs, but simply forgoing your Starbucks coffee each day will easily make up the difference. Go through your food spending and see if you can identify which splurges are putting you in the red. Get rid of the non-essentials altogether or find a way to make them at home. Buy a good-quality reusable mug or water bottle and fill it up before you leave the house in the morning. Eat real food rather than expensive protein powders and supplements. Don't waste money on those items that you could easily do without.

7 Skip the fillet steak

A great way to save money on animal foods is choosing cheaper cuts of meat such as brisket, chuck, shin, and so on, and offal (liver, heart, and so on). These not only contain important nutrients that balance out those found in lean meats like steak and chicken breast (as we discussed in Chapter 9); they're also some of the most tender and delicious cuts when slow cooking methods are used. Many people who can't otherwise afford grass-fed meat can afford these cuts. And it's especially important to buy organ meats from organic, grass-fed animals. These unpopular cuts often cost just a few pounds per pound (450g) and deliver an enormous nutritional benefit that will make a significant difference to your overall health.

Need extra help with your dietary changes?

If you're still having difficulty, don't worry. I know how frustrating that can be, but the truth is that making huge dietary and lifestyle changes can be hard, and sometimes it doesn't go so smoothly. This doesn't mean that the Personal Paleo Diet isn't a good choice for you; it just means that you may need a little extra support.

To that end, I've created a Paleo Troubleshooting Guide, which you can download at ChrisKresser.com/PPC. It will help you break through the most common challenges that keep people from succeeding with Paleo, such as low energy and sugar cravings, digestive distress and poor detox capacity.

GETTING THE SUPPORT YOU NEED TO SUCCEED

Having a strong network of social support is essential for long-term success when it comes to making big dietary and lifestyle changes. Developing a Personal Paleo Diet can be a challenge even when you do have family and friends behind you, but it's much harder if you're going it alone. Here are some ideas for how to build that support network.

Bringing the family on board

If you live with family members, eating Paleo can be really tough if they're not – especially if you're not the one preparing the meals! Bringing your family on board is one of the best ways of easing your transition. But how do you do that? After all, not everyone in your family may be as enthusiastic about 'going Paleo' as you are. Here are some tips:

Offer to take charge Change is hard. Sometimes the resistance towards switching to Paleo is mostly about fear of the extra work involved in getting to grips with new recipes, new ingredients to buy at the shops and new ways of putting meals and snacks together. Even if you haven't historically been the primary meal planner and preparer, consider assuming this role – at least during the transition. Use the recipes and meal plans in Chapter 21 and on my website to help you along.

Take it easy When you're living alone, it might be easy to change your diet radically for next to nothing, but when you're living with several family members, it's often more complicated. And sometimes, the more pressure you put on others to change, the more they'll resist. Consider starting with one Paleo meal a day (dinner is usually best). Once you've got that under your belt, you can move to lunch, then breakfast, then snacks. Before long you'll be where you want to be, but you won't have alienated your family in the process.

Start with the 'biggies' As an alternative to the 'one meal at a time' approach, you might instead consider choosing one particular change at a time; for example, you could decide to eliminate sugar first, then gluten, then industrial seed oils (eliminating packaged/processed foods and eating out less) and then grains, until you end up on a Personal Paleo Diet.

Find Paleo substitutes for your family's favourite meals Your family doesn't have to give up pizza, pancakes and other favourite foods for ever; simply substitute them with delicious Paleo versions! See the recipes in this book and on my website.

If you have young kids, different strategies may apply. This is especially true if your child has a health problem you are trying to address with a Paleo approach. Here are some additional things to consider with young children:

- Depriving a child of their favourite junk foods isn't child abuse – although they may certainly do their best to make you feel that way. I often hear parents say things like, 'My kid would never give up his Pasta 'n' Sauce Macaroni Cheese.' Trust me – they won't starve if you stop feeding them this stuff. You may have some epic battles initially, but if you hold your ground, eventually they'll get hungry enough to eat what you've put in front of them. This may sound harsh, but when your child's health is at stake, it's actually the most loving action you can take.

- Kids don't need 'kids' food' – they need good food. Big Food has been wildly successful in convincing us that babies and kids need special foods (usually packaged, processed and refined) that are different from what parents eat. The reality is that kids need real, unprocessed food even more than adults do, because they're still growing and developing. The sooner you let go of the idea of 'kids' food', the better off you'll be. You won't have to prepare separate snacks and meals for your kids, and they'll naturally begin to eat the right foods – because they are available.

- Young kids don't have the same prejudices against foods as many of us do; for example, adults may think of cod liver oil as 'disgusting', but a young toddler has no such pre-conception. When our daughter Sylvie was a toddler, she actually asked for unflavoured fermented cod liver oil after meals. And we couldn't keep her away from the raw sauerkraut!

I know it can seem especially hard to make the transition with young kids, but know that thousands of parents have gone before you, and it's absolutely possible with a little perseverance and planning. And don't try to do it alone! Join the forum at ChrisKresser.com/PPC to get some support from other parents who are on the other side.

Enlisting the support of your friends

Regardless of whether you live alone or with family, enlisting the support of your friends is another way to ease the transition into Paleo and increase your chances for success. Here are some tips for doing that:

Find a 'Paleo pal' See if any of your friends are interested in doing the 30-Day Reset with you. That way you'll have someone to share your challenges and successes with. And once they experience the results, they're a lot more likely to stick with Paleo over the long term, which means you'll have at least one friend who's with you.

Lead by example The best way to get your friends interested in Paleo is to 'speak softly but carry a big stick'. Proselytising and being pushy usually just create resistance and may end up jeopardising your friendship. But if they watch you drop 30 pounds in two months, your skin clear up and your energy level and mood improve dramatically, they'll start asking questions.

Educate them – gently If you sense that your friend is interested, rather than telling them all about Paleo yourself, consider giving them a book (like this one) as a gift. Sometimes the information is better received when it comes from a third party.

Find some new friends If the people you hang out with aren't really interested in improving their health at all, it's probably time for you to find some new friends who are. One of the best ways to do that is to join a gym, participate in group exercise or sports, or join – or create – a Paleo meet-up group in your local area. There are hundreds of these groups now around the world. See Paleo-Diet.meetup.com for a listing, or simply Google the term 'Paleo Meet-up' with the name of your city or town.

Online support

In addition to family and friends, tap into online support resources such as these:

ChrisKresser.com/PPC

Visit ChrisKresser.com/PPC to register for free bonus chapters, programme-enhancing tools, resources, guides and ongoing education and support to help you meet your health and wellness goals. There's also a forum where you can interact with people from around the world who are following the Personal Paleo Diet approach.

ChrisKresser.com

Check out my website and blog for regular articles on nutrition and health, recipes, book reviews, a lively discussion forum, recommended programmes and products, and an online store with hand-picked supplements that I use every day in my clinical practice.

Revolution Health Radio

Don't miss my podcast, available on my website and iTunes, where I discuss my latest research, provide practical advice on how to use nutrition to prevent and reverse disease, interview expert guests on a wide range of health-related topics and answer listeners' questions. A transcript of each show is available for those who prefer reading to listening.

Other Paleo websites and forums

There are several fantastic websites and forums that cover various aspects of the Paleo approach. I've listed some of my favourites on my website.

Finding a Paleo-friendly healthcare provider

Finding a health-care provider who understands and endorses the Paleo approach is another important step in making the transition successfully. Fortunately, that has become much easier now with two online directories of Paleo-oriented clinicians (doctors, naturopaths, chiropractors, acupuncturists, and so on):

- The Paleo Physicians Network (PaleoPhysiciansNetwork.com)
- Primal Docs (PrimalDocs.com)

Both of these networks list practitioners in many countries worldwide and both are growing quickly with new practitioners added on a weekly basis.

In addition to seeking out a Paleo-oriented clinician, I'd also suggest finding one that practises functional medicine. Functional medicine is neither conventional nor alternative medicine. It's a combination of the best elements of both and it represents the future of medicine. For more information on the differences between functional and conventional medicine, see my website, where you'll also find a list of questions that you can ask your healthcare provider to determine if they're 'Paleo-friendly'.

CHAPTER 20

Personalise Your Paleo Diet and Code for Specific Health Conditions

This chapter contains some basic nutritional and lifestyle strategies for ten of the most common health conditions we face today. At ChrisKresser.com/PPC, you'll find a free bonus chapter for each health condition discussed below, with more background information and detailed recommendations for supplements (including dosage and brand recommendations) that may be beneficial. You'll also find an interactive quiz that will help you identify which of these bonus chapters you may benefit from reading, based on your particular symptoms.

WEIGHT LOSS

Diet

Start with the low-carbohydrate version of the 30-Day Reset that I recommended during Step 1. You can find specific instructions on page 58. If you've already tried this, follow the suggestions below:

- **Eat more protein** Aim for as much as 25–35 per cent of calories from protein until you reach your target weight.

- **Don't snack** Snacking can lead to overeating and may cause hormonal shifts that aren't supportive of weight loss.

- **Go dairy-free** Many of my patients find it easier to lose weight when they aren't eating dairy – with the exception of small amounts of butter and ghee.

- **Reduce calorie density** by adding extra vegetables (both non-starchy and starchy) to your meals.

- **Eat all your food within an eight-hour period each day** This is called 'intermittent fasting'. See page 356 to learn how to do it.

Lifestyle

Several lifestyle factors contribute to weight gain, including:

- Sitting too much and not moving enough.

- Not getting enough sleep or poor sleep quality.

- Too much exposure to artificial light at night.

- Chronic stress and adrenal fatigue.

- Poor gut health.

Be sure to read Chapters 10, 12, 13 and 14, plus the bonus chapters on adrenal fatigue and digestive conditions on the website, for more information on these topics.

HIGH CHOLESTEROL AND HEART DISEASE

Diet

The basic Personal Paleo Diet I've suggested in this book is inherently a 'heart-healthy' diet. That said, you can make your diet even more heart-healthy by making sure you get enough of the following seven foods and macronutrients:

1 **Cold-water oily fish and shellfish** Aim for 450g of oily fish and/or oysters and mussels a week.

2 **Monounsaturated fat** Try adding a handful of macadamia nuts, a quarter or half an avocado, or a tablespoon of olive oil to your diet daily.

3 **Antioxidant-rich foods** 'Eat the rainbow' by choosing a variety of colours of fruits and vegetables, and don't forget that animal products like organ meats, muscle meats, eggs and grass-fed dairy are also rich in antioxidants.

4 **Polyphenol-rich foods** These include green tea, blueberries, extra virgin olive oil, red wine, citrus fruits, hibiscus tea, dark chocolate, turmeric and other herbs and spices.

5 **Nuts** Aim for a handful of tree nuts such as almonds, Brazil nuts, cashew nuts, chestnuts and hazelnuts each day. Be careful not to overeat nuts.

6 **Fermented foods** Add 1–2 tablespoons of raw sauerkraut or kimchi to each meal and 125ml of beetroot kvaas or kombucha and 125ml of yoghurt or kefir daily.

7 **Soluble fibre** Eat a wide range of fruits and vegetables every day, especially starchy tubers like sweet potatoes and yams, which are particularly high in soluble fibre.

Lifestyle

- **Meditation** Chronic stress significantly increases the risk of heart disease, and stress-management practices such as meditation have been shown to reduce deaths from heart disease. See Chapter 14 and the website for recommendations.

- **Sleep** Chronic insomnia doubles the risk of heart attack and stroke. See Chapter 13 for recommendations on improving sleep.

- **Physical activity** Exercise improves metabolic and cardiovascular function in several ways and extends lifespan. Remember: your goal should be not only to exercise more, but to sit less. See Chapter 12 for recommendations.

HIGH BLOOD PRESSURE

Diet

- **Strictly avoid refined sugar.**

- **Increase potassium intake** See the bonus chapter on high blood pressure for a chart of potassium-rich foods.

- **Eat 450g of cold-water, oily fish and/or shellfish** such as oysters and mussels per week.

- **Increase magnesium intake** Nuts, seeds, spinach, beetroot greens and chocolate are the highest food sources of magnesium on a Personal Paleo Diet.

- **Eat a 4cm serving of dark chocolate** (more than 80 per cent cocoa content) a day.

- **Drink two to three cups of hibiscus tea** each day.

- **Add wakame** (seaweed) to soups and stews, or re-hydrate it and eat it on its own.

See the bonus chapter on blood pressure on the website for important information about salt. You might be surprised by what you learn!

Lifestyle

- **Weight loss** Excess body fat can increase blood pressure, and reducing it can lower blood pressure. See above as well as the bonus chapter on weight loss on my website for specific recommendations.

- **Physical activity** Endurance exercise, strength training, high-intensity interval training and simply moving around more during the day (outside of a distinct exercise period) have all been shown to significantly reduce blood pressure. For specific recommendations on physical activity, see Chapter 12.

- **Sleep** Short sleep duration, poor sleep quality and sleep apnoea increase the risk that you'll develop high blood pressure. See Chapter 13 for tips on improving your sleep.

- **Ultraviolet light (via sunshine or tanning beds)** Ultraviolet light increases the production of a chemical in our bodies called nitric oxide, which helps our blood vessels to relax and lowers blood pressure. See Chapter 16 for specific recommendations for ultraviolet light exposure.

See the bonus chapter on the website for several other important lifestyle modifications for lowering blood pressure.

GERD, IBS, IBD AND OTHER DIGESTIVE PROBLEMS

Diet

- Follow a low-FODMAP (fermentable oligosaccharide, di-saccharide, monosaccharide and polyols) diet. See the bonus chapter on digestive conditions on my website for a detailed description and printable cheat sheets.

- Reduce your consumption of non-starchy vegetables high in insoluble fibre and prepare them with methods designed to make them more digestible (including fermentation). See page 196–197 for details.

- Consume 125–500ml of bone broth per day, in soups, stocks, stews or sauces. You can also drink it like tea.

- Eat plenty of fermentable fibre in the form of fruit and starchy vegetables such as potato, sweet potato, plantain, yuca (cassava/manioc), taro, celeriac and parsnip. (If you have GERD, heartburn or inflammatory bowel disease, you may need to limit these foods for a period of time.)

- Consume fermented foods such as sauerkraut, kimchi, beet-root kvaas, kefir (dairy or water) and yoghurt. Although milk (in kefir and yoghurt) and cabbage (in sauerkraut and kimchi) are both high in FODMAPs, fermentation breaks them down and makes these foods tolerable for most people with digestive issues.

- Limit alcohol consumption to four to six drinks per week, or avoid it altogether if you have significant gut issues.

Lifestyle

- **Manage stress** In plain language, stress wreaks havoc on the gut. See Chapter 14 for recommendations on stress management.

- **Gut-directed hypnotherapy** Gut-directed hypnotherapy is a form of self-hypnosis specifically designed to alleviate the symptoms of IBS and other functional gut disorders. It is one of the single most effective treatments for IBS. See my website for a specific recommendations for a home-based, audio instruction programme.

- **Sleep** Disturbed sleep interferes with gut functions in several ways, and many IBS patients notice an increase in their symptoms when they don't sleep well. See Chapter 13 for recommendations on improving sleep.

DIABETES AND OTHER BLOOD SUGAR DISORDERS

Diet

- **Adjust carbohydrate intake** Using a device called a glucometer to measure your blood sugar after meals, you can determine exactly how much carbohydrate is safe for you to eat. See the bonus chapter on blood sugar disorders as well as the cheat sheet on blood sugar testing on my website for detailed instructions.

- **Eat more protein** Higher-protein diets seem to have a stabilising effect on blood sugar – regardless of whether you have a tendency towards high or low blood sugar. Aim for between 25–30 per cent of total calories from protein (160–195g per day on a 2,600 calorie diet, or 125–150g per day on a 2,000 calorie diet).

- **Eat fermented foods and fermentable fibres** There's a strong connection between gut health and metabolic health. See Chapter 10 and the bonus chapter on digestive conditions on my website for more information.

- **If your blood sugar is too high,** avoid snacking and consider intermittent fasting (see page 356 to learn how to do it).

- **If your blood sugar is too low,** don't go more than two to three hours without eating, eat a high-protein (for example, at least 40g of protein) breakfast within 30 minutes of waking up and eat a snack before bed. See the section below and the bonus chapter on my website on adrenal fatigue syndrome for more detailed recommendations.

Lifestyle

- **Physical activity** Getting adequate exercise and sitting less are crucial for regulating blood sugar. See Chapter 12 for recommendations.

- **Sleep** Sleep deprivation impairs metabolic function and blood sugar control by several mechanisms. See page 273 for a recap of sleep recommendations.

- **Stress management** Stress reduces blood sugar control, promotes inflammation (a primary cause of blood sugar-related problems) and leads to low levels of cortisol (which can further disrupt blood sugar control). See page 291 for a recap of stress-management recommendations.

ANXIETY, DEPRESSION AND COGNITIVE DISORDERS

Diet

- **Low-FODMAP diet** See the bonus chapter on digestive conditions on my website for more info.

- **Glycine-rich foods** Balance your intake of lean proteins (for example, lean red meat, boneless, skinless chicken breast, and so on) with more gelatinous cuts of meat (for example, oxtail, shanks, brisket, shin, chuck steak, and so on), bone broth and egg yolks.

- **Fermented foods** See Chapter 10 for more information and the Fermented Foods Guide on my website for instructions on how to make fermented foods at home.

- **The GAPS (Gut And Psychology Syndrome) diet** The GAPS diet is a therapeutic approach to treating psychological and behavioural conditions by improving gut health. See my website for an outline of the various stages of the diet, along with recommendations for books, websites and how to find a GAPS-certified practitioner to work with.

Lifestyle

- **Sleep** There are few things more important to maintaining brain function than sleep. See page 273 for a recap of sleep recommendations.

- **Stress management** A regular stress-management programme is a must for those suffering from brain disorders. See page 291 for a recap of stress-management recommendations.

- **Physical activity** Movement and exercise promote healthy brain function in several important ways. See page 257 for a recap of recommendations to increase your physical activity.

- **Nature** Natural environments have restorative effects, reduce stress and improve our outlook on life. See page 328 for a recap of recommendations for reconnecting with nature.

- **Light therapy** Bright-light therapy involves sitting in front of, or near to, a device that emits artificial light that mimics natural outdoor light. It is particularly effective for seasonal affective disorder but has also shown positive results for non-seasonal depression, postpartum depression and bipolar disorder. See the bonus chapter and resources on my website for dosage and device recommendations.

THYROID DISORDERS

Diet

There are four primary dietary concerns for people with thyroid problems:

1 Limiting intake of goitrogens – foods and chemicals that increase the need for iodine in small amounts and can damage the thyroid gland in large amounts.

2 Ensuring adequate intake of iodine and selenium, which are crucial nutrients for thyroid function.

3 Being aware of foods that potentially trigger an immune response (if you have one of the autoimmune forms of thyroid disease).

4 Avoiding very low-carb and low-protein diets, which may decrease thyroid function by inhibiting the conversion of the less active form of thyroid hormone (T4) into the more active form (T3).

Please see the bonus chapter on thyroid disorders on the website for a detailed explanation of each of these topics, including a list of goitrogenic chemicals and foods, and foods highest in iodine and selenium.

Lifestyle

- **Stress management** Chronic stress impairs thyroid function in numerous ways. See page 291 for a recap of stress-management recommendations.

- Gut health. There's a strong – but little-known – connection between gut health and thyroid function. See Chapter 10 and the bonus chapter on digestive conditions on my website for detailed information about healing your gut.

- Ultraviolet light (via sun or UVA/UVB tanning beds) may help put the brakes on an overactive immune system. See Chapter 16 for specific recommendations.

AUTOIMMUNE DISEASE

Diet

There are three approaches to addressing autoimmunity through diet:

1 Remove foods that may trigger or exacerbate an immune response.

2 Increase your intake of nutrients that promote optimal immune function.

3 Increase your intake of foods that support healthy gut microbiota.

Please see the bonus chapter on autoimmune disease on the website for a detailed discussion of each of these approaches.

Lifestyle

- **Physical activity** Regular physical activity and exercise improve immune function via several different mechanisms. See Chapter 12 for tips on how to increase your physical activity and sit less.

- **Acupuncture** helps to bring the immune system back into balance. I recommend getting acupuncture two to three times a week for the first month and then at least once a week thereafter. Find a fully qualified practitioner from the British Acupuncture Council or Australian Acupuncture and Chinese Medicine Association website.

- **Pleasure and connection** release chemicals called endorphins that help to regulate the immune system. See Chapter 15 for specific recommendations.

- **Ultraviolet light** Exposure to sunlight (or UVA/UVB light in tanning beds) appears to be especially important for those with autoimmune disease. See Chapter 16 for specific recommendations.

ADRENAL FATIGUE SYNDROME

You won't find adrenal fatigue syndrome (AFS) listed in medical textbooks, and if you ask your doctor about it he or she will probably just shrug or tell you to stop paying so much attention to health information on the internet. Yet there's no doubt in my mind that this is a legitimate, common and potentially very serious condition. I see it every day in my work with patients and I've experienced it myself. Please see the bonus chapter on adrenal fatigue syndrome on the website for more information on this condition.

Diet

- **Eat a moderate-carbohydrate diet** I suggest between 15–30 per cent of calories from carbohydrate. Start with 20 per cent as a target and experiment with slightly higher and lower amounts to see what works best for you.

- **Eat adequate protein, especially in the morning** Eat at least 15 per cent of calories from protein, and start the day with a high-protein (that is, more than 40g of protein) breakfast.

- **Eat frequently throughout the day** Try not to go more than two to three hours without eating. You can either eat five to six small meals spaced throughout the day, or three regular meals with snacks in between. Snacks and meals should always have at least some protein and fat (never carbohydrates alone).

- **Avoid excess dietary potassium** Excess potassium can lower blood pressure, and many people with AFS already have low blood pressure to begin with. See the bonus chapter on blood pressure on my website for a list of high-potassium foods.

- **Ensure adequate sodium intake** Sodium increases aldosterone, which is often low in AFS. If your adrenal fatigue is pronounced, or if you have low blood pressure or strong salt cravings, I suggest starting each day with a full glass of water with ½–1 teaspoon of sea salt and using salt liberally on food, to taste. Monitor your blood pressure occasionally to make sure it remains in a healthy range.

- **Avoid caffeine and alcohol** Both caffeine and alcohol place additional stress on the body. It's best to avoid caffeine entirely and limit alcohol consumption to two to three drinks per week (or eliminate entirely) until your adrenals recover.

Lifestyle

- **Get plenty of sleep and rest** This is by far the most important recommendation for adrenal fatigue. See page 273 for a recap of recommendations for sleep.

- **Manage your stress** Along with poor sleep, psychological and emotional stress are primary contributors to AFS, and managing stress is a crucial part of the recovery process. In fact, I have never seen someone fully recover from AFS without paying significant attention to stress management. See Chapter 14 for specific recommendations on stress management.

- **Moderate your physical activity** Not enough physical activity can contribute to AFS, but overtraining is actually a more common cause. I see this particularly in my patients who are high-level athletes or CrossFit enthusiasts. See the box 'Are you overtraining' on page 251 for more on this topic, including a list of signs and symptoms of overtraining.

- **Go outside** Spending regular time outdoors in a natural environment is especially important for those with AFS. See Chapter 16 for specific recommendations.

- **Cultivate pleasure, have fun and connect with others** Pleasure, play and social connection are all deeply nourishing and restorative on both a physical and an emotional level and can provide a powerful antidote to the symptoms of AFS. See Chapters 15 and 17 for specific recommendations.

SKIN DISORDERS

The skin is influenced by other organs in the body and this is especially true of the brain and the gut; scientists coined the term 'gut–brain–skin axis' to describe the interconnection between these three systems. See the bonus chapter on skin disorders on the website for important background information on the gut–brain–skin axis and more detail on how to intervene when it is not functioning optimally.

Diet

I use one of two diets with my patients with skin conditions, depending on their particular presentation of signs and symptoms:

- Low-histamine diet
- Low-FODMAP diet

See the bonus chapter on skin conditions on my website to determine which is right for you and for more information on each of the diets. I also list several nutrients that are important for healthy skin. Fortunately, if you're following a Personal Paleo Diet approach, you'll naturally obtain adequate amounts of these nutrients.

Lifestyle

- **Stress management** Stress is associated with numerous skin conditions, including psoriasis, dermatitis, alopecia, urticaria, vitiligo, acne and herpes simplex virus. See Chapter 14 for specific recommendations, and read the section on adrenal fatigue syndrome on pages 402–404 for additional tips.

- **Physical activity** If you have a skin problem as well as symptoms of adrenal fatigue syndrome, I suggest taking more gentle forms of exercise such as walking, cycling and yoga, along with strength training two to three times a week. Avoid strenuous workouts until your adrenals recover.

- **Sleep** Chronic sleep deprivation promotes inflammation and disrupts hormones, both of which can trigger or exacerbate skin conditions. See Chapter 13 for recommendations on improving sleep.

- **Ultraviolet light** from sunlight or UVA/UVB tanning beds has been shown to improve certain skin conditions, such as psoriasis, vitiligo, acne, eczema, dermatitis and lichen planus.

CHAPTER 21

Seven-day Meal Plan
and Recipes

I've provided a lot of guidance throughout the book about what to eat, what not to eat and how to determine your own Personal Paleo Diet. But all of this information really comes alive in the meal plan and recipes in this chapter, where you'll discover just how easy it is to eat delicious, satisfying and healthy meals with this approach.

To get you started, I've provided a one-week meal plan with recipes. At ChrisKresser.com/PPC, you'll find an additional three weeks of meal plans and recipes. Finally, I've provided shopping lists for each week that you can print out and take to the shops with you.

Although I list new recipes for every meal, I realise that it won't be possible for the vast majority of people to cook from scratch at every single mealtime. This is where leftovers and planning in advance come in. If you work outside the home, consider doubling up the recipes the night before so that you'll have enough to bring with you for lunch the next day. Another helpful strategy is to set aside a few hours at the weekend to pre-pare snacks, soup, stocks and/or larger meals that you can eat throughout the week. With a little bit of advance preparation, it's entirely possible to eat this way without spending hours in the kitchen each day!

Bon appétit!

ONE-WEEK MEAL PLAN

Day 1:
Breakfast: Baked Eggs en Cocotte Florentine-style
Lunch: Butternut Squash Frittata with Salad
Snack: Nori Crisps
Dinner: Beef Rendang
Side dish: Roasted Carrots and Garlic

Day 2:
Breakfast: Poached Eggs with Swiss Chard
Lunch: Beefburgers with Mushrooms Provençale-style
Snack: Nori Crisps
Dinner: Grilled Tuna Steaks with Chinese Five Spices
Side dish: Cabbage, Pak Choi and Shiitake Mushrooms

Day 3:
Breakfast: Green Smoothie
Lunch: Cod with Coriander Red Pepper Sauce and Sautéed
    Broccoli
Snack: Hard-boiled Eggs with (or without) Avocado
Dinner: Tom Kha Gai
Side dish: Thai Basil Aubergine

Day 4:
Breakfast: Parsnip Fritters with Sausage
Lunch: Tuna, Ginger and Avocado Salad
Snack: Hard-boiled Eggs with (or without) Avocado
Dinner: Spanish Roasted Pork Loin Adobado
Side dish: Cauliflower Hash

Day 5:
Breakfast: Smoked Salmon with Eggs and Asparagus
Lunch: Greek Turkey with Courgette Noodles
Snack: Kale Crisps
Dinner: Chicken Tikka Masala
Side dish: Green Salad with Shallot Vinaigrette

Day 6:
Breakfast: Celeriac and Bacon Hash
Lunch: Chicken, Tarragon and Grapefruit Salad
Snack: Kale Crisps
Dinner: Rosemary Lamb Chops
Side dish: Sweet Potato Wedges

Day 7:
Breakfast: Cauliflower-stuffed Acorn Squash
Lunch: Salmon Fillets with Raspberry Vinaigrette Salad
Snack: Guacamole with Carrot Crisps
Dinner: Rustic Meatball and Tomato Stew
Side dish: Kale and Squash Salad

Recipe notes

- You'll see 'traditional fat of choice' listed as an ingredient in several recipes. This means you're free to use any of the saturated or monounsaturated fats listed in Chapter 5. If you're cooking at medium heat or above, I suggest choosing fats with a smoke point above 180°C. These include ghee, extra light (not extra virgin) olive oil, palm oil, expeller-pressed (not extra virgin) coconut oil, macadamia oil, beef tallow, duck fat and lard.

- If you're following the autoimmune or low-carb/high blood sugar version of the 30-Day Reset, please see ChrisKresser.com/PPC for specific meal plans for those approaches.

- You'll see nuts used in some of the recipes as a garnish or optional ingredient. In Chapter 3 I explained that it's best to soak and then either roast or dehydrate nuts before eating them in order to make them more digestible and improve the bioavailability of the nutrients they contain; however, when used in small quantities as part of a recipe, it's fine to simply use raw or roasted, unsoaked nuts to save time.

- I have purposely not included 'nutritional info' for the recipes. As I mentioned in Chapter 1, the 30-Day Reset is not about counting calories or macronutrients – it's about 'resetting' your body with the nutrient-dense, whole foods humans are adapted to eat. That said, if you're following a low-carb version of the 30-Day Reset, or if you'd simply like to know how much protein, fat or carbohydrate each recipe contains, you can enter the ingredients at NutritionData.com to find out.

- Vegetables and eggs listed in the recipes are medium unless otherwise stated.

THE RECIPES

Breakfasts

Baked Eggs en Cocotte Florentine-style

For this recipe you'll need two 250ml ramekins.

Serves: 2
Preparation time: 15 minutes
Cooking time: 15 minutes

1 tbsp traditional fat of choice
250g spinach
1 large garlic clove, crushed
125ml coconut milk
a pinch of freshly grated nutmeg
4 eggs
sea salt and freshly ground black pepper
1 tsp snipped chives, to garnish

Preheat the oven to 180°C/Gas 4. Heat the fat in a medium pan over a medium-high heat. Add the spinach, garlic, coconut milk and nutmeg, and season with salt and pepper. Cook until the spinach has wilted. Drain off the excess liquid.

Arrange the spinach mixture in the base of two 250ml ramekins. Crack two of the eggs into a small bowl and gently pour them into one ramekin. Repeat with the remaining two eggs. Bake in the oven until the eggs are cooked the way you like them – if you prefer soft-cooked eggs, 5 minutes should be enough. Serve garnished with chives.

Poached Eggs with Swiss Chard

To prepare chard, cut the leaves from the central stalk and coarsely chop them. The stalk should be peeled (this is preferable with many stalk vegetables such as celery, rhubarb, etc.) and chopped finely. Both stalks and leaves can then be cooked together. The eggs need to be as fresh as possible, as fresh eggs are best for poaching.

Serves: 2
Preparation time: 10 minutes
Cooking time: 15 minutes

1 tbsp traditional fat of choice
1 shallot, peeled and finely chopped
500g Swiss chard, chopped (see above)
a pinch of freshly grated nutmeg
1 tbsp cider vinegar
2 eggs
juice of ½ lemon
sea salt and freshly ground black pepper
2 tsp finely chopped fresh tarragon, to garnish (optional)

Heat the fat in a medium pan over a medium-high heat, add the shallot and cook for 3–5 minutes until lightly browned. Add the chard and nutmeg, and season with salt and pepper. Cook until the chard has wilted. Drain off the excess liquid, divide between two plates and keep warm.

Pour 1cm of boiling water into a pan and add the cider vinegar. Crack each egg into a small bowl. Reduce the water to a simmer and pour an egg into the water while vigorously stirring around the egg with a chopstick or kebab skewer. This forces the egg to the centre of the pan, helping to hold it together. Cook for 4 minutes, then remove the egg with a slotted spoon and put on top of a portion of warm chard. Repeat the process with the second egg. The white should be firm, but the yolk should be creamy, with a white film over it. Serve the chard and egg topped with a drizzle of lemon juice and a pinch of salt. Garnish with tarragon, if you like.

Green Smoothie

A quick, energising and delicious way to start the day. Note that raw spinach and kale contain compounds (for example, goitrogens, nitriles and oxalates) that may impair thyroid function if consumed in excess. If you have a thyroid issue, I suggest lightly steaming the kale and spinach first, and then cooling it before adding to the smoothie. This will at least partially inactivate the potentially harmful compounds.

Serves: 1
Preparation time: 5 minutes

250ml unsweetened almond milk
1 banana, or ½ mango, cut into chunks
125ml coconut milk
20g spinach
20g kale
1 tbsp almond butter (optional)

Put all the ingredients in a blender and process until smooth.

Parsnip Fritters with Sausage

The parsnip is a delicious, low-carb alternative to potatoes that can be cooked in many of the same ways. Keep in mind that parsnips cook very quickly and can easily become mushy if overcooked. These fritters (without the sausage) can also be served as a snack or side dish.

Serves: 2
Preparation time: 15 minutes
Cooking time: 20 minutes

500g parsnips, grated
1 egg
a pinch of sea salt
ground black pepper

For the sausage:

350g minced pork
½ tsp ground fennel seeds
¼ tsp sea salt
1 tsp Lard (see note below and page 448)
2 tsp chopped fresh parsley to garnish

Put the parsnips in a bowl and add the egg, salt and pepper to taste. Mix well, then shape into four equal-sized patties.

Mix together all the sausage ingredients, except the lard, and shape into patties. Heat the lard in a frying pan over a medium heat and fry the patties for 5 minutes on each side, or until thoroughly cooked through. Remove the patties from the pan.

Add the parsnip patties to the pan and cook until crisp on both sides. Return the sausage to the pan to heat through for 2 minutes, then serve the fritters and sausage garnished with parsley.

Note The lard can be prepared on the first day of Week 1.

Smoked Salmon with Eggs
and Asparagus

This Scandinavian-inspired dish can also be served cold with some sliced cucumber.

Serves: 2
Preparation time: 10 minutes
Cooking time: 15 minutes

10 asparagus stalks, tough ends snapped off and discarded
3 eggs
90ml full-fat coconut milk
2 tbsp Lard (see page 448)
120g smoked salmon, sliced
sea salt and freshly ground black pepper
2 tsp fresh chives, chopped to garnish

Put the asparagus in a pan of lightly salted boiling water and cook for 5 minutes, then refresh in cold water. Put the eggs in a bowl and beat with the coconut milk and pepper to taste. Heat the lard in a saucepan over a low heat, add the egg mixture and cook for 3–4 minutes, stirring gently from the base of the pan occasionally, until just set.

Arrange the scrambled eggs on the asparagus, then top with the smoked salmon and garnish with chives. Season the eggs with salt and serve.

Note When making scrambled eggs or omelettes, season with salt after cooking, otherwise the eggs will be rubbery. Also remember that the smoked salmon is already quite salty.

Celeriac and Bacon Hash

You can also make this with taro, which is usually available in Asian markets or the ethnic section of grocery stores. Make sure to peel away the purple layer of the taro, if present.

Serves: 2
Preparation time: 10 minutes
Cooking time: 15 minutes

450g celeriac, parsnip or taro, peeled and cut into small dice
1 tbsp Lard (see page 448)
8 bacon rashers, cut into 1cm pieces
1 onion, roughly chopped
2 tsp apple cider vinegar (optional)
sea salt and freshly ground black pepper
2 tsp chopped fresh parsley, to garnish

Put the celeriac in a pan of lightly salted, boiling water to cover, cover with a lid and cook for 3 minutes. Drain and leave to cool slightly.

Heat the lard in a medium pan over a medium heat, add the bacon and fry until crisp. Add the onion and cook for 5–7 minutes until browned. Add the celeriac, and season with salt and pepper. Fry for 8–10 minutes until crisp. Drizzle with vinegar, if you like. Serve garnished with parsley.

Cauliflower-stuffed Acorn Squash

This spicy squash dish can be served for brunch or prepared the day before and reheated, if you like. Shiitake mushrooms are a great touch, but you can use any mushroom variety or a mixture. Acorn squash is a smaller squash that is perfect for halving and stuffing. Look out for them at farmers' markets in the autumn – and you may also find them at your supermarket.

Serves: 8
Preparation time: 15 minutes
Cooking time: 30–45 minutes, plus cooling

4 acorn squash, unpeeled, halved and seeds removed
1 cauliflower, cut into florets
80ml Paleo Chicken Stock (see page 449)
2 tbsp traditional fat of choice
1 onion, finely chopped
4 celery sticks, finely chopped
150g shiitake mushrooms, or button, chestnut or mixed
     mushrooms, coarsely chopped
70g nuts of choice, chopped (optional)
1 tbsp cinnamon
2 tsp ground ginger
½ tsp freshly grated nutmeg
¼ tsp ground cloves
¼ tsp ground cardamom
sea salt and ground black pepper

Preheat the oven to 190°C/Gas 5. Put the acorn squash halves cut-side down in a large baking dish (or two dishes if necessary) and cook for 30–45 minutes, until a knife can be inserted into the flesh easily. Allow to cool enough to handle.

Meanwhile, put the cauliflower florets into a food processor and pulse until they look like rice. Tip the cauliflower into a pan with the chicken stock, cover and cook over a medium-low heat for 5 minutes, or until just softened. Remove from the heat.

While the cauliflower is cooking, heat the fat in a medium pan over a medium heat and fry the onion and celery for 10 minutes, or until translucent. Add the mushrooms and cook for 5–10 minutes until softened. Add the nuts, if using, and the spices, and cook, stirring, for a few more minutes to allow the flavours to mix.

Scoop out a small amount of flesh from around the edge of each squash to make the opening a little larger. Mix the scooped squash into the cauliflower mixture. Season with salt and pepper. Fill the acorn squash halves with the cauliflower stuffing until heaped. Serve.

Lunches

Butternut Squash Frittata

This works for lunch – and also for breakfast or dinner.

Serves: 6
Preparation time: 20 minutes
Cooking time: 30 minutes

1 tbsp traditional fat of choice
½ red onion, chopped
675g butternut squash, peeled and cut into 2.5cm cubes
7 eggs
80ml coconut milk
4 tbsp chopped fresh parsley
sea salt and freshly ground black pepper
salad leaves and Shallot Vinaigrette (see page 451), to serve

Preheat the oven to 190°C/Gas 5. Heat the fat in a heavy, ovenproof frying pan over a medium heat, then add the onion, ½ tsp salt and ¼ tsp pepper, and cook for 5 minutes, or until the onions are translucent. Add the squash cubes and continue cooking for 10 minutes, stirring lightly, until the squash is cooked through but retains its shape – do not let it turn mushy. Set aside.

In a large bowl, whisk the eggs, coconut milk, parsley, ½ tsp salt and ¼ tsp pepper. Pour the eggs into the frying pan with the squash and put it in the oven. Bake for 10 minutes, or until the eggs are just set. If the top is not browned, put the frying pan under a hot grill for 1–2 minutes. Cool briefly, cut into wedges and serve, accompanied by the salad leaves tossed with shallot vinaigrette.

Beefburgers with Mushrooms Provençale-style

'Provençale' traditionally involves tomatoes, basil, thyme and other herbs, but it can also refer to a rich mix of garlic, parsley and extra virgin olive oil. Use any mix of mushrooms you like.

Serves: 2
Preparation time: 5 minutes
Cooking time: 15 minutes

450g minced beef, preferably grass-fed
1 tbsp Lard (see page 448)
450g mixed mushrooms
½ tsp sea salt
juice of 1 lemon
4 large garlic cloves, crushed
1 tbsp extra virgin olive oil
4 tbsp chopped fresh parsley, plus 2 tsp chopped parsley to
   garnish
freshly ground black pepper

Divide the beef into two portions and shape into burgers. Season with salt and pepper, if you like. Heat the lard in a frying pan over a medium heat and fry the burgers for 4–5 minutes on each side. Remove from the pan and keep warm.

Add the mushrooms to the frying pan and season with the salt and pepper to taste. Fry until browned, then stir in the lemon juice. Add the garlic, oil and parsley, and cook for 3 minutes. Serve the burgers topped with the mushrooms and garnished with parsley.

Cod with Coriander Red Pepper Sauce and Sautéed Broccoli

A simple-to-prepare dish with the subtle, flavourful mix of coriander and ginger.

Serves: 2
Preparation time: 15 minutes
Cooking time: 30 minutes

1 head of broccoli, florets only, broken into 4cm pieces
2 tbsp traditional fat of choice
½ red onion, chopped
2 tsp fresh root ginger, peeled and grated
3 large garlic cloves, crushed
1 large red pepper, deseeded and chopped
2 tsp ground coriander
2 cod fillets, 175–225g each
1 bay leaf (optional)
1 tbsp lime juice
sea salt and freshly ground black pepper
2 tbsp finely chopped fresh coriander, to garnish (optional)

Put the broccoli in a pan of boiling, salted water and cook for 5 minutes, then refresh with cold water. Set aside.

In a medium pan, heat 1 tbsp of the fat over a medium-low heat. Add the onion and gently cook for 5 minutes. Add the ginger and cook for 3 minutes more. Stir in the garlic and cook for 1 minute. Add the red pepper and coriander, and cook, stirring occasionally, for 10 minutes, or until the pepper is softened. Season with salt.

Meanwhile, season the cod with salt and pepper, and lay the fillets in a pan. Cover with water and add a bay leaf, if you like. Bring to the boil, then reduce the heat to low, cover the pan and simmer for 8 minutes, or until the cod is fork-tender.

Remove from the cooking liquid with a slotted spoon and keep warm.

Heat the remaining fat in a medium pan over a medium heat, add the broccoli and cook for 5 minutes. When the pepper sauce is cooked through, turn off the heat and stir in the lime juice. Serve the cod fillets with the broccoli, then pour the sauce next to the fish. Garnish with coriander, if you like.

Tuna, Ginger and Avocado Salad

A refreshing, easy and quick salad.

Serves: 2
Preparation time: 10 minutes

185g can tuna in brine, drained
2 avocados, peeled, pitted and roughly chopped
1cm piece fresh root ginger, peeled and grated
1 small shallot, finely chopped
1 tbsp lime juice
4 tbsp Paleo Mayonnaise (see page 450)
sea salt and freshly ground black pepper
2 tsp chopped fresh coriander, to garnish
mixed salad leaves, to serve

Put all the ingredients in a bowl and gently mix together. Season with salt and pepper. Garnish with coriander and serve with the salad leaves.

Greek Turkey with Courgette Noodles

Greek flavours combine to provide a nice twist to a 'pasta' sauce.

Serves: 4
Preparation time: 20 minutes
Cooking time: 25 minutes

6 courgettes, cut into strips about 3mm thick
2 tbsp traditional fat of choice
4 tbsp red onion, finely chopped
1 large garlic clove, crushed
450g minced turkey
4 tbsp Kalamata olives, pitted and chopped
2 tbsp sun-dried tomatoes in oil, drained and chopped
2 tbsp finely chopped fresh parsley
sea salt

Toss the courgette 'noodles' in 1 tbsp salt, and leave to drain in a colander for 20 minutes. Plunge into a pan of boiling water for 1 minute, then remove the noodles, refresh them in cold water and set aside.

Heat 1 tbsp of the fat in a frying pan over a medium heat and add the onion and garlic. Cook for 5 minutes, stirring continuously. Add the turkey, and stir well to combine. Cook for 10 minutes, or until the turkey is cooked through and the onion is softened.

Add the olives, tomatoes and parsley and stir well, then cook for 5 minutes. Meanwhile, heat the remaining fat in a frying pan over a high heat and fry the courgette noodles for 2 minutes, stirring occasionally. Serve the turkey on top of the noodles.

Chicken, Tarragon and Grapefruit Salad

Tarragon goes famously with chicken, fish, salads and sauces. Fresh herbs are always preferable, but if you have to substitute dried, use half the amount called for in the recipe. If you can find a pomelo – an Asian citrus fruit similar to grapefruit – use that instead of the grapefruit for an extra-special taste.

Serves: 2
Preparation time: 10 minutes, plus 1–2 hours marinating
Cooking time: 20 minutes

2 boneless chicken breasts, about 175g each
125ml extra virgin olive oil
2 tbsp cider vinegar
1 shallot, finely chopped
2 tsp Dijon mustard
1 medium head cos or romaine lettuce, roughly torn
1 small red onion, halved and thinly sliced
1 large red grapefruit, peeled and segmented
4 tbsp black olives, pitted and halved (optional)
salt and freshly ground black pepper
2 tbsp finely chopped fresh tarragon, or 1 tbsp dried, plus
    tarragon sprigs to garnish

Put 4 tbsp salt in a jug, and add 1 litre water, then stir until dissolved. Put the chicken breasts in a shallow dish and pour over the brine. Leave to marinate for 1–2 hours. Preheat the grill to low, then grill the chicken for 10 minutes on each side. Remove the breasts from the heat and thinly slice them lengthways.

Put the oil in a small bowl and add the vinegar, shallot and mustard. Season with ½ tsp salt and add pepper to taste, and combine well using a fork. Divide the lettuce between two plates and top with the sliced onion and grapefruit segments, chicken and black olives. Add the tarragon to the dressing and pour over the salad, then garnish with the tarragon sprigs.

Salmon Fillets with Raspberry Vinaigrette Salad

Adding fried salmon fillets to this light but satisfying salad transforms it into a complete meal. This recipe makes enough vinaigrette for six to eight servings. Store the extra dressing in an airtight container in the fridge for up to one week.

Serves: 2
Preparation time: 15 minutes
Cooking time: 15 minutes

2 salmon fillets, about 175–225g each
1 tbsp traditional fat of choice
sea salt and freshly ground black pepper

For the raspberry vinaigrette salad:
85g raspberries
1½ tbsp balsamic vinegar
¼ tsp Dijon mustard or mustard powder
4 tbsp extra light olive oil
2 tsp fresh thyme leaves
salad leaves for 2 people
70g pecan nuts or walnuts, toasted and chopped, or 2
    bacon rashers, cooked and cut into small pieces
your choice of vegetables or salad toppings, such as grated
    carrots and quartered, hard-boiled eggs

To make the salad dressing, put the raspberries, vinegar and mustard into a blender and process until smooth. Transfer to a small bowl. Whisk in the olive oil and thyme, then set aside.

Season the salmon fillets. Heat the fat in a medium frying pan over a medium-high heat, then add the salmon fillets and cook for 5 minutes on each side, or until cooked through.

Meanwhile, toss the salad leaves and nuts in a large salad bowl with 4 tbsp of the vinaigrette and your choice of salad ingredients. Serve the salmon fillets with the salad.

Dinners

Beef Rendang

This slow-cooked, Indonesian-inspired stew uses ingredients easily found in the market or supermarket and has a quick preparation time. Look for dried kaffir lime leaves in the spice section if you can't locate fresh leaves. Lemongrass can usually be found in the fresh vegetables section.

Serves: 2–4
Preparation time: 15 minutes
Cooking time: 4 hours

6 shallots or 1½ red onions, roughly chopped
4 large garlic cloves, crushed
1½ tbsp fresh root ginger, peeled and grated
2 red chillies, deseeded and roughly chopped
5 cloves
3 kaffir lime leaves, fresh or dried
900g stewing beef, cubed
375ml coconut milk
1 tsp turmeric
1 tsp ground coriander
1 tsp ground cumin
½ tsp ground cinnamon
¼ tsp freshly grated nutmeg
¼ tsp sea salt, or to taste
3 lemongrass stalks, tough outer layer discarded

Preheat the oven to 150°C/Gas 2. Put the shallots in a food processor or blender and add the garlic, ginger, chillies, cloves and dried kaffir lime leaves, if using. Pulse until combined into a purée and set aside. (Alternatively, grind by hand using a mortar and pestle.)

Put the beef in a flameproof casserole and add the coconut milk. Stir in the spice mixture, then stir in the turmeric, coriander, cumin, cinnamon, nutmeg and salt.

Cut off the stem end and the green tops of the lemongrass stalks to make each 25cm long. Put the stalks on a chopping board and bang them with a heavy kitchen tool such as pestle to release the flavour. Put the lemongrass in the casserole. If you are using fresh kaffir lime leaves, bruise them using a mortar and pestle, and add them to the casserole.

Put the casserole, uncovered, on the hob over a medium heat and bring gently to the boil. Cover and put in the oven. Cook for 3 hours, stirring once or twice. Carefully bring the casserole back to the hob and uncover. Using tongs, remove the lemongrass and fresh kaffir lime leaves, if using, and discard. Bring the stew to a simmer over a low heat. Cook for 45 minutes, stirring frequently, until the meat is tender and the sauce has reduced by half. Stir constantly towards the end of the cooking process. Serve with Roasted Carrots and Garlic (see page 436).

Grilled Tuna Steaks with Chinese Five Spices

You can find Chinese five-spice powder in Asian markets or the supermarket spice section.

Serves: 2
Preparation time: 5 minutes, plus 30 minutes marinating and preparing the cabbage side dish
Cooking time: 10 minutes

1½ tbsp Chinese five-spice powder
2 tbsp coconut oil
1 tsp sea salt
juice of 1 lemon
2 tuna steaks, 2.5cm thick, about 225g each
1 tbsp chopped fresh coriander, to garnish
Cabbage, Pak Choi and Shiitake Mushrooms (see page 437),
    to serve

Put the spice powder in a bowl and add the oil, salt and lemon juice. Mix to make a paste and use to rub on both sides of the tuna steaks. Leave to marinate for 30 minutes.

Preheat the grill to medium and cook the steaks for 5 minutes on each side. Garnish the tuna with coriander and serve with the Cabbage, Pak Choi and Shiitake Mushrooms.

Tom Kha Gai

Made with real bone broth and coconut milk, Tom Kha Gai –
a creamy, flavourful, savoury soup – is surprisingly nutrient
dense. Move over chicken noodle soup – when it comes to
comfort foods ideal for colds or sore throats, this Thai
coconut soup is the champion.

Serves: 4
Preparation time: 5 minutes
Cooking time: 20 minutes

750ml Paleo Chicken Stock (see page 449)
750ml coconut milk
2–3 lemongrass stalks, to taste, tough outer leaves discarded
4 kaffir lime leaves, fresh or dried, each torn into four pieces
2 or more Thai bird chillies or other chillies of choice, stalks
    discarded, and pod lightly crushed (optional)
1–2 handfuls shiitake or oyster mushrooms (or any other
    mushrooms), thinly sliced
½ tsp sea salt
2 tbsp fish sauce
450g cooked chicken, shredded
juice of 1 lime
1 spring onion, thinly sliced
1 tbsp chopped fresh coriander

Bring the stock to the boil, then reduce to a simmer. Skim off
any foam that rises to the top, then add the coconut milk,
lemongrass, kaffir lime leaves, chillies (if using), mushrooms
and salt. Reduce the heat to a simmer and cook for 15 minutes.

Season to taste with fish sauce. Remove the kaffir lime leaves,
lemongrass and chillies, and add the chicken. Heat through for
5 minutes, then ladle the soup into bowls or mugs. Squeeze
over some lime juice and top with the spring onion and
coriander. Serve with Thai Basil Aubergine (see page 438).

Spanish Roasted Pork Loin Adobado

This savoury pork dish is irresistible.

Serves: 4
Preparation time: 15 minutes, plus 8–24 hours marinating
Cooking time: 1–1½ hours

1 tbsp paprika
6 large garlic cloves, crushed
1 tsp ground cumin
2 tsp chopped fresh thyme or 1 tsp dried
2 tsp dried oregano
½ tsp sea salt
125ml cider vinegar
900g–1.4kg boneless pork loin joint
3 tbsp Lard (see page 448) or traditional fat of choice (if
    needed)
4 tsp chopped fresh parsley
freshly ground black pepper

Put the paprika in a bowl and add the garlic, cumin, thyme, oregano, salt, vinegar and black pepper to taste. Whisk together to combine. Put the pork in a ceramic or glass dish large enough for it to fit snugly inside. Spread the spice mixture over the meat to cover thoroughly on all sides. Cover the bowl and chill in the fridge for 8–24 hours.

Bring the pork to room temperature for 20 minutes before cooking. Preheat the oven to 180°C/Gas 4. Put the pork, fat side up, on a rack in a roasting tin (if you don't have a rack, it's also fine to put it directly in the tin). If the meat has no fat on it, dot the lard over the top of the meat.

Cook for 45–60 minutes until cooked through and the juices run clear. (The internal temperature should be 60°C.) If the top isn't browned sufficiently, put the roast under a hot grill for a minute or two. Remove from the oven and allow the roast to rest for 10 minutes. Carve into thick or thin slices, as you prefer. Garnish with parsley. Serve with Cauliflower Hash (see page 439).

Chicken Tikka Masala

This marinated chicken dish is cooked on skewers and then added to a rich sauce. Use bamboo skewers, if you have them, or grill the chicken directly on the grill rack.

Serves: 4
Preparation time: 20 minutes, plus 1–3 hours marinating
Cooking time: 30 minutes

4 boneless, skinless chicken breasts, cut into 4cm chunks
4 tbsp chopped coriander, to garnish

For the marinade:

250ml coconut milk
2 tsp garam masala
2 tsp ground coriander
2 tbsp paprika
2cm fresh root ginger, peeled and grated
4 large garlic cloves, crushed

For the sauce:

2 tbsp coconut oil
1 onion, finely chopped
2 garlic cloves, crushed
2cm fresh root ginger, peeled and grated
1 chilli (such as serrano or jalapeño), deseeded and finely
   chopped
1 tsp paprika
1 tsp ground coriander

1 tbsp tomato purée
500ml tomatoes, finely diced
125ml coconut cream
1½ tsp garam masala
sea salt

To make the marinade, put all the ingredients in a bowl and mix well. Put the chicken in a dish or bowl and pour over the marinade. Mix to coat well. Cover and chill for 1–3 hours.

Soak eight wooden skewers for 30 minutes–1 hour. Meanwhile, make the sauce. Heat the coconut oil in a large pan over a medium heat. Add the onion and cook for 5 minutes, or until softened. Add the garlic, ginger, chilli, paprika, coriander and tomato purée, and stir well for 1 minute. Add the tomatoes, then reduce the heat to medium-low. Cover the pan and simmer for 15 minutes, stirring occasionally.

While the sauce simmers, preheat the grill to medium-high. Thread the marinated chicken onto the skewers (or arrange in a single layer in the grill rack). Grill, turning occasionally, for 6–8 minutes on each side until lightly browned.

Transfer the sauce in the pan to a blender or food processor and process until smooth. Return the sauce to the pan. Add the coconut cream to the sauce and stir well.

Remove the chicken from the skewers. Stir the chicken into the sauce and cook for 5–8 minutes. Stir in the garam masala, add salt to taste and serve, garnished with the coriander. Serve with Green Salad with Shallot Vinaigrette (see page 440).

Rosemary Lamb Chops

This recipe needs only 6 lamb loin chops, so try to get fully pastured, organic lamb if you can find it.

Serves: 2
Preparation time: 5 minutes, plus 1–3 hours marinating
Cooking time: 10 minutes, plus resting

2 tbsp traditional fat of choice
4 garlic cloves, crushed
1 tbsp finely chopped fresh rosemary
6 lamb loin chops
sea salt and freshly ground black pepper

Melt the fat in a small pan over a medium heat, then remove from the heat. Add the garlic, rosemary and season with pepper, then combine well. Add the lamb chops, and turn them in the mixture to make sure the meat is well coated with marinade on all sides. Leave to marinate for 1–3 hours.

Heat a heavy frying pan over a medium heat. Sprinkle the chops with salt on both sides. Once the pan is hot (you should hear a sizzle when the meat is dropped in), sear the chops for 3–4 minutes on each side, until a golden-brown crust develops. (Alternatively, grill the chops for 5 minutes on each side, or until cooked to your liking.) Transfer the chops to a plate and allow them to rest for 5 minutes before serving. Serve with the Sweet Potato Wedges (see page 440).

Rustic Meatball and Tomato Stew

'Rustic' in this recipe means that you keep the tomatoes, celery and carrots in large pieces to retain their shape and visual appeal.

Serves: 4
Preparation time: 15 minutes
Cooking time: 1 hour 10 minutes

680g minced beef (preferably grass-fed)
1 onion, finely chopped
2 large garlic cloves, crushed
1 tsp fennel seeds, coarsely ground, or 1 tsp ground fennel
2 eggs
5 tbsp extra virgin olive oil
salt and freshly ground black pepper to taste

For the stew:

1 onion, cut into 8 wedges
4 garlic cloves, crushed
500ml Beef Bone Broth (see page 447)
4 carrots, sliced diagonally into 5cm pieces
2 large celery stalks, sliced diagonally into 5cm pieces
¼ tsp crushed chillies (optional)
400g can whole plum tomatoes, drained
1 tbsp balsamic vinegar
4 tbsp chopped fresh basil, to garnish

Put the beef in a bowl and add the onion, garlic, fennel, eggs and 2 tbsp of the oil. Season with 1 tsp salt and some pepper. Mix well. Heat the remaining oil in a pan and fry a small portion of the mixture to taste test for salt. Add more salt if needed. Shape into golf-ball-sized meatballs and fry for 10 minutes until firm and well browned on all sides without over-cooking. You may have to do this in batches. Remove the meatballs and set aside. Do not clean the pan.

To make the stew, in the same pan briefly fry the onion and garlic over a low heat for 10 minutes. Add the bone broth, bring it to the boil and add the carrots, celery, chillies and 1 tsp salt, or to taste. Cover and reduce the heat to a simmer. Cook for 10 minutes or until the carrots and celery are tender. Add the meatballs, tomatoes and vinegar, then simmer, uncovered, for 15 minutes. Adjust the seasoning and serve in soup bowls, garnished with the basil. Serve with Kale and Squash Salad (see page 441).

Side dishes

Roasted Carrots and Garlic

I like to use duck fat for maximum taste, but any traditional fat of your choice will do. Whichever fat you choose, warm it to a liquid state before tossing it with the carrots.

Serves: 4
Preparation time: 10 minutes
Cooking time: 35 minutes

2 tbsp duck fat or traditional fat of choice, plus extra if
    needed
680g carrots, peeled and quartered
1 garlic bulb, cloves separated and peeled but left whole
2 tbsp chopped fresh rosemary
sea salt

Preheat the oven to 200°C/Gas 6. Melt the fat in a roasting tin. Put the carrots in the roasting tin and add the garlic cloves. Sprinkle with salt and shake the tin to toss the carrots and garlic in the fat to coat. Spread out evenly. Roast for 15 minutes, then remove the tin and stir the vegetables.

If the vegetables seem dry, add a little more fat. Roast for 15 minutes, then check that the vegetables are cooked. The garlic should be browning slightly and the carrots should be fork-tender. Stir again and sprinkle with rosemary. Roast for a further 5 minutes, then remove from the oven and leave to cool slightly before serving.

Cabbage, Pak Choi and Shiitake Mushrooms

Umeboshi plum vinegar from Japan (available in Asian markets or specialist shops and supermarkets) adds a great touch to this dish, but you can also use any other vinegar of your choice. Use as much or as little garlic as you like.

Serves: 4
Preparation time: 10 minutes
Cooking time: 30 minutes

3 tbsp coconut oil
3–6 garlic cloves, to taste, crushed
2 tbsp fresh root ginger, peeled and grated
450g cabbage, roughly chopped
225g shiitake mushrooms, sliced
210g pak choi, cut into 1cm slices
1 tsp umeboshi plum vinegar
sea salt and freshly ground black pepper

Heat the oil in a large pan over a medium-low heat. Add the garlic and ginger, and cook for 2 minutes, stirring, or until fragrant. Add the cabbage and mushrooms, then cook for 10 minutes, stirring frequently.

Reduce the heat to low, add the pak choi and cook for 15 minutes more, stirring. Turn off the heat and stir in the vinegar. Season to taste with salt and pepper. Remove the vegetables with a slotted spoon to drain off the liquid, and serve.

Thai Basil Aubergine

The Thai basil and chilli pepper in this recipe give the aubergine an exotic twist. In Thailand, the aubergines are green and long, unlike the big purple aubergines found in the UK. You may be able to locate Thai aubergines and Thai basil in an Asian market but, if not, regular aubergines and basil work perfectly well.

Serves: 4
Preparation time: 5 minutes
Cooking time: 15 minutes

1.2kg aubergines
1 tbsp coconut oil
1 chilli, deseeded and thinly sliced, or a pinch of crushed
  chillies
2 garlic cloves, chopped
2 tbsp fish sauce
1 handful Thai basil leaves, or fresh basil

Cut the aubergines into chunky 4cm irregular shapes for easy turning in the pan. Using a steamer basket over a pan of simmering water, steam the aubergines for 5 minutes, or until softened.

Heat a pan or wok over a medium heat. Add the oil, chilli and garlic. Cook, stirring, for 5 minutes, or until the garlic turns light golden brown. Add the steamed aubergine and stir, cooking for a few minutes to blend the flavours. Stir in the fish sauce and heat through. Add the basil and turn off the heat immediately, so that the basil retains its colour, then serve.

Cauliflower Hash

This side dish is a hearty accompaniment to roast meats and chicken.

Serves: 4
Preparation time: 5 minutes
Cooking time: 25 minutes, plus cooling

1 large cauliflower
1 onion, peeled and finely chopped
2 bay leaves
2 garlic cloves
2 tsp fresh thyme
4 cloves
3 tbsp bacon dripping or traditional fat of choice
sea salt and freshly ground black pepper
3 tbsp chopped fresh parsley, to garnish

Cut off the base of the cauliflower to remove any green leaves, and cut out the main stem and tough base core. Put the cauliflower, base side up, in a large pan and add enough water to cover. Add the onion, bay leaves, garlic, thyme and cloves, then bring to the boil. Reduce the heat and simmer for 10 minutes.

Remove the cauliflower, drain, cool and coarsely chop. The cauliflower should have a crumbly consistency. Heat the bacon dripping in a medium pan over a medium-high heat. Add the cauliflower and cook, stirring occasionally, for 10 minutes. Season to taste with salt and pepper and serve garnished with chopped fresh parsley.

Green Salad with Shallot Vinaigrette

This salad uses romaine lettuce, which retains its crispness, but any lettuce or mixed salad leaves will do. Always make sure your salad leaves (and herbs) are well dried after washing – a salad spinner is a good and inexpensive investment.

Serves: 2
Preparation time: 5 minutes

125ml Shallot Vinaigrette (see page 451)
1 small head romaine or cos lettuce, torn into pieces

Pour the vinaigrette into a large salad bowl, then add the lettuce and gently toss together. Serve immediately.

Sweet Potato Wedges

Salty, sweet and spicy, these are great with a main dish or on their own for a snack.

Serves: 4
Preparation time: 5 minutes
Cooking time: 30 minutes

3 sweet potatoes (peeled optional)
3 tbsp melted coconut oil or Lard (see page 448), plus extra
   if needed
1½ tsp paprika, or to taste
1½ tsp cumin, or to taste
⅓ tsp cayenne, or to taste
1 tbsp salt, or to taste

Preheat the oven to 220°C/Gas 7. Cut the sweet potatoes in half widthways and then in half again lengthways. Cut these chunks evenly into wedges, about 1cm thick – they should be uniform for even baking.

Put the wedges in a mixing bowl, and add the melted coconut oil or lard and the spices and salt. Toss and mix very well until the potatoes are evenly coated.

Transfer the potatoes to a roasting tin and bake for 15 minutes, then stir and toss them, adding more oil if needed and more spices if you like. Cook for 15–30 minutes, depending on the size of wedges, until cooked through and lightly golden.

Kale and Squash Salad

I love kale and squash in any recipe, but the lemony bacon dressing here really makes the flavours pop. Use butternut, acorn or nutty-flavoured Japanese kabocha squash, which you can sometimes find in farmers' markets in the autumn.

Serves: 2–3
Preparation time: 10 minutes
Cooking time: 1 hour

680g butternut squash, peeled, deseeded and cut into 2cm
    cubes
5 bacon rashers, chopped
450g kale, finely sliced
3 tbsp lemon juice
1 tbsp finely sliced fresh chives
1 tbsp finely chopped fresh sage
70–100g toasted walnuts or pecan nuts, to taste
sea salt and freshly ground black pepper

Preheat the oven to 180°C/Gas 4. Put the squash cubes in an ovenproof dish and add the bacon. Roast for 1 hour, stirring well every 15 minutes.

Put the kale in a large mixing bowl and add salt to taste. Strongly massage the salt into the kale for 1 minute. Add

2 tbsp of the lemon juice and continue massaging the kale leaves for 1 minute. Set aside until ready to assemble the salad.

When the squash is tender and the bacon crispy, remove the dish and carefully drain off the bacon fat into a small bowl (there should be about 3 tbsp). Whisk the fat with the remaining lemon juice.

Drain the kale in a colander and squeeze out the remaining moisture. Tip the kale into a salad bowl and add the squash, bacon, chives, sage and walnuts. Toss with the lemon and bacon dressing, season with salt and pepper, and serve.

Snacks

Nori Crisps

You'll save money making your own nori crisps instead of paying for ready-made versions – plus, it's really easy to do.

Makes: enough snacks for 2 days for 2 people
Preparation time: 5 minutes
Cooking time: 15 minutes, plus cooling

9 nori sheets, untoasted or toasted
2 tbsp extra virgin olive oil
sea salt to taste
optional seasonings of your choice, such as onion powder,
    garlic powder or sesame seeds

Preheat the oven to 180°C/Gas 4. Cut the nori sheets into squares with a knife or kitchen scissors, or into smaller pieces if you prefer (for easy storage). Put the nori on a baking sheet in a single layer. Lightly brush the nori on one side with oil, using a pastry brush or your fingers. Sprinkle the oiled side of the nori with salt and the powdered seasonings of your choice.

Bake for 15 minutes, or until the nori chips become dry and crispy and just begin to pucker a little. Cool on a wire rack and serve or store in an airtight container for up to five days.

Hard-boiled Eggs with Avocado

Simple seasonings of salt and pepper bring out the flavours in this satisfying combination. One or two eggs and half an avocado make a healthy and filling snack.

Makes: enough snacks for 2 days for 2 people
Preparation time: 5 minutes
Cooking time: 12 minutes, plus cooling

6 eggs
3 ripe avocados
sea salt and freshly ground black pepper

Pour boiling water into a large pan and put on the hob over a high heat. If you have an egg piercer, pierce the eggs at the wide end. Using a spoon, lower the eggs into the water and return the water to the boil. Time the eggs for 10 minutes, then tip out the water and pour cold water into the pan. Tip out the cold water and refill with fresh cold water. Leave the eggs to cool in the water, and then drain. Store the eggs in their shells in the fridge for up to two days.

When ready to eat, peel off the shells and cut the eggs in half. Cut an avocado in half and leave the pit in one half. Peel off the skin from the other half and slice the flesh. Serve the avocado with the egg, sprinkled with salt and pepper to taste. Store the remaining avocado with the pit intact for up to one day. Prepare the avocado only when you are ready to eat your snack, as it will turn grey (oxidise) once cut. You can also brush some lemon juice over the cut side of the half you are not using straight away to stop the oxidisation.

Kale Crisps

The secret of success with this nutrient-rich snack is to make the kale crisps as crispy as possible.

Makes: enough for 2 days of snacks for 2 people
Preparation time: 5 minutes
Cooking time: 12–15 minutes, plus cooling

2 large bunches of kale, central stems removed
4 tbsp traditional fat of choice, melted
1 tbsp cider vinegar
sea salt and freshly ground black pepper

Preheat the oven to 150°C/Gas 2. Cut the kale leaves into large, uniform pieces. In a mixing bowl combine the kale, melted fat and vinegar until the kale is well coated. Season with salt and pepper to taste.

Spread the kale on a baking tray (you may have to do this in two batches) and bake for 12–15 minutes, tossing the kale crisps at least once to help dry them out. Remove from the oven and leave to cool on a wire rack. Serve or store in an airtight container for up to five days.

Guacamole with Carrot Crisps

This easy snack can be prepared up to two days in advance. If you have unripe avocados, put them in a paper bag with half an apple, close the bag and leave for two to three days to ripen.

Makes: enough for 2 days of snacks for 2 people
Preparation time: 10 minutes

4 ripe avocados
2 tbsp lemon juice
1 tbsp very finely chopped onion
4 tbsp coconut cream
½ tsp sea salt
freshly ground black pepper to taste
900g carrots, peeled

Cut the avocados in half, remove the pits and scoop out the flesh. Put all the ingredients, except the carrots, in a bowl and mash with a fork to combine well.

Slice the carrots on the diagonal into 'crisps'. Serve the guacamole with the carrot crisps.

To store guacamole, cover it with clingfilm to keep it from turning grey (oxidising), lightly pressing the wrap onto the surface of the guacamole to 'seal' it. The guacamole can be stored in the fridge, but eat it quickly, because it will stay fresh for only two to three days. The carrot chips can be stored in a bowl of water, covered so that they won't dry out in the fridge for up to one day.

Basics

Beef Bone Broth

This richly flavoured broth makes an excellent stock for cooking or drinking. The best bones to use are marrow bones combined with any other beef joint bones, such as knuckle. Any scraps of meat, whether cooked or uncooked, can also be added.

Makes: about 4 litres
Preparation time: 10 minutes
Cooking time: 3½ hours, plus cooling

1.8kg beef bones (preferably marrow and knuckle bones)
2 onions, halved
4 carrots, cut into large pieces
2 bay leaves
2 tsp fresh thyme leaves
4 cloves
4 celery sticks, chopped
1 large handful of parsley leaves

Preheat the oven to 200°C/Gas 6. Put the bones, onions and carrots in a roasting tin and roast for 15 minutes or until very well browned. Pour water into the tin to a depth of 1cm so that any dripping won't burn and stick to the base of the tin.

Transfer the bones to a large pan and pour in the liquid from the roasting tin, scraping the base. Add 5½ litres water, and all the remaining ingredients, to a pan. Bring the liquid to the boil, then reduce the heat to low. Cover and simmer for 3 hours. (Alternatively, cook in a slow cooker on Low for 6 hours.)

Strain the stock and leave to cool. When the stock is completely cold, pour it into 1 litre storage jars, then seal and store in the fridge for later use. It should keep for about a week. You can also freeze it in bulk or in individual portions in freezer bags.

Lard

Home-rendered lard is easy to make, particularly if you make one or two practice batches. You'll use this traditional fat in many Paleo recipes, so it's worth learning how to prepare it yourself. The trick is not to burn the lard. If made on the first day of Week 1, this recipe will make more than enough for the full Seven-Day Meal Plan. Glass Kilner jars, or other fully sealable glass jars, are useful for storing the fat.

Makes: about 850g
Preparation time: 5 minutes
Cooking time: about 1 hour, plus cooling

2.3kg pork back fat, with skin, cut into 2.5cm cubes

Heat the pork fat in a large pan over a medium-low heat and stir frequently for about 1 hour. If you use too low a heat setting, little will happen during the cooking; however, too high a heat will cause sticking and burning. Aim for medium-low and stir frequently; this is a slow-cooking process. Eventually, 5mm of rendered liquid fat will gather at the base of the pan and you will see the cubes start to change colour from pink to tan. Keep stirring to prevent sticking and to keep the heat even throughout the pieces.

Soon the liquid will begin to accumulate to cover the cubes. Once all the cubes are submerged, stirring is no longer necessary for even cooking, but it may be necessary to prevent sticking. Avoid too high a heat, because if the lard is burned it will be ruined. The fat should never smoke or even come close to smoking.

When the cubes have lost much of their original size and are light brown (not burned), they will have turned into cracklings and you are ready to strain the lard. You can dry the cracklings on kitchen paper and eat them, of course!

Being very careful because the lard is very hot, strain the mixture through a fine mesh sieve into a 1 litre glass storage jar. The fat should be the colour of apple juice. Leave to cool, then cover and store in the fridge. Once chilled and solidified, the fat should be white in colour. (If it is brown once solid, this means that the lard has burned and it should not be used.) The lard will keep for several weeks in the fridge.

Paleo Chicken Stock

Chicken stock is used for everything from soups to sauces, stews and fried dishes. It goes well not only with poultry but also with pork, veal and eggs. The ingredients and preparation are simple but it takes time. Be patient and let it simmer for several hours to bring out the full flavour of the ingredients. You can either use the carcass from a roasted chicken after you have removed all the meat, or buy a chicken, cut off the breasts and leg joints to use in another dish, and then use the remaining carcass to make the stock.

Makes: about 3.75 litres
Preparation time: 15 minutes
Cooking time: 3 hours, plus cooling

1 chicken, about 1.3–1.8kg, breasts and leg joints removed
   and used for another dish
2 onions, halved
4 carrots, cut into large chunks
2 bay leaves
4 fresh thyme sprigs or 1 tbsp dried thyme
4 celery sticks, cut into large pieces
4 cloves
1 bunch of fresh parsley

Put the chicken carcass (all the bones and the meat and wings remaining on the carcass) into a large pan and add all the remaining ingredients and 4.25 litres water. Bring to the boil over a high heat, then reduce the heat and simmer, covered, for 3 hours. (Alternatively, cook in a slow cooker on Low for 6 hours.)

Leave to cool slightly, then strain the stock through a sieve. Strain again, through wet muslin, to remove all the fine particles. When the stock is at room temperature, put the pan in the fridge for a few hours for the fat to harden on the surface.

Skim off the fat and use for cooking. The fat and stock will keep for up to a week in a tightly sealed glass jar.

Paleo Mayonnaise

An essential base for many cold sauces, mayonnaise should always be served cold. Very fresh organic, and preferably pastured, eggs are a must for this recipe. The oil should have a neutral taste, which is why olive oil is not recommended for basic mayonnaise.

Makes: 500ml
Preparation time: 10 minutes

2 pastured/organic egg yolks
1 tbsp Dijon mustard
½ tsp sea salt
⅛ tsp white pepper
2 tsp lemon juice
375ml avocado or macadamia nut oil

All the ingredients and equipment must be at room temperature. Put the eggs in a ceramic or stainless steel bowl (do not use glass or plastic) and add the mustard, salt, pepper and lemon juice. Whisk until smooth. (You can use a blender, but the container must be steel; a bowl is actually preferable.)

Tip: put a folded wet tea towel beneath the bowl to prevent it from moving while you're whisking.

While continuing to whisk, start adding the oil in a very thin stream at first. When the mixture starts to cling to the sides of the bowl, then – and only then – add the remaining oil in a slow stream, whisking the whole time. Fresh mayonnaise can be stored in a bowl covered with clingfilm in the fridge for up to three days.

Shallot Vinaigrette

A little shallot goes a long way, as it is actually more aromatic than both garlic and onions. The quantity of vinegar used is very much a question of personal taste, so add it in stages, keeping in mind that the Dijon mustard contains vinegar as well. You don't need to use extra virgin olive oil in this recipe, as the taste of the shallots is the priority here.

Makes: 1 litre
Preparation time: 10 minutes

750ml olive oil
2 shallots, finely chopped
3 tbsp Dijon mustard
1½ tsp sea salt
250ml cider vinegar
freshly ground black pepper

Put all the ingredients, except the vinegar, in a bowl and season with pepper to taste. Whisk together, then add the vinegar slowly, occasionally tasting for acidity.

Pour the vinaigrette into a glass container with a lid and store in the fridge. Vinaigrette will keep for at least three weeks. Before use, give it a good shake, as the oil and vinegar tend to separate.

Index